Sports Nutrition Needs for Child and Adolescent Athletes

Sports Nutrition Needs for Child and Adolescent Athletes

Edited by
Chad M. Kerksick
Lindenwood University
St. Charles, Missouri, USA

Elizabeth Fox
Assistant Director of Sports Nutrition
University of Florida, Gainesville, USA

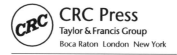

CRC Press is an imprint of the
Taylor & Francis Group, an **informa** business

CRC Press
Taylor & Francis Group
6000 Broken Sound Parkway NW, Suite 300
Boca Raton, FL 33487-2742

© 2016 by Taylor & Francis Group, LLC
CRC Press is an imprint of Taylor & Francis Group, an Informa business

No claim to original U.S. Government works

Printed on acid-free paper
Version Date: 20160324

International Standard Book Number-13: 978-1-4665-7974-3 (Hardback)

This book contains information obtained from authentic and highly regarded sources. Reasonable efforts have been made to publish reliable data and information, but the author and publisher cannot assume responsibility for the validity of all materials or the consequences of their use. The authors and publishers have attempted to trace the copyright holders of all material reproduced in this publication and apologize to copyright holders if permission to publish in this form has not been obtained. If any copyright material has not been acknowledged please write and let us know so we may rectify in any future reprint.

Except as permitted under U.S. Copyright Law, no part of this book may be reprinted, reproduced, transmitted, or utilized in any form by any electronic, mechanical, or other means, now known or hereafter invented, including photocopying, microfilming, and recording, or in any information storage or retrieval system, without written permission from the publishers.

For permission to photocopy or use material electronically from this work, please access www.copyright.com (http://www.copyright.com/) or contact the Copyright Clearance Center, Inc. (CCC), 222 Rosewood Drive, Danvers, MA 01923, 978-750-8400. CCC is a not-for-profit organization that provides licenses and registration for a variety of users. For organizations that have been granted a photocopy license by the CCC, a separate system of payment has been arranged.

Trademark Notice: Product or corporate names may be trademarks or registered trademarks, and are used only for identification and explanation without intent to infringe.

Library of Congress Cataloging-in-Publication Data

Names: Kerksick, Chad M., editor. | Fox, Elizabeth (Dietician), editor.
Title: Sports nutrition needs for child and adolescent athletes / [edited by] Chad M. Kerksick and Elizabeth Fox.
Description: Boca Raton : Taylor & Francis, 2016. | Includes bibliographical references and index.
Identifiers: LCCN 2016010471 | ISBN 9781466579743 (hardback : alk. paper)
Subjects: | MESH: Sports Nutritional Physiological Phenomena | Child Nutritional Physiological Phenomena | Athletic Performance--physiology | Sports--physiology
Classification: LCC RJ133 | NLM QT 263 | DDC 613.7/043--dc23
LC record available at http://lccn.loc.gov/2016010471

Visit the Taylor & Francis Web site at
http://www.taylorandfrancis.com

and the CRC Press Web site at
http://www.crcpress.com

On a personal level, I dedicate this book to Adrien, Camden, and Emery:

Adrien: You represent all that is great in my life. I could not ask for a better partner in all things life has thrown at us. Simply saying "I love you" does not fully portray my feelings for the continual support you provide to projects such as these that demand so much of my time and energy. I love you!

Camden: You changed your father in countless ways. Your mother and I love you dearly and will move mountains for you. You are the reason why this book became important to me.

Emery: When this book hits print, you will be working toward your second birthday. Your parents were dubious whether another child could fill our hearts with as much love as your sister, but you managed to accomplish that task with impressive ease. I love you and look forward to seeing the path you will carve.

Camden and Emery: My aspirations for you are to be strong, confident women who know themselves and are courageous enough to pursue whatever their hearts are guiding them to do. If you grow up to have the class and perspective on life that your mother does, you will do great things! Just like your parents, you will have a set of parents who will do everything they can to make your life as rich and fulfilling as possible.

On a professional level, I dedicate this book to the five original founders of the International Society of Sports Nutrition: Anthony Almada, Jose Antonio, Douglas Kalman, Susan Kleiner and Richard Kreider who continue to inspire me and many others with their energy and passion for educating, teaching and researching all aspects of the field of sports nutrition.

Chad

I dedicate this book to my parents, Tom and Cheryl Fox; my husband Brandon; my siblings, Gerry and his wife Kate, Mary and her wife Stephanie, Therese, and John; to my nephew Jackson and goddaughter Elizabeth, and to our beloved family dog, Rocky. You have all inspired me to work hard, dream big, and never give up. Thank you for your years of love, support, and advice.

Elizabeth

Contents

Preface ix
Editors xi
Contributors xiii

SECTION I Nutritional Foundation

Chapter 1 Sport Nutrition and Youth 3
  Elizabeth Fox and Chad M. Kerksick

Chapter 2 Energy Needs and Body Composition Considerations 17
  Ann L. Gibson and Michelle Kulovitz Alencar

Chapter 3 Carbohydrate Needs of the Young Athlete 35
  Julia K. Zakrzewski and Keith Tolfrey

Chapter 4 Protein Needs of Young Athletes 59
  Kurt A. Escobar, Trisha A. McLain, and Chad M. Kerksick

Chapter 5 Fat Needs 77
  Trisha A. McLain and Carole A. Conn

Chapter 6 Vitamin and Mineral Needs 99
  Brad Schoenfeld and Alan Aragon

Chapter 7 The Importance of Proper Fluid and Hydration 113
  Gabriela Tomedi Leites and Flavia Meyer

SECTION II Special Considerations in Child and Adolescent Athletes

Chapter 8 Effects of Caffeine, Nicotine, Alcohol, and Marijuana on Exercise Performance 135
  Dominik H. Pesta, Siddhartha S. Angadi, Martin Burtscher, and Christian K. Roberts

Chapter 9 Drugs, Steroids, and Youth 153
  Andrew Jagim and Jonathan Mike

Chapter 10 Clinical Considerations for the Child and Adolescent Athlete 173
Jessika Brown, Elizabeth Yakes Jimenez, Carole A. Conn, and Christine M. Mermier

Chapter 11 Nutrition and the Overweight Athlete 193
Elizabeth Fox

Chapter 12 Nutrition and the Weight-Conscious Athlete 203
Roger A. Vaughan and Christine M. Mermier

Chapter 13 Dietary Supplement Considerations for the Young Athlete 219
Paul E. Luebbers

Chapter 14 Exercise Prescription and Strength and Conditioning Considerations 239
Adriana Coletta, Kyle Levers, Elfego Galvan, and Richard B. Kreider

SECTION III A Hands-on, Practical Approach

Chapter 15 How to Fuel Your Day 265
Jennifer McDaniel and Elizabeth Fox

Chapter 16 How to Fuel Your Workouts and Games 281
Jennifer McDaniel and Elizabeth Fox

Index 291

Preface

While massive amounts of empirical research are published each year on responses and adaptations to exercise and nutrition, a relative lack of this data is focused on children and adolescents. As a result, two primary goals have guided us through the development of this book. First, to generate a scientifically grounded volume that was written by exercise and nutrition experts on a variety of topics centered on the needs of children and adolescent athletes. In doing this, many contributors to this book through phone calls, E-mails, and conversations indicated to us their concerns about the relative lack of literature and the fact that they were forced to use data from adult or young college-aged (18–25 years) participants. Thus, our second goal is for other scientists and practitioners to read the information gathered and for them to be motivated and inspired to conduct more research using children and adolescent athletes. Whether or not these two goals were realized will be left for the readers and critiques to determine and any fault of this book to accomplish these goals falls squarely upon our shoulders. Lastly, it is important for readers and other colleagues to understand the challenge to capture all available and relevant literature on these topics. Collectively, we apologize for any colleague's work we may have overlooked.

In developing the organization of this book, we created three unique and independent sections:

- *Nutritional Foundation*—This section outlines chapters devoted to a broad overview of sport participation and nutrient needs (Chapter 1), followed by critically important chapters that emphasize concepts related to energy needs and body composition goals (Chapter 2), macronutrient metabolism as well as age-specific requirements and recommendations (Chapters 3, 4, and 5, respectively), and a chapter devoted to vitamin and mineral needs (Chapter 6). Finally, the first section concludes with a chapter discussing the importance of fluid and proper hydration (Chapter 7).
- *Special Considerations in Child and Adolescent Athletes*—While the first section is intended to offer a comprehensive look at topics that relate to nearly every athlete, the second section focuses on topics that are more specific. For example, Chapter 8 highlights in a very detailed and scientific manner, the impact of common recreational drugs on exercise performance. Chapter 9 furthers this discussion into topics related to steroid use in youth and to associated dangers. Chapter 10 was prepared by a highly qualified group of clinical nutrition experts and covers key elements of working with diabetic and other clinically relevant populations. Chapters 11 and 12 provide discussions that relate to overweight and weight-conscious athletes, respectively. Chapter 13 takes a detailed approach at discussing the use of many popular dietary supplements by child and adolescent athletes, a situation that according to survey research is all too common. Finally, Chapter 14 was included to provide a scientifically derived discussion on exercise prescription considerations for young athletes to ensure their safety while training.
- *A Hands-On, Practical Approach*—This is the "How-To" section. In many respects, Chapters 15 and 16 might be the most "useful" chapters for coaches, athletes, researchers, or health care practitioners who read this book. Both chapters use an easy-to-understand approach to discuss and apply situations that can challenge athletes, their parents, and coaches by making sure young athletes are well fueled and recovered for all sporting situations.

In closing, it is worth mentioning up front that across all chapters a child or adolescent athlete has been defined by chronological age. All contributors certainly recognize the potential for a wide range of biological difference within the same age of athletes. That being said, a child athlete was defined as an athlete between the ages of 7 and 12 years while an adolescent athlete was defined as an athlete 13–17 years of age.

Editors

Chad M. Kerksick, PhD, is currently an assistant professor of exercise science in the Exercise Science department in the School of Sport, Recreation and Exercise Sciences at Lindenwood University. Dr. Kerksick's primary research interests include sports nutrition as well as the biochemical, cellular, and molecular adaptations relative to various forms of exercise and nutrition interventions, primarily those that promote muscle hypertrophy and prevent muscle atrophy in healthy as well as clinical populations.

Elizabeth Fox earned her master's in nutrition and physical performance at Saint Louis University. She is a registered dietitian and a board-certified specialist in sports dietetics (CSSD). She currently works as the assistant director of sports nutrition for the University Athletic Association at the University of Florida. Fox is active as a writer of nutrition and sports nutrition and continues to collaborate with colleagues on topics related to sports nutrition and human performance.

Contributors

Siddhartha S. Angadi
School of Nutrition and Health Promotion
Arizona State University
Phoenix, Arizona

Alan Aragon
Department of Family and Consumer Sciences
California State University, Northridge
Northridge, California

Jessika Brown
Sandia National Laboratory and Eating
    Disorders Treatment Center
Albuquerque, New Mexico

Martin Burtscher
Department of Sports Science, Medical Section
University Innsbruck
Innsbruck, Austria

Adriana Coletta
Department of Health and Kinesiology
Texas A&M University
College Station, Texas

Carole A. Conn
Department of Individual, Family,
    and Community Education: Nutrition
    and Dietetics
University of New Mexico
Albuquerque, New Mexico

Kurt A. Escobar
Department of Health, Exercise,
    and Sports Sciences
University of New Mexico
Albuquerque, New Mexico

Elizabeth Fox
University Athletic Association
University of Florida
Gainesville, Florida

Elfego Galvan
Department of Health and Kinesiology
Texas A&M University
College Station, Texas

Ann L. Gibson
Department of Health, Exercise,
    and Sports Sciences
University of New Mexico
Albuquerque, New Mexico

Andrew Jagim
Department of Exercise and Sport Sciences
University of Wisconsin—La Crosse
La Crosse, Wisconsin

Chad M. Kerksick
School of Sport, Recreation, and Exercise
    Sciences
Lindenwood University
St. Charles, Missouri

Richard B. Kreider
Department of Health and Kinesiology
Texas A&M University
College Station, Texas

Michelle Kulovitz Alencar
Department of Kinesiology—Fitness
California State University, Long Beach
Long Beach, California

Kyle Levers
Department of Health and Kinesiology
Texas A&M University
College Station, Texas

Paul E. Luebbers
Health, Physical Education, and Recreation
    Department
Emporia State University
Emporia, Kansas

Jennifer McDaniel
McDaniel Nutrition Therapy, LLC
Clayton, Missouri

Trisha A. McLain
Department of Health, Exercise, and Sports
    Sciences
University of New Mexico
Albuquerque, New Mexico

Christine M. Mermier
Department of Health, Exercise, and Sports Sciences
University of New Mexico
Albuquerque, New Mexico

Flavia Meyer
Department of Physical Education
Federal University of Rio Grande do Sul (UFRGS)
Porto Alegre, Brazil

Jonathan Mike
School of Sport, Recreation, and Exercise Sciences
Lindenwood University
St. Charles, Missouri

Dominik H. Pesta
Department of Internal Medicine
Yale University School of Medicine
New Haven, Connecticut

Christian K. Roberts
Translational Sciences Section, School of Nursing
University of California
Los Angeles, California

Brad Schoenfeld
Department of Health Sciences
Lehman College, CUNY
Bronx, New York

Keith Tolfrey
School of Sport, Exercise, and Health Sciences
Loughborough University
Loughborough, United Kingdom

Gabriela Tomedi Leites
Child Health and Exercise Medicine Program
McMaster University
Hamilton, Canada

Roger A. Vaughn
Department of Exercise Science
High Point University
High Point, North Carolina

Elizabeth Yakes Jimenez
Department of Individual, Family and Community Education: Nutrition and Dietetics
University of New Mexico
Albuquerque, New Mexico

Julia K. Zakrzewski
Department of Sport Science and Physical Activity
University of Bedfordshire
Bedford, United Kingdom

Section I

Nutritional Foundation

1 Sport Nutrition and Youth

Elizabeth Fox and Chad M. Kerksick

CONTENTS

Abstract 3
1.1 Introduction 4
  1.1.1 Child and Adolescents Defined 5
  1.1.2 Youth Sport Participation 6
  1.1.3 Dietary Status and Dietary Challenges of Young People 6
1.2 Optimal Energy 6
1.3 Macronutrient Considerations 8
  1.3.1 Carbohydrates 8
  1.3.2 Protein 9
  1.3.3 Fat 10
1.4 Fluid Status and Fluid Needs 11
1.5 Micronutrient Concerns and Considerations 11
1.6 Dietary Supplement Use in Youth and Adolescent Athletes 12
1.7 Conclusions 13
References 13

ABSTRACT

The number of child and adolescent athletes participating in sports has climbed substantially in the past several decades. In many situations, athletes participate in more than one sport and as a result undergo significant amounts of exercise stress throughout the year. As the training load and physical stress increases due to higher amounts of participation, the need and concern for adequate nutrition also increases. Across the board, young athletes require more energy (calories) in their diet as a direct consequence of the extra energy expended while participating in sports and other activities. Carbohydrates should be considered a primary fuel source for exercising athletes with many reports recommending carbohydrate intake to be around 4–6 grams of carbohydrate per kilogram of body mass each day. To facilitate recovery, repair, and growth of a new tissue, adequate protein is needed and again studies report that exercising athletes have greater dietary protein needs than age-matched nonexercising children or adolescents; protein intakes of 1.2–1.8 grams of protein per kilogram of body mass each day are recommended. Finally, dietary intake of fat is an important consideration due to the many important functions for dietary fat. A primary consequence of exercise and competition is metabolic heat production whereby the human body responds by increasing its rate of sweat production in an attempt to cool the body. For these reasons, fluid intake and hydration are important considerations for young athletes. Adequate intake of key micronutrients is of utmost importance as many vitamins or minerals can become deficient if extreme dietary restrictions or patterns are followed. Finally, the number of child and adolescent athletes exposed to and intrigued by dietary supplements is impressive and in the overwhelming majority of situations, athletes should first focus on learning how to use food in their diet to fuel their activities and to promote growth and recovery. In the end, sports and other types of organized activities are intended to be fun and recreational for children and adolescents offering opportunities for them to grow physically, emotionally, and psychologically. Adequate dietary habits can be and should be an important adjunct to facilitate these outcomes for all kids who participate in sports.

1.1 INTRODUCTION

Sporting activity is an excellent way for children to develop motor skills and coordination, improving their fitness and health in addition to developing important "life" skills related to interacting with other people, teamwork, communication, hardship, and sacrifice. From a health perspective, the daily pattern of activity in children has changed immensely and the ways in which children go about their day have changed. For example, a 2011 report by kids and gaming indicated that the percentage of 2–17-year olds who regularly play various technology-based games increased by 12.9%; when compared to 2009, those figures have increased from 9% of all kids in the ages of 2–17 years (NPD 2011). In what is viewed by many to be highly related to these data, activity levels exhibit a consistent decline across adolescence, whereby less than three out of every 10 U.S. high school students participate in the recommended 60 minutes of daily physical activity (Figure 1.1) (Centers for Disease Control 2012). Moreover, Lee and colleagues in 2007 reported that middle school students log an average of 40 minutes of physical activity each day, again, less than the recommended amounts (Lee et al. 2007). While other factors remain as to why physical activity is declining, these data contribute to a myriad of factors that unfortunately has resulted in childhood obesity becoming an epidemic that spans the globe. To this point, approximately 17% or 12.5 million, U.S. children and adolescents between the ages of 2 and 19 are classified as obese (with a body mass index [BMI] greater than the 95th percentile), while nearly 155 million school-aged children worldwide are considered overweight or obese (Ogden et al. 2014). These data are particularly problematic because obese boys are 11% less likely to be physically active when compared to normal or even overweight boys, while obese and overweight girls are 5% less likely to get the recommended amounts of physical activity when compared to normal weight girls (Figure 1.2) (Centers for Disease Control 2012).

Documented benefits of physical activity in children and adolescents are widespread and include both physiological and psychological components. For example, improved levels of cardiovascular fitness and bone health, decreases in the risk for chronic diseases, such as hypertension and obesity (Lee et al. 2007; Lowry et al. 2013), and reduced symptoms of depression and anxiety (Eime et al. 2013), are all supported benefits of regular physical activity in youth. Promotion, maintenance, and

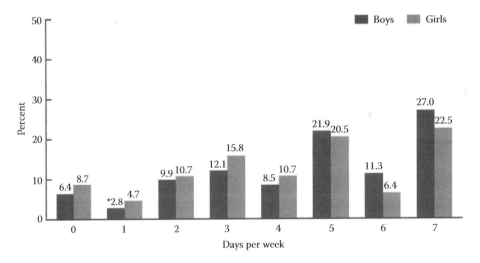

FIGURE 1.1 Percentage of youth who were physically active, by number of days per week and sex: United States, 2012. *Does not meet the standard of statistical reliability and precision. Physical activity in this figure was defined as engaging in any kind of moderate-to-vigorous physical activity, including activities both in school and outside of school that increased heart rate and made breathing harder some of the time for at least 60 minutes. Data shown are weighted percentages. (Adapted from Centers for Disease Control [CDC]/National Center for Health Statistics [NCHS], National Health and Nutrition Examination Survey, and National Youth Fitness Survey, 2012. http://www.cdc.gov/nchs/data/databriefs/db141.htm.)

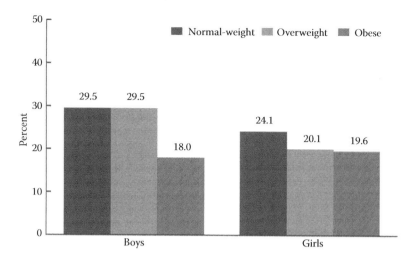

FIGURE 1.2 Percentage of youth who were physically active, by weight status and sex: United States, 2012. Physical activity in this figure was defined as engaging in any kind of moderate-to-vigorous physical activity, including activities both in school and outside of school that increased heart rate and made breathing harder some of the time for at least 60 minutes. (Adapted from CDC/NCHS, National Health and Nutrition Examination Survey, and National Youth Fitness Survey, 2012. http://www.cdc.gov/nchs/data/databriefs/db141.htm.)

improvement of activity levels are critical, as studies have found that both leisure time physical activity and physical fitness in childhood and adolescence predict these attributes well into adulthood (Barnekow-Bergkvist et al. 1998; Dennison et al. 1988; Tammelin et al. 2003; Telama 2009). In addition to improvements in health and physical fitness, participation in sports and other physical activities promotes the development of positive sociocultural skills, creativity, and other attributes that are as much emotional and psychological as they are physical. This chapter serves as a broad introduction to many salient topics regarding the nutrition needs and considerations of child and adolescent competitors. In addition to this chapter, other reviews prepared on the topic are available (Desbrow et al. 2014; Hoch et al. 2008; Meyer et al. 2007; Unnithan and Goulopoulou 2004).

1.1.1 Child and Adolescents Defined

Owing to the myriad of biological changes that occur throughout childhood and into adolescence, it would be helpful to review how the terms "child" and "adolescent" are commonly defined, particularly in the context of athletes or competitors. Commonly and what is used throughout this book is that children are defined as those in the age group of 7–12 years while adolescents are 13–18 years. From a clinical perspective, Tanner stages are the most commonly used scale to assess the physical development of children, adolescents, and adults. James Tanner, a British physician, came up with the scale that used primary and secondary sex characteristics to determine the development state of the individual. For both males and females, five Tanner stages exist with stage I representing the youngest or least biological development while stage V represents adult or full biological development. Natural variation in biological development makes it impossible to definitely state what Tanner stages are represented by these ages. The majority of research indicates that Tanner stages II–IV are widely represented from these ages with some individuals being stage V if the athlete population is in their late teenage years.

Desbrow and a team of sports dietitian colleagues from Australia published a position statement in 2014 focusing on adolescent athletes (Desbrow et al. 2014). In their summary, they incorporated how much training the young athlete was taking part in to classify them. Briefly, an "active adolescent athlete" was defined as "an adolescent aged 12–18 years, who applies foundational movement skills in a sports specific context, and may be associated with commitment to training, skill development and/or formal engagement in competition" (p. 571). In a similar light, a "competitive adolescent athlete" was defined as "an adolescent aged athlete between 12–18 years who demonstrates gifts/talents in the physical, physiological or movement domains which may indicate future potential in high performance sport" (p. 571). Such athletes are likely engaged in sustained practice through high-training volumes.

1.1.2 Youth Sport Participation

For many children and adolescents, participation in activities in the form of individual and team sports is their primary source of physical activity. In consideration of the available statistics on obesity prevalence, it is somewhat paradoxical that participation in organized sports from 1992 to 2002 in the United States increased in children by 8.4% and adolescents by 15.4% (Petrie et al. 2004). Across Europe, approximately 53%–98% of children aged 6–11 years are at least occasionally involved in sports with similar participation numbers found in adolescents between 12 and 16 years of age (Petrie et al. 2004). In accordance, the National Council of Youth Sports reported in 2008 that the overall number of boys and girls participating in sports was greater than those children surveyed in both 1997 and 2000, respectively (National Council of Youth Sports 2008). More recent statistics show more divergent activity patterns particularly when considered at the individual sport level, at least in the United States, but for the most part sport participation has held steady. Importantly, a recent 2013 study involving 1421 children reported that children involved in sports were more physically active (Tomlin et al. 2013). Similarly and when viewed strictly from an energy balance perspective, it should come as no surprise that participation in organized sports at a young age has consistently been shown to be inversely related to BMI (Nikolaidis 2012; Tomlin et al. 2013).

1.1.3 Dietary Status and Dietary Challenges of Young People

When examining the trends witnessed for physical activity in child and adolescent populations, similar patterns are evident regarding dietary intake. In this respect, multiple studies examining the typical dietary intake of nonathlete adolescents consistently report that many fail to consume recommended amounts of fruits, vegetables, dairy, and whole grains, while also consuming more than enough "energy dense" foods such as fast food as well as sugary foods and beverages (Magarey et al. 2001; Munoz et al. 1997; Neumark-Sztainer et al. 1996; Yngve et al. 2005).

Much like data seen regarding physical activity and BMI levels, multiple studies report that adolescents who are involved in sports many times have better-quality diets than age-matched nonathlete adolescents (Cavadini et al. 2000; Pate et al. 2000; Tomlin et al. 2013), but not all populations fit with this conclusion. For example, studies highlighting the diet of adolescent athletes, especially female athletes in weight-conscious sports, suggest that various aspects of their daily diet may be limited in quantities of essential minerals, carbohydrates, and calories (Beals 2002; Bergen-Cico and Short 1992; Cupisti et al. 2002; Lindholm et al. 1995; Ruiz et al. 2005; Ziegler et al. 1999). As a final thought, one must consider these data and outcomes as impacted by a number of factors including gender, socioeconomic status of the family or child, type of sport and age of the athlete, and as a result more data are needed to conclusively determine the impact of sport participation on diet quality in children and adolescents.

1.2 OPTIMAL ENERGY

The need for adequate energy is requisite to ensure proper growth, development, and maturation. Moreover, the appropriate balance of energy intake against expenditure points toward concerns on both ends of the energy balance equation. Deficiency of energy results in poor recovery and training quality, menstrual dysfunction, and impacted growth and development, while excessive energy puts children at risk for developing obesity, diabetes, and other metabolic complications. While it is accepted that athletic children and adolescents have greater energy needs when compared to nonathletic age-matched youth (Rodriguez et al. 2009), the magnitude of this difference is anything but straightforward. Determining daily energy requirements for physically active youth requires the calculation of total energy expenditure (TEE), which consists of resting energy expenditure (REE), energy required for growth and menstruation, energy required for daily physical activity and exercise, as well as digestive energy demands. A limited number of scientific studies have directly measured energy expenditure in young athletes. Using the doubly labeled water approach, eight male adolescent speed skaters were estimated to have a TEE of 16.8 ± 3.8 MJ/day or 4012 ± 908 kcals/day (Ekelund et al. 2002). A small group (6 girls, 10 boys) of high school-aged (16.5 ± 1.6 years) athletes were estimated to have TEE levels of 3196 ± 590 kcals/day using an activity log and 3012 ± 518 kcals/day using a SenseWear armband (Aerenhouts et al. 2011). Interestingly and in relation to the previous sections in this chapter, total energy intake (2569 ± 508 kcals/day) in these young athletes was lower than the TEE measurements suggesting that the diet was not providing enough calories to match what was being expended.

Accurate determination of TEE is complicated and as a result, the determination of REE is commonly made by nutritionists and researchers to determine daily caloric needs. Measurement of REE using indirect calorimetry is preferred, but prediction of REE using population-specific equations is suitable and most convenient due to its relative ease of calculation. REE is representative of daily caloric needs as it accounts for 65%–70% of an individual's TEE level. While a number of REE prediction equations exist, the Institute of Medicine (IOM) has developed REE predictive equations for both obese and nonobese children (Institute of Medicine 2002), and these equations, or other validated *youth-specific equations*, should be used when measurement of REE is not possible as a general guide and starting point to determine daily caloric needs. In this respect, one must appreciate that factors such as age, gender, body composition, and puberty are all factors that influence REE in children and adolescents while also understanding that calculations used to predict energy needs in adults are typically not entirely applicable to children. Consequently, the determined value is best considered as a guide or starting point.

Once REE is determined, it must be converted into values of TEE, commonly through multiplication with a predetermined factor that represents physical activity level (PAL). An examination of 574 measurements of TEE revealed that PAL values range from 1.2 × REE in completely sedentary adults and can reach 4.5 × REE in populations of elite endurance runners (Black et al. 1996). Unfortunately, PAL values used for adults may not be suitable for youth due to differences in efficiency of movements and metabolic development among other factors; researchers recently published a recommended PAL range of 1.75–2.05 when calculating TEE in adolescent athletes (Carlsohn et al. 2011).

All this information comes together in Table 1.1 that outlines the estimated daily caloric needs as a function of gender, age, and activity level (Table 1.1). To further aid coaches, parents, and practitioners in determining adequate energy needs, several questions should be considered, including (a) what is their age and gender? (b) how much training (days/total time) is being performed daily? (c) what is the typical intensity and duration of this training? (d) what is the athlete's fitness and body composition level? and (e) what are their energy demands later in the day or in subsequent days? As a very general guideline, if total energy is adequate, the athlete will have a hard time recovering, may experience reductions in performance, and could even experience increases in heart rate and poor sleep quality. If total energy intake is too high, the athlete will experience weight gain along with decrements in body composition that ultimately will negatively impact performance. As a rudimentary starting point, youth athletes should aim to include 2–3 servings from the milk group, 2–3 servings from the meat group, 4 servings from the vegetable group, 3 servings from the fruit group, and 9 servings from the bread/grain group daily (Steen 1994), but again, actual requirements will be influenced by factors of age, body mass, gender, and activity level. While somewhat beyond the scope of this chapter, recommended snacks and feeding strategies are provided in Chapters 15 and 16 of this book.

TABLE 1.1
Estimated Daily Caloric Needs[a] According to Age, Gender, and Activity Level

Gender	Age (Years)	Sedentary[b]	Moderately Active[c]	Active[d]
Female[e]	2–3	1000	1000–1400	1000–1400
	4–8	1200	1400–1600	1400–1800
	9–13	1600	1600–2000	1800–2200
	14–18	1800	2000	2400
	19–30	2000	2000–2200	2400
	31–50	1800	2000	2200
	51+	1600	1800	2000–2200
Male	2–3	1000	1000–1400	1000–1400
	4–8	1400	1400–1600	1600–2000
	9–13	1800	1800–2200	2000–2600
	14–18	2200	2400–2800	2800–3200
	19–30	2400	2600–2800	3000
	31–50	2200	2400–2600	2800–3000
	51+	2000	2200–2400	2400–2800

Source: Adapted from the Institute of Medicine Dietary Reference Intakes Report for Macronutrients in 2002. Institute of Medicine. 2002. *Dietary Reference Intakes for Energy, Carbohydrate, Fiber, Fat, Fatty Acids, Cholesterol, Protein, and Amino Acids.* Washington, DC: The National Academies Press.

[a] Based on estimated energy requirement (EER) equations, using reference heights (average), and reference weights (healthy) for each age–gender group. For children and adolescents, reference height and weight may vary, but the reference adult man is 5′10″ and 154 pounds (70 kg). The reference woman is 5′4″ and 126 pounds (60 kg).
[b] Sedentary means a lifestyle that includes only the light physical activity associated with typical day-to-day life.
[c] Moderately active means a lifestyle that includes physical activity equivalent to walking about 1.5–3 miles per day at 3–4 miles/hour, in addition to the light physical activity associated with typical day-to-day life.
[d] Active means a lifestyle that includes physical activity equivalent to walking more than 3 miles per day at 3–4 miles/hour, in addition to the light physical activity associated with typical day-to-day life.
[e] Does not account for women who are pregnant, lactating, or nursing.

1.3 MACRONUTRIENT CONSIDERATIONS

1.3.1 CARBOHYDRATES

The majority of an athlete's caloric intake, young or not, should come from carbohydrate. Carbohydrate is the body's predominant fuel source during most activities, and therefore is the cornerstone of a well-balanced diet for any athlete. Unfortunately, few longitudinal studies exist that examine carbohydrate recommendations or intake during exercise in youth athletes. It is well recognized that active children and adolescents have much greater carbohydrate needs than the dietary reference intake (DRI) of 100 grams of carbohydrate per day, as this level is sufficient for blood glucose provision exclusively to the brain (Petrie et al. 2004). In fact, available research indicates that young athletes participating in heavy exercise can utilize 1.0–1.5 grams of carbohydrate per kilogram of body mass per hour. At this rate, a 50-kg athlete would completely expend this minimum value for carbohydrate in less than 2 hours of activity! As a result, carbohydrate needs may indeed be closer to 200–500 grams of carbohydrate per day for young athletes (Petrie et al. 2004). Accordingly, many authors recommend carbohydrate intakes of 50%–60% of total calories (Bass and Inge 2000; Cavadini et al. 2000; Petrie et al. 2004; Rodriguez et al. 2009; Steen 1996a, b), a value that is similar to recommended levels for adult athletes.

A recent review on carbohydrate intake and young athletes suggests that determining carbohydrate requirements for child and adolescent athletes are very intricate and are influenced by many metabolic and physiological changes that occur during growth and development (Petrie et al. 2004). During adolescence, fat oxidation is greater compared to an adult athlete, most likely due to a limited glycolytic capacity (Eriksson 1972; Eriksson and Saltin 1974), lower blood lactate concentrations during exercise (Armstrong and Welsman 1994), and decreased glucose tolerance (Amiel et al. 1986; Moran et al. 1999). Furthermore, age can influence glycogen concentrations whereby younger boys (~11.5 years) were found to have lower glycogen concentrations than both older (12.5–13.5 years) and adolescent boys (15.5 years) at rest (Eriksson et al. 1971). Due to lower muscle glycogen stores found in children and adolescents, it is not currently recommended for children to carbohydrate load and instead, they are advised to consistently and judiciously deliver carbohydrate-containing foods surrounding the competitive exercise bout (Rodriguez et al. 2009).

Nutritional surveys of athletes 12–18 years of age show that males consume about 6–9 grams of carbohydrate per kilogram of body mass per day (Chen et al. 1989; Leblanc et al. 2002) and female athletes consume around 3–5.5 grams of carbohydrate per kilogram of body mass per day (Cupisti et al. 2002; Papadopoulou et al. 2002; Wiita and Stombaugh 1996). Until further research is attempted and more conclusive recommendations on daily carbohydrate needs of youth athletes can be made, child and adolescent athletes should aim to consume at least 50% of their calories from carbohydrate (oftentimes equating to 4–6 grams of carbohydrate per kilogram of body mass per day), with the focus on nutrient-dense carbohydrate choices, such as whole grains, fruits and vegetables, and low-fat dairy, with limited amounts of refined sugars (<10%).

1.3.2 Protein

Dietary carbohydrate is needed in the athlete's diet as a fuel source and for energy production, while adequate protein is important for tissue growth and repair, hormone and enzyme production, and nutrient transfer in the blood (Cotunga et al. 2005). Adult (nonathlete) protein recommendations are 12%–15% of total energy intake, which oftentimes equates to 0.8–1.2 grams of protein per kilogram of body mass per day (Petrie et al. 2004), but athletic or highly active counterparts are well accepted to require greater amounts, that is, 1.2–1.8 grams of protein per kilogram of body mass per day (Buford et al. 2007; Maughan and Burke 2002; Rodriguez et al. 2009). The World Health Organization recommends a protein intake of 0.85–0.92 grams of protein per kilogram of body mass per day for individuals who are 3–18 years, but published research indicates that this amount is not adequate for adolescent athletes (Boisseau et al. 2007). Recommended amounts for adults (1.2–1.8 g/kg/day) are likely more appropriate for child and adolescent athletes, but recommendations and final amounts should be made on an individual basis, and account for age, gender, training status and schedule, and weight goals. Moreover, using available reference weights for adolescents, this recommended protein intake also falls in line with the more general recommendation of consuming a diet that provides protein as 12%–15% of the total calories consumed (assuming adequate energy is delivered overall). Finally, a key perspective should also consider that for most athletes in the Western world, protein needs even in these greater amounts are routinely met by a diet that adequately provides necessary energy in an appropriately balanced diet (Jeukendrup and Cronin 2011).

Dietary survey methods have found that protein intakes vary among youth athletes. Female gymnasts (artistic, rhythmic, and ballet) in one study averaged 1.8 ± 0.8–2.3 ± 1.2 g/kg/day (Soric et al. 2008), while another study on adolescent male tennis players found that 88% and 63% of the 10–13-year olds, and 14–18-year olds, respectively, consumed greater than 1.5 g/kg/day (Juzwiak et al. 2008). Furthermore, Ruiz et al. (2005) found that age was a predictor of protein intake in soccer players of different ages, where 14–16.6-year olds had an intake of 2.03–2.14 g/kg/day, compared to the 20-year-old athletes, who consumed around 1.81 g/kg/day (Ruiz et al. 2005). Overall, most studies conclude that youth athletes consume enough protein to meet their needs (Nemet and Eliakim 2009). An interesting point to consider, however, was brought forward by Horswill and others in 1990 when they reported that adolescent wrestlers exhibited reductions in their overall protein status as their season progressed, even though their reported intake levels seemed adequate (Horswill et al. 1990). This finding highlights the need for coaches, nutritionists, dietitians, and parents to watch closely for other signs of inadequate protein status (e.g., fatigue, losing weight, losing strength, lack of recovery, etc.), particularly in young sporting populations that may be restricting the overall energy intake to make weight, lose fat, etc., as is commonly done in wrestling at all levels and many other sports. To this point, high-risk athletes for inadequate protein intakes include vegetarian or vegan athletes, and athletes attempting to lose weight or maintain a lower body weight for performance such as wrestlers, dancers, cheer, and divers. As a broad recommendation, young athletes are recommended to consume a variety of protein sources, including lean meats, fish, nuts and seeds, legumes, low-fat dairy, and eggs in amounts that are approximately 12%–15% of their daily caloric intake or relative amounts that correspond to 1.2–1.8 grams of protein per kilogram of body mass per day.

1.3.3 Fat

Much like carbohydrate and protein, fat plays a critical role in overall physiology including energy production, facilitation of fat-soluble vitamin absorption and assimilation, and an insulator and stabilizer of cell membranes. Analysis of the type of fat in a young athlete's diet is just as important as the total amount of fat. Linoleic acid (an omega-6 fatty acid) and alpha-linolenic acid (an omega-3 fatty acid) are the two essential fatty acids that play a critical role in growth and development, cell signaling, and inflammation. The adequate intake (AI) for males of 9–13 years of age is 12 grams per day and 1.2 grams per day of linoleic and alpha-linolenic acid, and 10 grams per day and 1.0 grams per day of linoleic and alpha-linolenic acid for females of 9–13 years of age (Institute of Medicine 2002), respectively. Fatty fish, flaxseed, oils, nut, seeds, and green leafy vegetables are all great food sources of these essential fats, and should be included daily.

Nutrition experts recommend that young athletes consume between 20% and 35% of total calories from fat (Bonci 2010; Petrie et al. 2004; Purcell and Paediatric Sports Canadian Paediatric Society, and Section Exercise Medicine 2013), with less than 10% from saturated fat (Rodriguez et al. 2009), no more than 10% from polyunsaturated fat, and 10%–15% from monounsaturated fat; this distribution of fat calories should meet the essential fatty acid recommendations provided above. Furthermore, athletes attempting to lose weight or make weight for performance should be cautious to restrict dietary fat too much as studies indicate that diets with less than 15% of their calories from fat negatively impact performance as well as health outcomes (Rodriguez et al. 2009). Alternatively, diets that routinely provide fat intakes that exceed 40% can put the athlete at risk for consuming too many calories overall and gaining weight or minimally not ingesting enough carbohydrate (and potentially protein) to fuel optimal performance and recovery. Studies show that most young athletes' fat intakes, as estimated by 3–7-day food logs, fall close to or within the recommended range. Specifically, adolescent female volleyball players in one study consumed around 26% of their calories from fat (Beals 2002). Canadian female soccer players in another study averaged a fat intake of 29.9% of calories (Gibson et al. 2011), and a mix of 15–19-year-old male and female competitive athletes recorded 33%–35% of their calories from fat (Elmadfa and Rupp 1994).

One study, by Martinez et al. (2011), focused on both the type of fat and relative contribution to daily fat consumption and found that young, male amateur swimmers consumed approximately 33.9% of calories from fat, with 17.6% of those calories from unsaturated fats, and 12.5% from saturated fats (Martinez et al. 2011). The female swimmers recorded 37.5% of total calories from fat, with around 21% and 13.6% of calories from unsaturated and saturated fats, respectively. Dietary prescriptions by nutritionists and dietitians commonly focus more on adequate delivery of carbohydrate and protein, which oftentimes results in adequate levels of fat being delivered, particularly if the overall energy intake is appropriate. Owing to other healthful considerations, the majority of ingested fat should come from unsaturated versions, which also works to ensure that many other important micronutrients are ingested in adequate amounts, a point discussed in Section 1.3.3 of this chapter.

1.4 FLUID STATUS AND FLUID NEEDS

Alongside the importance of AI of the macronutrients, adequate fluid intake and hydration are critical considerations. Maintaining appropriate fluid intake is important for health, safety, and performance reasons; daily fluid turnover in young populations has been estimated and reported to be ~1.6 liters per day, which is a value that is anywhere from 50% to 75% of the required amounts for adults (Ballauff et al. 1988). Exercise and sporting activity increases metabolic heat production and leads to an increased loss of fluid (and to a lesser extent, electrolytes) in the form of sweat. Lack of adequate rehydration can challenge thermoregulatory processes and in the event the situation persists, further dehydration will occur eventually leading to heat injuries (i.e., exhaustion or stroke) and potentially death. Previous reports have indicated that sweat rates in adults can range from 0.3 to 5.0 liters per hour (Petrie et al. 2004; Rodriguez et al. 2009), but these values are largely impacted by fitness, acclimation, body composition, clothing worn, and the environment. Children typically sweat less than adults due to immature development of physiological sweating mechanisms (Bergeron et al. 2005), which further adds to their thermal demand and the need for appropriate reporting of fluid intake and loss (Harrell et al. 2005).

While the availability of controlled literature examining the impact of dehydration on children and adolescent athletes is scant, data do suggest that team sport performance is negatively impacted when dehydrated (Baker et al. 2007) as is specific skill performance in adolescent basketball players who lost 2% of their body mass due to dehydration (Dougherty et al. 2006). Other research reported that a 2.9% loss of body mass occurred in adolescent soccer athletes as they completed a soccer-specific drill, which corresponded with a decrease in sport-specific performance (Rico-Sanz et al. 1996). All these factors point toward the need for parents, coaches, teachers, administrators, school health personnel, athletes, and sporting body representatives to be aware of the many factors that can combine to threaten the health of a young athlete who is exercising in the heat.

In the end, no one factor can ultimately predict heat-related outcomes, but daily tracking of body mass, education regarding urine color, and the adoption of a regimented hydration schedule can go a long way toward helping to prevent future heat-related injuries. Table 1.2 provides recommended fluid intake levels for child-aged athletes during and after exercise and sporting activity (Rowland 2011). Again, these values should be considered as a starting point and adjusted according to changes in body mass before and after a practice or competition, urine color, and overall readiness by the athlete.

1.5 MICRONUTRIENT CONCERNS AND CONSIDERATIONS

The micronutrients—vitamins and minerals—represent a wide variety of constituents within the body that impact its several functions. Particularly in the growing individual, adequate delivery of these nutrients is important. As a group, micronutrients are known to be intimately involved in bone health, immune function, metabolism, iron status, oxygen transport, and antioxidant activity (Institute of Medicine 2002; Rodriguez et al. 2009). For these reasons, daily needs must be met by

TABLE 1.2
Recommended Minimal Fluid Intake during and after Exercise in Child Athletes

Body Weight (kg)	Fluid Replacement during Exercise (mL/hour)	Fluid Replacement after Exercise (mL/hour)
25	325	100
30	390	120
35	455	140
40	520	160
45	585	180
50	650	200
55	715	220
60	780	240

Source: Used with permission from Rowland, T., *Sports Med.*, 41, 279–88, 2011.

the diet, which "typically" occurs in situations where an amount of calories is consumed that meets daily expenditure using a balanced dietary approach.

Micronutrient deficiency most commonly occurs when inadequate levels of energy are consumed in the diet. However, restricted patterns of energy intake and selective or complete restriction of various types of foods or food groups due to preferences or digestive insufficiencies may result in inadequate levels of certain micronutrients in the diet. Calcium, for example, is crucial in its involvement with healthy bone development and muscle contractions. Restriction of dairy and other calcium-containing foods, particularly in young females lays a precarious foundation for future bone development through their peak bone-growing years. Iron is another nutrient that due to dietary choices may be consumed in inadequate amounts whose overall status is tightly married to hemoglobin status and can subsequently impact oxygen transport and exercise performance (Rodriguez et al. 2009). Factors such as sporting activity can impact iron loss and when combined with the onset of menses and periodic loss of blood, the status of iron in young athletes (particularly females) should be of concern. Finally, the status and intake of electrolytes such as sodium and potassium may become threatened in young athletes who are exercising in hot and humid environments. Both nutrients are critically linked to optimal cell function and fortunately their replacement is easily facilitated by lightly salting of foods and consciously replacing lost fluid and electrolytes with a sports drink as opposed to nothing or plain water.

1.6 DIETARY SUPPLEMENT USE IN YOUTH AND ADOLESCENT ATHLETES

A number of published reports are available outlining the use of various food products and dietary supplements by grade school and high school-aged athletes. An excellent, detailed section has been prepared in Chapter 13 of this book with multiple reports consistently indicating that dietary supplement use is quite common in children and adolescents. For example, Metzl and investigators (Metzl et al. 2001) reported that creatine was used by 5.6% of 1103 young athletes with nearly all of them being boys who played strength-oriented sports such as football, wrestling, and hockey. Kayton et al. reported that 59% of 270 athletic, high school boys and girls regularly ingested sports drinks while 46% consumed a multivitamin (Kayton et al. 2002), a finding quite similar to that of McDowall and colleagues (McDowall 2007). In addition, creatine use was definite (21% in boys vs. 3% in girls) along with usage rates of protein supplements (8% and 1%, respectively for boys and girls). Finally, Hoffman et al. (2008) surveyed 3248 high school students throughout 12 states in the United States and reported usage rates of 59.3% for multivitamins, 31.5% for energy drinks,

15.3% for protein powders, and 7.2% for creatine. Not surprisingly, usage rates of energy drinks and protein powders showed general trends to increase as the children were older with an estimated 39.8% of 12th-grade boys consuming protein, 22% taking creatine, while 10th-grade boys (40.9%) and girls (27.8%) reported the highest rates of energy drink consumption.

Collectively, the results from these published reports clearly point toward the fact that young people are exposed to dietary supplements early in their lives and as they get older and into high school, the likelihood of them choosing to use a dietary supplement goes up markedly. While factors such as age and gender appear to strongly impact whether or not a young athlete has begun using a dietary supplement, other factors such as the type and number of sporting activities can influence the amount and type of supplement chosen. In the end, it is important for coaches, school administrative personnel, parents, athletes, and nutrition professionals to be aware of the likelihood that a high school or grade school individual is taking or has been exposed to dietary supplements. While definitive answers regarding the safety and efficacy of every dietary supplement in this population is beyond the scope of this chapter and others in this book, it should be highlighted that healthy diets and eating patterns are encouraged and should be the norm for nearly all athletes, irrespective of their age, but in particular those athletes who are still growing and developing physically and emotionally.

1.7 CONCLUSIONS

The rate of participation in sports from children and adolescents has experienced a steady increase for the past two to three decades. Higher rates of participation lead to increased dietary requirements in the form of more calories as well as greater required intakes of carbohydrate, protein, and fat. Parents, coaches, health-care providers, school administrators, and the young athletes themselves need to understand their body's increased requirements for nutrients and work to provide it through the diet. In addition to greater dietary needs, it is also important for all parties to understand that exercising results in appreciable amounts of fluid loss and inappropriate levels of hydration can compromise performance and more importantly a young athlete's health. Adequate delivery of all necessary micronutrients will encourage optimal health and dietary strategies that grossly restrict calories or entire food groups should be discouraged to ensure that adequate energy is delivered in the diet along with necessary levels of micronutrients. Through information provided in this chapter and across this book, care givers toward children and adolescents can learn a great deal that will help them plan and prepare snacks and meals to help young athletes compete in a fun and healthy manner.

REFERENCES

Aerenhouts, D., E. Zinzen, and P. Clarys. 2011. Energy expenditure and habitual physical activities in adolescent sprint athletes. *J Sports Sci Med* 10 (2):362–8.
Amiel, S. A., R. S. Sherwin, D. C. Simonson, A. A. Lauritano, and W. V. Tamborlane. 1986. Impaired insulin action in puberty. A contributing factor to poor glycemic control in adolescents with diabetes. *N Engl J Med* 315 (4):215–9. doi: 10.1056/NEJM198607243150402.
Armstrong, N. and J. R. Welsman. 1994. Assessment and interpretation of aerobic fitness in children and adolescents. *Exerc Sport Sci Rev* 22:435–76.
Baker, L. B., D. E. Conroy, and W. L. Kenney. 2007. Dehydration impairs vigilance-related attention in male basketball players. *Med Sci Sports Exerc* 39 (6):976–83. doi: 10.1097/mss.0b013e3180471ff2.
Ballauff, A., M. Kersting, and F. Manz. 1988. Do children have an adequate fluid intake? Water balance studies carried out at home. *Ann Nutr Metab* 32 (5–6):332–9.
Barnekow-Bergkvist, M., G. Hedberg, U. Janlert, and E. Jansson. 1998. Prediction of physical fitness and physical activity level in adulthood by physical performance and physical activity in adolescence—An 18-year follow-up study. *Scand J Med Sci Sports* 8 (5 Pt 1):299–308.
Bass, S. and K. Inge. 2000. Nutrition for special populations. In *Clinical Sports Nutrition,* L. Burke and V. Deakin (Eds), Australia: McGraw-Hill, pp. 554–593.

Beals, K. A. 2002. Eating behaviors, nutritional status, and menstrual function in elite female adolescent volleyball players. *J Am Diet Assoc* 102 (9):1293–6.

Bergen-Cico, D. K. and S. H. Short. 1992. Dietary intakes, energy expenditures, and anthropometric characteristics of adolescent female cross-country runners. *J Am Diet Assoc* 92 (5):611–2.

Bergeron, M. F., D. B. McKeag, D. J. Casa, P. M. Clarkson, R. W. Dick, E. R. Eichner, C. A. Horswill et al. 2005. Youth football: Heat stress and injury risk. *Med Sci Sports Exerc* 37 (8):1421–30.

Black, A. E., W. A. Coward, T. J. Cole, and A. M. Prentice. 1996. Human energy expenditure in affluent societies: An analysis of 574 doubly-labelled water measurements. *Eur J Clin Nutr* 50 (2):72–92.

Boisseau, N., M. Vermorel, M. Rance, P. Duche, and P. Patureau-Mirand. 2007. Protein requirements in male adolescent soccer players. *Eur J Appl Physiol* 100 (1):27–33. doi: 10.1007/s00421-007-0400-4.

Bonci, L. 2010. Sports nutrition for young athletes. *Pediatr Ann* 39 (5):300–6. doi: 10.3928/00904481-20100422-11.

Buford, T. W., R. B. Kreider, J. R. Stout, M. Greenwood, B. Campbell, M. Spano, T. Ziegenfuss, H. Lopez, J. Landis, and J. Antonio. 2007. International Society of Sports Nutrition position stand: Creatine supplementation and exercise. *J Int Soc Sports Nutr* 4:6. doi: 10.1186/1550-2783-4-6.

Carlsohn, A., F. Scharhag-Rosenberger, M. Cassel, J. Weber, A. de Guzman Guzman, and F. Mayer. 2011. Physical activity levels to estimate the energy requirement of adolescent athletes. *Pediatr Exerc Sci* 23 (2):261–9.

Cavadini, C., B. Decarli, J. Grin, F. Narring, and P. A. Michaud. 2000. Food habits and sport activity during adolescence: Differences between athletic and non-athletic teenagers in Switzerland. *Eur J Clin Nutr* 54 (Suppl 1):S16–20.

Centers for Disease Control. 2012. Physical Activity Guidelines for Americans. Accessed July 18, 2014. http://www.cdc.gov/physicalactivity/data/facts.html.

Chen, J. D., J. F. Wang, K. J. Li, Y. W. Zhao, S. W. Wang, Y. Jiao, and X. Y. Hou. 1989. Nutritional problems and measures in elite and amateur athletes. *Am J Clin Nutr* 49 (5 Suppl):1084–9.

Cotunga, N., C. E. Vickery, and S. McBee. 2005. Sports nutrition for young athletes. *J Sch Nurs* 21 (6):323–8.

Cupisti, A., C. D'Alessandro, S. Castrogiovanni, A. Barale, and E. Morelli. 2002. Nutrition knowledge and dietary composition in Italian adolescent female athletes and non-athletes. *Int J Sport Nutr Exerc Metab* 12 (2):207–19.

Dennison, B. A., J. H. Straus, E. D. Mellits, and E. Charney. 1988. Childhood physical fitness tests: Predictor of adult physical activity levels? *Pediatrics* 82 (3):324–30.

Desbrow, B., J. McCormack, L. M. Burke, G. R. Cox, K. Fallon, M. Hislop, R. Logan et al. 2014. Sports dietitians Australia position statement: Sports nutrition for the adolescent athlete. *Int J Sport Nutr Exerc Metab* 24 (5):570–84. doi: 10.1123/ijsnem.2014-0031.

Dougherty, K. A., L. B. Baker, M. Chow, and W. L. Kenney. 2006. Two percent dehydration impairs and six percent carbohydrate drink improves boys basketball skills. *Med Sci Sports Exerc* 38 (9):1650–8. doi: 10.1249/01.mss.0000227640.60736.8e.

Eime, R. M., J. A. Young, J. T. Harvey, M. J. Charity, and W. R. Payne. 2013. A systematic review of the psychological and social benefits of participation in sport for adults: Informing development of a conceptual model of health through sport. *Int J Behav Nutr Phys Act* 10:135. doi: 10.1186/1479-5868-10-135.

Ekelund, U., A. Yngve, K. Westerterp, and M. Sjostrom. 2002. Energy expenditure assessed by heart rate and doubly labeled water in young athletes. *Med Sci Sports Exerc* 34 (8):1360–6.

Elmadfa, I. and B. Rupp. 1994. Nutritional status of young athletes. *Bibl Nutr Dieta* 51:163–5.

Eriksson, B. O. 1972. Physical training, oxygen supply and muscle metabolism in 11–13-year old boys. *Acta Physiol Scand Suppl* 384:1–48.

Eriksson, B. O., J. Karlsson, and B. Saltin. 1971. Muscle metabolites during exercise in pubertal boys. *Acta Paediatr Scand Suppl* 217:154–7.

Eriksson, O. and B. Saltin. 1974. Muscle metabolism during exercise in boys aged 11 to 16 years compared to adults. *Acta Paediatr Belg* 28 (Suppl):257–65.

Gibson, J. C., L. Stuart-Hill, S. Martin, and C. Gaul. 2011. Nutrition status of junior elite Canadian female soccer athletes. *Int J Sport Nutr Exerc Metab* 21 (6):507–14.

Harrell, J. S., R. G. McMurray, C. D. Baggett, M. L. Pennell, P. F. Pearce, and S. I. Bangdiwala. 2005. Energy costs of physical activities in children and adolescents. *Med Sci Sports Exerc* 37 (2):329–36.

Hoch, A. Z., K. Goossen, and T. Kretschmer. 2008. Nutritional requirements of the child and teenage athlete. *Phys Med Rehabil Clin N Am* 19 (2):373–98, x. doi: 10.1016/j.pmr.2007.12.001.

Hoffman, J. R., A. D. Faigenbaum, N. A. Ratamess, R. Ross, J. Kang, and G. Tenenbaum. 2008. Nutritional supplementation and anabolic steroid use in adolescents. *Med Sci Sports Exerc* 40 (1):15–24. doi: 10.1249/mss.0b013e31815a5181.

Horswill, C. A., S. H. Park, and J. N. Roemmich. 1990. Changes in the protein nutritional status of adolescent wrestlers. *Med Sci Sports Exerc* 22 (5):599–604.

Institute of Medicine. 2002. *Dietary Reference Intakes for Energy, Carbohydrate, Fiber, Fat, Fatty Acids, Cholesterol, Protein, and Amino Acids*. Washington, DC: The National Academies Press.

Jeukendrup, A. and L. Cronin. 2011. Nutrition and elite young athletes. *Med Sport Sci* 56:47–58. doi: 10.1159/000320630.

Juzwiak, C. R., O. M. Amancio, M. S. Vitalle, M. M. Pinheiro, and V. L. Szejnfeld. 2008. Body composition and nutritional profile of male adolescent tennis players. *J Sports Sci* 26 (11):1209–17. doi: 10.1080/02640410801930192.

Kayton, S., R. W. Cullen, J. A. Memken, and R. Rutter. 2002. Supplement and ergogenic aid use by competitive male and female high school athletes. *Med Sci Sports Exerc* 34 (5):S193.

Leblanc, JCh, F. Le Gall, V. Grandjean, and P. Verger. 2002. Nutritional intake of French soccer players at the Clairefontaine training center. *Int J Sport Nutr Exerc Metab* 12 (3):268–80.

Lee, S. M., C. R. Burgeson, J. E. Fulton, and C. G. Spain. 2007. Physical education and physical activity: Results from the school health policies and programs study 2006. *J Sch Health* 77 (8):435–63. doi: 10.1111/j.1746-1561.2007.00229.x.

Lindholm, C., K. Hagenfeldt, and U. Hagman. 1995. A nutrition study in juvenile elite gymnasts. *Acta Paediatr* 84 (3):273–7.

Lowry, R., S. M. Lee, J. E. Fulton, Z. Demissie, and L. Kann. 2013. Obesity and other correlates of physical activity and sedentary behaviors among U.S. high school students. *J Obes* 2013:276318. doi: 10.1155/2013/276318.

Magarey, A., L. A. Daniels, and A. Smith. 2001. Fruit and vegetable intakes of Australians aged 2–18 years: An evaluation of the 1995 National Nutrition Survey data. *Aust N Z J Publ Health* 25 (2):155–61.

Martinez, S., B. N. Pasquarelli, D. Romaguera, C. Arasa, P. Tauler, and A. Aguilo. 2011. Anthropometric characteristics and nutritional profile of young amateur swimmers. *J Strength Cond Res* 25 (4):1126–33. doi: 10.1519/JSC.0b013e3181d4d3df.

Maughan, R. J. and L. M. Burke. 2002. *Sports Nutrition*. Maiden, MA: Blackwell Science.

McDowall, J. A. 2007. Supplement use by young athletes. *J Sports Sci Med* 6 (3):337–42.

Metzl, J. D., E. Small, S. R. Levine, and J. C. Gershel. 2001. Creatine use among young athletes. *Pediatrics* 108 (2):421–5.

Meyer, F., H. O'Connor, and S. M. Shirreffs. 2007. Nutrition for the young athlete. *J Sports Sci* 25 (Suppl 1):S73–82. doi: 10.1080/02640410701607338.

Moran, A., D. R. Jacobs Jr., J. Steinberger, C. P. Hong, R. Prineas, R. Luepker, and A. R. Sinaiko. 1999. Insulin resistance during puberty: Results from clamp studies in 357 children. *Diabetes* 48 (10):2039–44.

Munoz, K. A., S. M. Krebs-Smith, R. Ballard-Barbash, and L. E. Cleveland. 1997. Food intakes of U.S. children and adolescents compared with recommendations. *Pediatrics* 100 (3 Pt 1):323–9.

National Council of Youth Sports. 2008. *Report on Trends and Participation in Organized Youth Sports*. Market Research Report, NCYS Membership Survey, 2008 Edition.

Nemet, D. and A. Eliakim. 2009. Pediatric sports nutrition: An update. *Curr Opin Clin Nutr Metab Care* 12 (3):304–9. doi: 10.1097/MCO.0b013e32832a215b.

Neumark-Sztainer, D., M. Story, M. D. Resnick, and R. W. Blum. 1996. Correlates of inadequate fruit and vegetable consumption among adolescents. *Prev Med* 25 (5):497–505. doi: 10.1006/pmed.1996.0082.

Nikolaidis, P. T. 2012. Physical fitness is inversely related with body mass index and body fat percentage in soccer players aged 16–18 years. *Med Pregl* 65 (11–12):470–5.

NPD. 2011. Video Game Industry is adding 2–17 year-old gamers at a rate higher than that age's population growth. Accessed July 15, 2014. https://www.npd.com/wps/portal/npd/us/news/press-releases/pr_111011/.

Ogden, C. L., M. D. Carroll, B. K. Kit, and K. M. Flegal. 2014. Prevalence of childhood and adult obesity in the United States, 2011–2012. *J Am Med Assoc* 311 (8):806–14. doi: 10.1001/jama.2014.732.

Papadopoulou, S. K., S. D. Papadopoulou, and G. K. Gallos. 2002. Macro- and micro-nutrient intake of adolescent Greek female volleyball players. *Int J Sport Nutr Exerc Metab* 12 (1):73–80.

Pate, R. R., S. G. Trost, S. Levin, and M. Dowda. 2000. Sports participation and health-related behaviors among U.S. youth. *Arch Pediatr Adolesc Med* 154 (9):904–11.

Petrie, H. J., E. A. Stover, and C. A. Horswill. 2004. Nutritional concerns for the child and adolescent competitor. *Nutrition* 20 (7–8):620–31. doi: 10.1016/j.nut.2004.04.002.

Purcell, L. K. and Paediatric Sports Canadian Paediatric Society, and Section Exercise Medicine. 2013. Sport nutrition for young athletes. *Paediatr Child Health* 18 (4):200–5.

Rico-Sanz, J., W. R. Frontera, M. A. Rivera, A. Rivera-Brown, P. A. Mole, and C. N. Meredith. 1996. Effects of hyperhydration on total body water, temperature regulation and performance of elite young soccer players in a warm climate. *Int J Sports Med* 17 (2):85–91. doi: 10.1055/s-2007-972813.

Rodriguez, N. R., N. M. Di Marco, and S. Langley. 2009. American College of Sports Medicine position stand. Nutrition and athletic performance. *Med Sci Sports Exerc* 41 (3):709–31. doi: 10.1249/MSS.0b013e31890eb8600005768-200903000-00027 [pii].

Rowland, T. 2011. Fluid replacement requirements for child athletes. *Sports Med* 41 (4):279–88. doi: 10.2165/11584320-000000000-00000.

Ruiz, F., A. Irazusta, S. Gil, J. Irazusta, L. Casis, and J. Gil. 2005. Nutritional intake in soccer players of different ages. *J Sports Sci* 23 (3):235–42. doi: 10.1080/02640410410001730160.

Soric, M., M. Misigoj-Durakovic, and Z. Pedisic. 2008. Dietary intake and body composition of prepubescent female aesthetic athletes. *Int J Sport Nutr Exerc Metab* 18 (3):343–54.

Steen, S. N. 1994. Nutrition for young athletes. Special considerations. *Sports Med* 17 (3):152–62.

Steen, S. N. 1996a. Timely statement of the American Dietetic Association: Nutrition guidance for adolescent athletes in organized sports. *J Am Diet Assoc* 96 (6):611–2. doi: 10.1016/S0002-8223(96)00170-8.

Steen, S. N. 1996b. Timely statement of the American Dietetic Association: Nutrition guidance for child athletes in organized sports. *J Am Diet Assoc* 96 (6):610–1. doi: 10.1016/S0002-8223(96)00169-1.

Tammelin, T., S. Nayha, A. P. Hills, and M. R. Jarvelin. 2003. Adolescent participation in sports and adult physical activity. *Am J Prev Med* 24 (1):22–8.

Telama, R. 2009. Tracking of physical activity from childhood to adulthood: A review. *Obes Facts* 2 (3):187–95. doi: 10.1159/000222244.

Tomlin, D. L., S. K. Clarke, M. Day, H. A. McKay, and P. J. Naylor. 2013. Sports drink consumption and diet of children involved in organized sport. *J Int Soc Sports Nutr* 10 (1):38. doi: 10.1186/1550-2783-10-38.

Unnithan, V. B. and S. Goulopoulou. 2004. Nutrition for the pediatric athlete. *Curr Sports Med Rep* 3 (4):206–11.

Wiita, B. G. and I. A. Stombaugh. 1996. Nutrition knowledge, eating practices, and health of adolescent female runners: A 3-year longitudinal study. *Int J Sport Nutr* 6 (4):414–25.

Yngve, A., A. Wolf, E. Poortvliet, I. Elmadfa, J. Brug, B. Ehrenblad, B. Franchini et al. 2005. Fruit and vegetable intake in a sample of 11-year-old children in 9 European countries: The pro children cross-sectional survey. *Ann Nutr Metab* 49 (4):236–45. doi: 10.1159/000087247.

Ziegler, P. J., J. A. Nelson, and S. S. Jonnalagadda. 1999. Nutritional and physiological status of U.S. national figure skaters. *Int J Sport Nutr* 9 (4):345–60.

2 Energy Needs and Body Composition Considerations

Ann L. Gibson and Michelle Kulovitz Alencar

CONTENTS

Abstract 17
2.1 Energy Intake Considerations 17
    2.1.1 Estimating Energy Needs 18
    2.1.2 Macronutrient Recommendations 18
2.2 Body Composition Considerations 20
    2.2.1 Anthropometrics 20
    2.2.2 Body Water 24
    2.2.3 Multiple-Component Models 26
    2.2.4 Recommendations Regarding Body Fatness of Child and Adolescent Athletes 30
2.3 Summary and Conclusions 31
References 31

ABSTRACT

As exercise and sport participation by child and adolescent athletes continues to grow, the need for understanding energy requirements, caloric needs, as well as optimal body composition becomes vital to the performance and well-being of the athlete. Energy needs are expected to increase as activity level and intensity of the activity increase. Nonetheless, certain athletic groups may have an increased energy requirement in order to prevent shortfalls in their diet. Adequate intake that is sport-specific must be suitable for the developmental stage of the child or adolescent athlete and include the appropriate intake of carbohydrates, proteins, and fats. Furthermore, the concurrent complementary nutritional needs and body composition requirements are crucial to support the growing body as well as performance in sport. A variety of body composition methods are available, including field methods (e.g., anthropometrics, skinfold thickness, and bioelectrical impedance) as well as more accurate estimations from laboratory methods (e.g., multiple-component models, hydrodensitometry, and air-displacement plethysmography). However, the assumptions and utility of each of these methods must be considered with respect to a population of child or adolescent athletes using population-specific prediction equations. The considerations of both energy requirements and body composition recommendations for the child and adolescent athlete will be described in this chapter.

2.1 ENERGY INTAKE CONSIDERATIONS

Child and adolescent athlete involvement in sport continues to grow worldwide. Nutritional needs for optimal athletic performance include ensuring adequate energy intake encompassing proper carbohydrates, proteins, and fats to meet the demands of a growing and maturing body. Student athletes of various ages, including young adolescents, and their advisors often have misconceptions with regard to proper nutrition that can support their involvement in sport.

With the growing involvement of children and adolescents in sport, acute nutrient requirements change for this population in order to meet total daily energy needs. A critical component of success in sport begins with sufficient energy intake to support the absolute increase in caloric expenditure for activity completion and to facilitate development of strength, endurance, lean body mass, and health of any athlete. It is a common fact, especially in younger athletes, that participation in sport or regular physical activity naturally increases caloric consumption. However, as described in an excellent review by Petrie and colleagues (2004), certain groups of young athletes may be at risk for dietary deficits in energy intake. Groups that may be at risk include individual sport athletes when compared to team sport athletes, participants in weight-controlled sports, and endurance athletes, especially female distance runners. It is imperative that coaches, parents, school nurses, or anyone having any potential to influence the young athlete's nutritional intake focus upon the athlete meeting adequate daily energy requirements. When the athlete is not eating a well-balanced diet that meets their daily energy requirements, inadvertent impairments in the body's growth and maturation can occur; additionally, athletic performance and recovery may be hindered as well (Sundgot-Borgen et al. 2013).

2.1.1 Estimating Energy Needs

According to the Academy of Nutrition and Dietetics (AND) and the recent report from the *Pediatric Nutrition Care Manual* (http://www.nutritioncaremanual.org) (American Dietetic Association 2014), energy needs can be calculated based on four levels of physical activity: sedentary, low active, active, and very active (Cunningham 2010, American Dietetic Association 2014). The Food and Nutrition Board has recommended estimating energy intake based on equations that take into consideration factors such as age, reference height and body weight, and physical activity classification. Owing to the variability of these factors, it is difficult to establish energy requirements for any group of diverse young athletes. For example, the energy requirements of adolescents aged 9–13 years can range from 1415 kcal/day for sedentary children to over 3000 kcal/day for very active athletes (Petrie et al. 2004). The *Pediatric Nutrition Care Manual* and the Academy of Nutrition and Dietetics have provided a useful tool for coaches and/or nutrition professionals to aid in the estimation of energy needs (http://www.bcm.edu/cnrc/healthyeatingcalculator/eatingCal.html).

It is important to grasp that routine participation in sport or physical activity may elevate energy requirements independent of training demands. When daily caloric needs and caloric expenditure for physical activity were calculated for obese children, actual energy needs, when measured, were 12% more than estimated for the training session (Blaak et al. 1992). Additionally, nonobese, nonathletic children undergoing a 6-week training regimen increased their energy expenditure beyond what was expected (Bolster et al. 2001). With this understanding, caution and consideration of the individual athlete should underlie the estimation of energy requirements in this population. Estimations should take into account variability in seasonal exercise changes, including intensity, duration, and behavioral changes that may influence compensation or conservation of energy requirements; furthermore, adjustments for in-season versus off-season needs as well as requirements for the nontraining periods of the day must be considered (Petrie et al. 2004). For these reasons and others, a prudent recommendation is for a young athlete and their parent(s) to visit with either a licensed dietitian or an experienced nutritionist who has experience working with youth athletes.

2.1.2 Macronutrient Recommendations

Athletes of all ages have unique nutritional needs that should be based on individual energy requirements with an appropriate macronutrient breakdown. The macronutrients are energy-providing nutrients and include carbohydrates, proteins, and fats. Specific nutrient requirements will be described in more detail in other chapters of this book (Chapters 3, 4, and 5); however, it is important to highlight the basic recommendations for child or adolescent athletes in the context of energy goals.

Energy Needs and Body Composition Considerations

Athletes of all ages should consume adequate carbohydrates. Limited research exists providing specific carbohydrate needs for young athletes, and no definitive recommendations for carbohydrate intake of young athletes exist at this time. However, some authors have ventured to recommend similar intakes (50%–60% of total caloric intake) for both young athletes and normally active children (Petrie et al. 2004). It is crucial that coaches or nutrition professionals provide young athletes with recommendations for carbohydrate intake that reflects both the intensity and duration of the physical activity performed, and in some cases, the number of practices or competitive bouts completed by the athlete in a given time period. As exercise intensity increases, so does the need for carbohydrate as a fuel source for energy; however, young athletes may have differing substrate metabolism when compared to adult populations at a given relative intensity. A 1992 study investigated adolescent girls (10–12 years) during prolonged running on a treadmill (30 minutes at 70% VO_2 peak) (Martinez and Haymes 1992). After 25 minutes of exercise, data showed higher fat oxidation levels for the young girls as compared to adult females exercising at the same relative intensity. Similar findings were shown in boys compared to men; the boys had a greater fat oxidation during exercise intensities ranging between 50% and 70% VO_2 peak (Delamarche et al. 1992). Differences between adolescent athletes appear to lie within the type of sport in which the athlete is trained. For example, endurance-trained young athletes require higher carbohydrate intakes than do young non-endurance-trained athletes. More information surrounding carbohydrate considerations can be found in Chapter 3.

Dietary protein is involved in tissue synthesis and is vital for the natural growth and development of young athletes. Protein needs for athletes are higher than for the general population because of the increased rates of protein breakdown and synthesis. Similar to carbohydrate recommendations, dietary protein recommendations vary for young athletes. Protein requirements for endurance athletes undergoing heavy training range from 1.0 to 1.8 g/kg/day, whereas young athletes involved in high-intensity resistance exercise can require up to 2.4 g/kg/day to maintain a positive nitrogen balance (Phillips 2004, Boisseau et al. 2007). While ingesting adequate carbohydrates may help attenuate muscle protein breakdown, when amino acids are ingested or coupled with carbohydrates, improvement in net protein balance occurs. In general, it is recommended that athletes consume 10%–15% of their total daily energy intake from protein; however, analysis of an individual's dietary needs must be considered when providing recommendations on an individual basis and the coach and practitioner must understand that a combination of low energy intake by the athlete even at the above-recommended range can result in an adequate intake of dietary protein. For these reasons, protein intakes relative to the athlete's body weight (g/kg/day) help to eliminate these circumstances. These ranges of carbohydrate and protein appear to be acceptable for child and adolescent athletes as well (Maughan and Burke 2002). More information surrounding protein considerations can be found in Chapter 4.

Dietary fats are a fundamental fuel source for energy production during resting and exercising conditions. Dietary fat recommendations for young athletes are between 20% and 25% of total energy intake; there appears to be no benefit of reducing fat intake below 15% or increasing it beyond 30% (American Dietetic Association 2014). More research is needed with young athletes to investigate and better determine sport-specific macronutrient needs for this population; this topic is discussed in greater detail in Chapter 5.

Overall, most energy intake recommendations are based on adult populations due to the lack of scientific evidence available for child and adolescent athletes. Coaches and individuals providing nutritional guidance for young athletes should create individualized recommendations that encompass adequate energy, including appropriate carbohydrates, proteins, and fats, and take into account the age, gender, and specific physical activity requirements of the athlete. From this point, observing the athlete's body composition changes (explained below) against their energy level, performance, recovery ability, and their overall mood and attitude toward training and practice can help further determine the adequacy of an athlete's diet.

2.2 BODY COMPOSITION CONSIDERATIONS

Participation in sports confers numerous benefits to the athlete with body composition changes being primarily determined by the type of sport, be it contact, noncontact, or aesthetic in nature; training volume is also an important factor influencing body composition. In general, it is well known that high-impact or load-bearing sports improve bone mineral content, bone density, and muscularity while low- or no-impact endurance sports have more of a fat-mass reduction and cardioprotective effect. These benefits start accruing when the individual begins to undertake their sporting activities and training on a regular basis. This is true for children as well as for adults; however, the physiological adaptations for the child and adolescent athlete depend primarily on where the young person falls within the spectrum of development for their age and sex. Similarly, the demands of each type of sport underlie the extent and variety of training and energy required for optimal performance. Consequently, simultaneous matching of nutritional and body composition requirements are imperative to support both the healthy growth patterns and competitive aspirations of the child and adolescent athlete.

While the human body comprises a combination of 50 atoms (primarily oxygen, carbon, hydrogen, nitrogen, calcium, phosphorus, sulfur, potassium, sodium, chlorine, and magnesium) (Wang et al. 1992), the ability to assess each is only practical for research purposes. Exercise physiologists and nutritionists tend to focus their attention on an individual's bone, adipose, and muscular tissues. Loomba-Albrecht and Styne (2009) concisely identified that fat mass, fat-free mass (FFM), and bone mass offer clues reflective of the individual's hormonal status (i.e., prepubertal, postpubertal), genetics, race/ethnicity, and physical environment. To best understand how fat mass, FFM, and bone mass contribute to the whole of the human body, a body composition assessment is required, and a variety of assessment methods and models are available.

2.2.1 ANTHROPOMETRICS

Anthropometric assessment methods are quick, easy, inexpensive, and require varying degrees of technician skill. Anthropometrics provide information about bodily lengths, breadths, circumferences, subcutaneous fat distribution, area, volume, and weight. The resulting measurements may be used singly to provide a discrete value or in combination to serve as indices or estimations of regional distributions of the variables of interest. However, none of the anthropometric assessments can provide an accurate determination of body composition.

The anthropometric technique requiring the highest degree of technician skill is the skinfold (SKF) thickness assessment. It is also an invasive technique that requires the exposure and touching/grasping of the client's skin/subcutaneous fat at strategic anatomical locations. Understandably, for these reasons, ethical issues are present for the use of the SKF technique with children and adolescents and sensitivity toward these considerations and privacy of the young athlete are important. Cultural considerations should also be respected and accommodated. The assumptions underlying SKF are grounded in sex-specific fat distribution patterns, the ability to accurately estimate relative total body fatness percent body fat (% BF) from SKF measurements, and the relationship between body density (Db), age, and the sum of measurements from multiple SKF sites (Heyward and Wagner 2004). While numerous % BF estimation formulas exist for adults, the options for application within a sample of children or adolescents are fewer (Table 2.1). The association between Db and the sum of four SKF sites (Σ4SKF; triceps, abdomen, thigh, medial calf) for a sample of 317 subjects spanning the Tanner scale spectrum from prepubescent to adult was investigated by Slaughter and associates (1984). In addition to identifying developmental differences in the average Db (increasing with increasing Tanner scale) for all, they identified directional changes in the Σ4SKF (mm) with the males decreasing and the females increasing with maturation. The greatest changes in Db for males occurred between prepubescence and postpubescence while for females, the trend appeared to occur between prepubescence and pubescence. The medial calf and triceps

SKF sites were reported as being the most significant predictors of Db in their sample (Slaughter et al. 1984). Subsequent development of equations to estimate % BF from SKF (Slaughter et al. 1988) were developed with a sample of African American and Caucasian boys and girls ranging in age from 8 to 17 years. Found within both Tables 2.1 and 2.2 are Db equations that have been used in populations that include child and adolescent athletes. The equations found within Table 2.2 were

TABLE 2.1
Select Prediction Equations for SKF Thickness and BIA Inclusive of Children and Adolescents

Method	Sport	Sex (M/F)	Age (year)	Result	Equation	References
SKF	Varied	M	14–19	Db	$= 1.10647 - 0.00162(\text{subscap SKF}) - 0.00144(\text{ab SKF}) - 0.00077(\text{triceps SKF}) + 0.00071(\text{midax SKF})$	Forsyth and Sinning (1973)
SKF	Varied	M	18–29	Db	$= 1.112 - 0.00043499(\Sigma 7\text{SKF}) + 0.00000055(\Sigma 7\text{SKF})^2 - 0.00028826(\text{age})$	Jackson and Pollock (1978)
SKF	Varied adolescent athletes, high school wrestlers	M	14–19	Db	$= 1.0973 - 0.000815(\Sigma 3\text{SKF}) + 0.00000084(\Sigma 3\text{SKF})^2$	Lohman (1981) and as modified by Thorland et al. (1991) for high school wrestlers
SKF	Varied adolescent athletes (11–14 years), high school gymnasts	F	18–29	Db	$= 1.096095 - 0.0006952(\Sigma 4\text{SKF}) - 0.0000011(\Sigma 4\text{SKF})^2 - 0.0000714(\text{age})$	Jackson et al. (1980)
SKF	NR	M	8–17	% BF	$= 0.735 + (\Sigma 2\text{SKF}) + 1.0$	Slaughter et al. (1988)
SKF	NR	F	8–17	% BF	$= 0.610 + (\Sigma 4\text{SKF}) + 5.1$	Slaughter et al. (1988)
BIA (RJL 101A)	Dancers	F	18–27	FFM	$= 0.282(\text{Ht}) + 0.415(\text{BM}) - 0.037(R) + 0.096(Xc) - 9.734$	Fornetti et al. (1999)
BIA (RJL 106)	High school gymnasts	F	13–17	FFM	$= 0.52(\text{Ht}^2/R) + 0.29(\text{BM}) + 7.49$	Van Loan et al. (1990)
BIA (BIO-Z)	Elite distance runners	F	16–37	% BF	$= 7.32 - 0.572(\text{Ht}^2/R) + 0.664(\text{BM})$	Hannan et al. (1993)

Source: Adapted from Heyward, V.H. and Wagner, D.R. *Applied Body Composition Assessment*, Human Kinetics, Champaign, IL, 2004.

$\Sigma 7\text{SKF}$ = sum of SKF from the chest, midaxillary, triceps, subscapular, abdomen, anterior suprailiac, and thigh sites.
$\Sigma 4\text{SKF}$ = sum of SKF from the triceps, abdomen, anterior suprailiac, and thigh sites.
$\Sigma 3\text{SKF}$ = sum of SKF from the triceps, subscapular, and abdomen sites. $\Sigma 2\text{SKF}$ = sum of SKF from the triceps and medial calf sites.
NR = not reported.
Ht = height in cm; BM = body mass in kg; R = resistance in ohms; Xc = reactance in ohms.

TABLE 2.2
Select Population-Specific Db to Relative % BF Conversion Formulas Inclusive of Children, Adolescents, and Young Adult Athletes

Group	Age (year)	Sex	% BF Conversion	FFM Density (g/cc)
African American	9–17	F	$100 \times (5.24/Db) - 4.82$	1.088
	19–45	M	$100 \times (4.86/Db) - 4.39$	1.106
American Indian	18–60	F	$100 \times (4.81/Db) - 4.34$	1.108
	18–62	M	$100 \times (4.97/Db) - 4.52$	1.099
Japanese Native	18–48	F	$100 \times (4.76/Db) - 4.28$	1.111
		M	$100 \times (4.97/Db) - 4.52$	1.099
White	8–12	F	$100 \times (5.27/Db) - 4.85$	1.086
		M	$100 \times (5.27/Db) - 4.85$	1.086
	13–17	F	$100 \times (5.19/Db) - 4.76$	1.090
		M	$100 \times (5.12/Db) - 4.85$	1.092
	18–59	F	$100 \times (4.96/Db) - 4.51$	1.100
		M	$100 \times (4.96/Db) - 4.76$	1.090
Athletes (all sports)	18–22	F	$100 \times (4.97/Db) - 4.52$	1.099
		M	$100 \times (5.12/Db) - 4.68$	1.093

Source: Adapted from Heyward, V.H. and Wagner, D.R. *Applied Body Composition Assessment*, Human Kinetics, Champaign, IL, 2004.

Note: F = female; M = male; FFM = fat-free mass.

developed specifically with athletes whereas the Slaughter et al. (1988) equations found in Table 2.1 were not developed using just athletes, but have been used and reported by others who have used them for young athletes (Ibnziaten et al. 2002, Watts et al. 2003, Portal et al. 2010).

Probably the most commonly used anthropometric result is the body mass index (BMI). It is commonly used to identify a child as being overweight (≥85th percentile) or obese (≥95th percentile) for their age and sex (Centers for Disease Control and Prevention 2000). This technique is used for athletes and nonathletes alike. Although it is an easily acquired index that depicts a child's weight in relation to their height (kg/m^2), it cannot differentiate between fat mass and FFM. Similarly, BMI cannot account for the ethnic differences in the content of the FFM. Lohman and colleagues (1984) estimated the mineral contribution to FFM from the bone mineral content of the radius for a sample of prepubescent, pubescent, and postpubescent children (not identified as being athletes). They reported that for the males, American Black children had lower mineral contribution (5.19 ± 0.17%) compared to American White children (5.22 ± 0.17%) during prepubescence, but higher values during pubescence (5.68 ± 0.24% and 5.45 ± 0.18%, respectively) and postpubescence (6.26 ± 0.38% and 6.16 ± 0.41%, respectively). For the females, similar patterns were reported for prepubescence (5.10 ± 0.15% and 5.21 ± 0.15%) and postpubescence (5.87 ± 0.18% and 5.72 ± 0.22%), but not pubescence (5.33 ± 0.15% and 5.38 ± 0.23%) for the American Black and American White children, respectively. Ellis et al. (2000) identified differences in the total body water, potassium, and bone mineral content between American Black, American White, and Mexican-American adolescents (Ellis et al. 2000). American Black males consistently had the highest values throughout childhood (5–10 years) and adolescence (11–19 years) as compared to their American White and Mexican-American age-group peers. While ethnic differences were noted for the males, no consistent differences were reported for the females although the between-sex differences were most evident during adolescence (Ellis et al. 2000). An important point to highlight here is that any deviation from the

TABLE 2.3
Contribution of Select Constituents of FFM for Children and Adolescents

	Relative Contribution to FFM									
	Water (%)		Protein (%)		Mineral (%)		Potassium (g/kg)		FFM Density (g/cc)	
Age (year)	M	F	M	F	M	F	M	F	M	F
7–9	76.8	77.6	18.1	17.5	5.1	4.9	2.40	2.32	1.081	1.079
9–11	76.2	77.0	18.4	17.8	5.4	5.2	2.45	2.34	1.084	1.082
11–13	75.4	76.6	18.9	17.9	5.7	5.5	2.52	2.36	1.087	1.086
13–15	74.7	75.5	19.1	18.6	6.2	5.9	2.56	2.38	1.094	1.092
15–17	74.2	75.0	19.3	18.9	6.5	6.1	2.61	2.40	1.096	1.094
17–20	74.0	74.8	19.4	19.2	6.6	6.0	2.63	2.41	1.098	1.095

Source: Adapted from Lohman, T.G. 1986. *Exerc Sport Sci Rev* 14: 325–357 and Malina, R.M. 2005. Variation in body composition associated with sex and ethnicity. *Human Body Composition*. S.B. Heymsfeld, T.G. Lohman, Z. Wang and S.B. Going. Champaign, IL, Human Kinetics: 271–298.

Note: M = males; F = females. Values are compiled from a variety of studies and based on American White children.

assumed contribution of water, protein, and mineral content (Table 2.3) will affect the density of the FFM and, consequently, fat mass calculations.

In their continuing effort to promote healthy weight in young athletes, the American Academy of Pediatrics (2005) recommended that BMI results be interpreted with caution and highlighted the importance of augmenting BMI results by including at least one additional anthropometric measurement (American Academy of Pediatrics Committee on Sports Medicine and Fitness 2005). Evidence of the importance of the American Academy of Pediatrics policy statement is found in a recent study by Etchison and colleagues (2011) who evaluated the ability of BMI to correctly categorize athletes as being obese compared to SKF thickness assessment. Their primary finding was that using BMI alone misclassified the relative fat mass (% BF) of the adolescent athletes (15.24 ± 0.01 years, 165.25 ± 0.05 cm, 66.80 ± 0.09 kg, 22.88 ± 0.02 kg/m^2) in their study (Etchison et al. 2011). Over 13% (4470 of 33,595) of the sample athletes were classified as obese by BMI; however, when SKF thickness measurements were used, the number of athletes classified as obese dropped by 55% to 1999 (approximately 6% of the sample). In other words, of the athletes classified as obese by BMI, 62% were classified as not being obese based on the gender-specific three-site (male sites: chest, abdomen, and thigh; female sites: triceps, suprailiac, and thigh) SKF thickness equations of Jackson and Pollock (Jackson et al. 1980, Jackson and Pollock 2004). Etchison and colleagues defined obesity using the SKF technique as being >24% for males and >30% for females (Etchison et al. 2011). Klungland and Sundgot-Borgen (2012) also concluded that BMI was not valid for estimating or monitoring the body composition of the elite female athletes (13–39 years) in their study (Klungland Torstveit and Sundgot-Borgen 2012).

Therefore, while sole anthropometric evaluations of young athletes provide little insight into their body composition, they have been used to provide comparative information of athletes in sports such as rowing, tennis, sport rock climbing, rugby, and volleyball. Specifically, elite male junior rowers representing 41 of the countries participating in the 1997 World Junior Rowing Championships underwent anthropometric assessments and were found to have significantly (p < 0.01) higher weight, length, breadth (except bicristal), girth, and tricep SKF thickness dimensions compared to the nonfinalists. Compared to reference anthropometric values for Belgian school-age males (17.5–18.0 years), the rowers (15.1–18.6 years) were significantly (p < 0.01) taller and heavier; had greater biacromial diameters; had larger humerus and femur widths; had higher circumferences of the biceps, thigh, and calf; and had greater triceps and subscapular SKF thickness values (Bourgois et al. 2000). Sanchez-Munoz et al. (2007) assessed 57 male and 66 female elite junior tennis players participating in the 2005 and 2006 Davis Junior Cup and Fed Junior Cup competitions to compare 17 anthropometric variables of the athletes finishing in the top 12 to those finishing at lower rankings. Although there were no significant differences for the boys, the top 12 girls were significantly taller and had wider femoral and humeral breadths compared to the lower-ranked players ($p < 0.01$) (Sanchez-Munoz et al. 2007). In terms of somatotype, the boys, on average, were ectomesomorphic while the girls were endomesomorphic; however, somatotypes were similar among the two levels of rankings for the two sexes. Compared to a control group of children and adolescents participating in competitive basketball, swimming, soccer, cross-country skiing, and cross-country running, 90 sport rock climbers (13.5 ± 3.0 years, 5.11 d on the Yosemite decimal system scale for climbing ability) competing in the Junior Competition Climbers Association U.S. National Championship were found to be shorter, lighter, leaner, and more linear (higher biiliocristal/biacromial ratio) in stature ($p < 0.01$). Interestingly, the absolute BMI and BMI expressed as a percentile were similar between the climbers and nonclimbers (Watts et al. 2003). Gabbett et al. (2009) recruited elite (16.0 ± 0.2 years, 178.0 ± 5.9 cm, 77.5 ± 10.0 kg) National Rugby League club players (n = 28) and subelite (15.9 ± 0.6 years, 176.0 ± 6.0 cm, 74.3 ± 13.4 kg) junior rugby league club players (n = 36) and performed a variety of assessments, including height, weight, and sum of seven SKF thickness measurements. Players from each level of club play were further categorized into starters and nonstarters. Elite starters were found to be taller and heavier than the corresponding nonstarters. Subelite starters were also found to be taller, but were similar in weight to the subelite nonstarters. Positional differences were also investigated by club level. For the elite players, the hit-up forwards were significantly ($p < 0.05$) fatter than the adjustables and heavier than the adjustables and outside backs. At the subelite level, a similar trend in significant differences by position was reported; although, both the adjustables and outside backs were significantly leaner than the hit-up forwards ($p < 0.05$) (Gabbett et al. 2009). For a small sample of elite adolescent Israeli volleyball players (14 males, 15 females; 13–18 years) representing the national team, BMI was reported as lacking validity for body composition estimation as compared to two-component (2C) models (Portal et al. 2010).

2.2.2 Body Water

Anthropometric methods and bioelectrical impedance analysis (BIA) are known as field methods of body composition estimation as the requisite technology is portable, the measurements are quick, technical skill is generally minimal, and many people can be assessed in a short period of time. BIA requires the introduction of a low-level (~50 kHz) electrical current into the body; single-frequency BIA is a noninvasive technique that can be used to estimate extracellular water (ECW) volume and, ultimately, FFM. Alternatively, multiple-frequency analyzers utilize one lower and one higher frequency level (i.e., 250 kHz). Bioelectrical impedance spectroscopy is similar to multiple-frequency analysis with the exception that currents representing the spectrum of frequencies (i.e., 5 kHz to 1 MHz) are introduced. Regardless of the technique used to introduce electrical currents, the currents are introduced via a pair of electrodes with the drop in current frequencies recorded by a pair of sensing electrodes. The original configuration of electrodes was tetrapolar with one pair of gel electrodes at the hand and wrist with the other pair of gel electrodes at the foot and ankle (wrist-to-ankle) on the right side of the body. This standard tetrapolar configuration requires the client to be in a supine position, with hands pronated, on a nonconductive surface; the arms and legs must be slightly abducted to avoid contact between body parts. Vertical analyzers have also been developed, which allow for ECW estimation with the client either holding (hand-to-hand or upper body analyzer) or standing barefoot (leg-to-leg or lower body analyzer) on the analyzer. This style of analyzer utilizes plate electrodes embedded into the handles or scale platform, respectively. The upper and lower body analyzers are collectively known as segmental analyzers since they derive their measurement of electrical current resistance in a specific segment of the body instead of throughout the entire length of the body (wrist-to-ankle configuration). The newest analyzers combine upper- and lower-body analyzer features and include embedded electrodes in both the handles and scale platform for a total of eight electrodes; this style of analyzer provides the opportunity to include both the right and left sides of the body in addition to the upper- and lower-body segments for a whole body assessment.

Caution must be exercised, however, when interpreting the results from BIA and bioelectrical impedance spectroscopy as many analyzers utilize a proprietary conversion formula and display results for % BF and FFM without any explanation as to what constant pertaining to the hydration of FFM (% water) was used. In addition to this important bit of information, the client's level of hydration will also directly affect the results. Since electricity is conducted by water and electrolytes contained therein, being in a dehydrated state will increase the resistance of the body tissues to the current. Consequently, the result will produce a higher estimation of % BF than if the client is adequately hydrated (i.e., euhydrated). Given the age- and sex-specific differences in the relative contribution of water to the FFM as shown in Table 2.3, it is important to understand how BIA and bioelectrical impedance spectroscopy equations were created and validated. The age- and sex-specific hydration constants of FFM (Table 2.3) have been reported to provide the most valid estimations of total body water as compared to the deuterium oxide reference for adolescent athletes (Quiterio et al. 2009).

Clarys and associates (2011) utilized segmental BIA and an underwater weighing reference measure in their study of 30 adolescent judo athletes having an average age of 16.3 ± 1.3 years. Unfortunately, they did not specify whether the residual volume was measured or estimated. Regardless, they reported a significant correlation and no mean difference between upper-body BIA (17.7 ± 3.3% BF) and underwater weighing (16.4 ± 5.6% BF) for the 13 girls (r = 0.77). The lower-body BIA results (22.1 ± 4.5% BF) were higher than both the upper-body BIA and underwater weighing results; the correlation between the lower-body BIA and underwater weighing results was both nonsignificant (p > 0.05) and moderately strong (r = 0.49). For the boys, values for 14 of the participants were attained via upper-body BIA (9.3 ± 5.1% BF) whereas values for all 17 participants were recorded via lower-body BIA (9.7 ± 3.7% BF) and underwater weighing (7.2 ± 4.5% BF). However, the correlations for both segmental BIA estimations of percent fat (% fat) were weak (r = 0.22, lower-body) or moderately strong (r = 0.47, upper-body) in relation to the underwater weighing reference; yet, no significant differences between the means were reported for the boys (Clarys et al. 2011). The authors emphasized that sex-specific fat distribution patterns and musculoskeletal adaptations to judo training most likely explain the similarities and differences between the methods, and it is worth noting that these general conclusions are likely to be present with analyses involving other athletes.

Most of the tetrapolar BIA estimation equations for FFM have been validated using underwater weighing in conjunction with residual volume measurements as the reference value, while a few have been validated using an isotope dilution reference. The electrical frequencies used by bioelectrical impedance spectroscopy analyzers allow an estimation of ECW and total body water through the introduction of the low-level and higher-level frequencies, respectively. The current of the higher-level frequencies passes through cell membranes, whereas the lower-level frequencies (≤100 kHz) cannot penetrate them (Moon 2013). Once total body water and ECW are known, the intracellular water volume can be computed by subtracting ECW from total body water. The intracellular water has been used as a proxy for body cell mass in adults. Alternatively, isotope dilution (i.e., deuterium oxide and sodium bromide) techniques can be used to more accurately measure total body and extracellular water, respectively, but do require more expensive and complicated assessment techniques.

In addition to being the gold standard for measuring the various water compartments, the dilution method has also been used to estimate total energy expenditure. Ebine and colleagues (2000) used doubly labeled water to measure the daily energy expenditure of Japanese national synchronized swimmers over a 6-day period. The junior swimmers (n = 5; 17.6 ± 1.1 years, 52.8 ± 2.3 kg), expended a total of 11.5 ± 2.95 MJ/d (2747 ± 705 kcal) as determined by isotope dilution. Their energy intake (7-day food recall), on average, was 9.82 ± 1.71 MJ/d (2345 ± 408 kcal), resulting in what the authors concluded was an underreporting of energy intake as there was no change in body mass over the course of the study. In comparison to the recommended daily allowance (RDA) for energy intake for the Japanese women, the results were found to be statistically similar for the group. The authors highlighted their finding of interindividual variability in the ability of RDAs and self-reported food recalls to match the total energy expenditure requirement and cautioned against using RDA as an accurate estimation of an elite athlete's total energy requirement (Ebine et al. 2000).

2.2.3 Multiple-Component Models

Multiple-component models of body composition assessment provide more accurate estimations of an individual's FFM and fat mass; they also serve as the preferred reference measure for prediction equation development. FFM is traditionally defined as being comprised of water, protein, and mineral. Each of these constituents has its own density, which is believed to be known and additive; it is also assumed that the relative proportions of the constituents are constant (Behnke et al. 1995). Mineral is the densest of these three constituents while water is the least dense. The relative (%) contribution of each constituent varies with age, ethnicity/race, and physical activity. In contrast to what is known about constituent density, the relative proportion of water is the highest while mineral is the lowest (Table 2.3). The more constituents of the FFM that are directly measured, the more accurate the estimation of the corresponding fat mass.

The 2C model categorizes the body as being fat mass and FFM. The 2C model is the basis of underwater weighing or hydrodensitometry. It is also the basis of air-displacement plethysmography. Consequently, the majority of body composition estimation equations based on anthropometric assessments (e.g., SKF thicknesses or circumferences) were developed using a densitometric method (usually underwater weighing) as the reference measure of Db and rely on the assumptions underlying the 2C model (Heyward and Wagner 2004). However, both densitometric methods have inherent errors, thereby making the prediction equations designed and validated using them nothing more than an estimate. Regardless, 2C model equations tend to produce accurate estimations of % BF if the individual tested meets the model assumptions. While the concept of Db (body mass/body volume) is universal, the resulting Db values must be converted to % BF via either a population-specific or generalized conversion formula. However, the population-specific Db to % BF conversion formulas that included children and adolescents in the samples are limited (Table 2.2) and require that the professional selects a suitable conversion formula based on the density of the FFM. An athlete-specific Db to % BF conversion formula does exist, but it was developed on college-aged individuals (men and women; 18–22 years) making it inappropriate for use with younger athletes who have yet to attain chemical maturity (FFM composition resembling that of adults: 73.8% water, 19.4% protein, 6.8% mineral) (Siri 1961, Brozek et al. 1963). Lohman and associates (1984) identified that appropriate relative contributions of mineral and water were 5.4% and 76.6%, respectively, for prepubescent children (Lohman et al. 1984). This results in a FFM density calculated as 1.084 grams/cubic centimeter (g/cc) thereby making the Keys and Brozek (1953) Db to % BF conversion formula [% BF = (100 × 5.30/Db) − 4.89] (Keys and Brozek 1953) more appropriate for prepubescent children as compared to the conversion formulas of Siri (1961) and Brozek et al. (1963); the latter two formulas assume that FFM density is 1.10 g/cc. Again, caution is warranted since the prepubescent children referenced in the Lohman study were not specified as being athletes; furthermore, training and nutritional habits of young athletes have changed substantially since 1984. For example, a study of elite junior rowers from the 1997 (n = 603) and 2007 (n = 398) Junior World Rowing Championships revealed that although there were no significant differences in body mass between the groups, the 2007 rowers were found to be significantly taller by 1.0 cm (males) and 2.1 cm (females). Interestingly, in both time periods, the finalists were found to be both taller and heavier compared to the nonfinalists (Rakovac et al. 2011).

Three-component (3C) models were created to reduce the number of unknown variables contributing to the FFM. Siri's (1961) 3C model computes fat mass from measurements of total body water, body volume, and body mass (Siri 1961); Lohman's (1986) 3C model computes fat mass from measurements of mineral, body volume, and body mass (Lohman 1986). Both the Siri and Lohman models utilize a body volume derived from underwater weighing at measured residual volume and are beneficial if the individual being measured is believed to deviate from the assumed proportion of water or mineral, respectively. Dual-energy x-ray absorptiometry (DXA) is the newest 3C model and estimates bone mineral, lean soft tissue, and fat (Ellis 2000). Of the three 3C models discussed here, DXA requires the least exertion by the client. If the primary interest is in obtaining the most accurate estimate of bone mineral content or bone mineral density, then DXA is the recommended method. DXA is receiving substantial interest as a reference measure of total body and regional fat mass and FFM, especially for children and youth, because it does not rely on the assumptions of the 2C model. Nevertheless, caution is urged when interpreting results. DXA is an automated x-ray-based system; when software upgrades are made, the prediction results have been reported to vary (Plank 2005); furthermore, measurements of the same person on DXA machines from the different manufacturers have been shown to differ as well (Plank 2005). Changing scan modes during a longitudinal study has also introduced bone mineral area, bone mineral content, and bone mineral density differences of 3.4%, 7.6%, and 3.1%, respectively, for a sample of girls (10–13 years; Tanner stage I–III) assessed with a GE Lunar Prodigy densitometer (Cheng et al. 2005). Pediatric assessment software modules are available and should form the basis of DXA scans of the child and adolescent athletes, and should be mentioned if used in studies of children and adolescents. Regardless, literature searches for the body composition of child and adolescent athletes yield far more studies based on DXA than on underwater weighing or air-displacement plethysmography.

Four-component (4C) models further increase the accuracy of body composition estimations by measuring total body water, bone mineral, body mass, and body volume. The third constituent of FFM, protein, can then be calculated by subtracting the water and mineral from the FFM (% protein = 100% FFM − [% water + % mineral]). For these models, water is usually measured via isotope dilution, bone mineral by DXA, and body volume by underwater weighing; although, there has been some interest in utilizing air-displacement plethysmography for the body volume measure. The popular two-site SKF thickness equation was created using a 4C reference measure with underwater weighing at measured residual volume for body volume; however, the individual % BF prediction error by this SKF equation ranges from ±8%–10% (Slaughter et al. 1988).

While each measured component increases the accuracy of the body composition estimation, it must be noted that it also increases the opportunity for measurement error, especially if the client does not meet the assumptions underlying the methods or models, the client does not match the demographics of the sample for which the equations were designed, or the technician was not attentive to detail. More than four components can be measured if there is access to the technology. Multiple-component models are expensive and time-intensive for both the athlete and the evaluator to implement compared to 2C models (Moon 2013). So, the practitioner needs to carefully weigh the costs and benefits for the young athlete. However, if using a 2C model for assessing the body composition of a child or adolescent athlete, it is important to use a prediction equation that was validated using a multiple-component model to improve the individual predictive accuracy.

Silva and colleagues (2006) compared the predictive accuracy of DXA (Hologic QDR-1500) and air-displacement plethysmography to a five-component (5C) (total body water, body volume, bone mineral, soft tissue mineral, and body mass) reference measure for a sample of young, sports club athletes (32 girls: 15.1 ± 0.3 years, 165.0 ± 13.0 cm, 56.2 ± 14.2 kg, 20.2 ± 2.6 kg/m^2; 46 boys: 15.3 ± 1.2 years, 180.0 ± 12.0 cm, 71.5 ± 12.3 kg, 22.0 ± 2.5 kg/m^2). The athletes, 82% of whom were post-pubescent, represented the sports of judo, swimming, rugby, gymnastics, and basketball. The authors concluded that neither air-displacement plethysmography nor DXA produced individual estimates of % BF that were narrow enough to be considered precise when compared to a 5C reference. Further toward this point, DXA overestimated % BF for both groups ($p < 0.05$), but the estimation difference was larger for the girls (3.69 ± 2.89% BF) than the boys (1.04 ± 2.7% BF). For air-displacement plethysmography, the only significant difference was a 1.65 ± 1.53% underestimation of % BF for the girls with no statistically significant difference between that reported for boys using air-displacement plethysmography. In terms of proportions of the FFM constituents, the girls had significantly lower water (70.9 ± 1.2%) and higher protein (22.8 ± 1.6%) fractions compared to the boys (water: 72.4 ± 1.7%; protein: 21.5 ± 1.5%); $p < 0.05$. Consequently, the girls had a higher ($p < 0.05$) FFM density (1.105 ± 0.004 g/cc) than did their male counterparts (1.100 ± 0.007 g/cc) whose FFM density matched the assumed FFM density of the 2C model. When the air-displacement plethysmography Db to % BF conversion formula was switched from the default Siri (1961) formula (a formula that was derived from an adult sample) to include Lohman's age-adjusted conversion factors (1986), air-displacement plethysmography significantly underestimated ($p < 0.05$) the reference % BF by 4.04 ± 1.63% and 1.70 ± 2.7% for the girls and boys, respectively. Nevertheless, the authors concluded that although statistically significant differences were reported, the clinical, or practical, differences for air-displacement plethysmography are acceptable for the adolescent in that study if the default Siri Db equation to % BF equation is used, but is not suitable if age-adjustments by Lohman are used (Silva et al. 2006).

In addition to improving sport skill and establishing a competitive edge of their young athletes, coaches and parents are wise to monitor the health and physical development trajectory of the child and adolescent. While annual monitoring of body composition of child and adolescent athletes is recommended, understanding what comprises the FFM is crucial and multiple component models of body composition assessment are helpful in this regard. Additionally, body fatness operates on a continuum with health and performance issues being affected at both ends of the spectrum. High levels of fatness typically are the result of physical activity levels that are too low and an energy intake that is too high. Not surprisingly, rates of overweightness, obesity, and poor fitness in children continue to climb. For these reasons, concerns related to high levels of body fatness in young athletes are more pertinent today than they were several decades ago (Centers for Disease Control 2012, Fakhouri et al. 2014). However, low levels of body fatness are of concern given their association with conditions such as fluid or electrolyte abnormalities, bone fractures, reproductive disorders, endothelial dysfunction, and disordered eating.

Studying both the bone integrity and geometry of young athletes provides clues to nutritional, hormonal, and energy balance status and an extensive review of bone health in the adolescent athlete has been previously published (Tenforde and Fredericson 2011). The comprehensive review by Javed and colleagues (2013) details the screening and management of the female athlete triad (comprised eating disorders, amenorrhea, and low bone mineral density); their review provides an in-depth coverage of topics ranging from the pathophysiology and consequences to educational strategies for the athlete and their healthcare practitioners (Javed et al. 2013). In accordance with Wolff's law, bone adapts to stresses applied to it in healthy individuals. Weight-bearing or impact sports place stresses on bone via musculoskeletal attachments and direct support of external loads; alternatively, no-impact sports induce smaller stresses on bone. The peri-pubertal period appears to be an optimal window in which bone density can be favorably enhanced (Loomba-Albrecht and Styne 2009, Going and Farr 2010, Maimoun et al. 2013). As a result, it is not surprising that post-menarcheal female competitive swimmers (15.9 ± 2 years, 164.9 ± 6.9 cm, 56.8 ± 5.9 kg) had a lower bone mineral density (DXA: Hologic QDR 4500-series) than did soccer (16.2 ± 0.7 years, 165.0 ± 5.8 cm, 57.1 ± 6.1 kg) players (1.03 ± 0.05 g/cc and 1.19 ± 0.07 g/cc, respectively) with soccer players having significantly higher bone mineral density values in the lumbar spine, hip, trochanter, intertrochanter, and femoral neck (Ferry et al. 2013). Similarly, for female athletes (13.83 ± 1.97 years), the artistic gymnasts had areal bone mineral density (DXA: Hologic QDR 4500A) values that were higher at all sites when compared to age-paired swimmers (Maimoun et al. 2013). In a comparison of male road cyclists and age-matched recreationally active controls, Olmedillas and associates (2011) found that after adjusting for height and lean mass, the bone mineral density (DXA: Hologic

QDR Explorer) of the controls (16.7 ± 2.1 years, 176.1 ± 8.9 cm, 74.4 ± 16.8 kg) was significantly higher than that of the cyclists (16.9 ± 1.9 years, 173.2 ± 6.7 cm, 61.3 ± 7.7 kg) for the pelvis, hip, leg, and whole body; interestingly, these differences were magnified when older (17+ years) cyclists were compared against controls than when comparing younger participants to age-matched, less-active controls (Olmedillas et al. 2011). Elite junior Olympic weightlifters (17.4 ± 1.4 years) were found to have bone mineral density values of the lumbar spine, Wards triangle, trochanter, and femoral neck that were significantly higher than age-matched controls; the junior weightlifters also had lumbar spine and femoral neck bone mineral density values comparable to adult (20–39 years) references (Conroy et al. 1993).

As mentioned previously, the low level of body fat associated with years of high-volume training begun in the prepubertal years is believed to delay the onset of menses. Female rowers competing in the 1997 FISA World Junior Rowing Championships were found to have a significantly different age of menarche depending on when, in relation to menarche, they began their training; those who began training prior to menses entered menarche 1 year later (mean age of menses: 13.4 years) than those who began training after menarche (Claessens et al. 2003). Likewise, intense, high-volume training in the postpubertal years may contribute to athletic amenhorrea (Javed et al. 2013) and lower bone mineral density (Olmedillas et al. 2011).

Whether it is the sheer volume of exercise, hormonal irregularities, or disordered eating patterns that may develop following caloric restriction (either self-imposed based on perception of the ideal body or based on recommendations by coaches or trainers), low levels of body fat can adversely affect bone health, because bone mineralization is estrogen-dependent. Unfortunately, many young female athletes are unaware of the connection between menstrual status and bone health. Feldmann and colleagues (2011), in addition to citing statistics regarding awareness of this link in female college-aged athletes, conducted an investigation of 103 high school athletes (14.3–18.6 years, 3.8 ± 1.54 years post-menarche) on the girls' track and field team. The results revealed that, on average, the girls had little knowledge about the relationship between training intensity, bone health, and menstrual status even though approximately one-third of them reported menstrual irregularities. While 48.5% knew they were too young to have weak bones, 38.8% knew that skipping menstrual cycles was not normal; only 8.7% knew that menstrual irregularities decreased bone integrity. The authors indicated that it was the high mileage runners who were more knowledgeable about menstrual irregularities and bone status (Feldmann et al. 2011).

Competitive tennis is a rigorous, weight-bearing sport that, for females, is played in an attire that exposes a substantial amount of the body. Coelho et al. (2013), finding no published research on the topic, sought to determine whether adolescent, Brazilian female tennis players were at risk for developing disordered eating habits and female athlete triad. Body composition was assessed via DXA (GE Lunar Prodigy Plus Advanced); a nutritionist evaluated 3-day food recall logs, and questionnaires were used to assess menstrual status and eating/body image attitudes. Recognizing the continuum of female athlete triad, Coelho and colleagues (2013) identified two categories for their participants. Stage I, or moderately severe, was defined as having low bone mineral density (−1.0 Z-score units), low energy availability (<45 kcal/kg of FFM per day), and menstrual irregularity. Stage II, or severe, was defined as having a bone mineral density score that was −2.0 Z-score units, disordered eating, and being amenorrheic. Of the 24 tennis players, 1 met all 3, 11 met 2, and 98% met 1 of the criteria for Stage I. Whereas in terms of Stage II classification, only 1 player met 2 and 13 met 1 of the 3 criteria. Of note, regardless of the significant differences between the athletes (14.77 ± 2.16 years, 52.28 ± 7.74 kg, 159.50 ± 6.06 cm) and age-group sedentary controls (15.41 ± 1.86 years, 54.41 ± 9.15 kg, 156.29 ± 5.73 cm) for % BF (lower), FFM (higher), and hours spent exercising (higher), there were no significant differences in total body or lumbar spine bone mineral density. Among the numerous conclusions offered, the authors commented that the athletes' low energy availability influenced the athletes' bone mineral density since those with low bone mineral density (at least −1.0 Z-score units) were positive for low energy availability (Coelho et al. 2013). Similarly, female Brazilian swimmers (11–19 years) underwent DXA (GE Lunar Prodigy Plus Advanced) scans and answered questionnaires regarding their eating patterns (Ferreira et al. 2013). Thirty-four of the 77 female swimmers were positive for disordered eating. Of the younger group (11–14 years), those who were classified as having disordered eating were significantly heavier (53.7 kg) and fatter (27.5% BF) than those who were negative for disordered eating (46.6 kg and 23.4% BF, respectively). In the 15–19-year-old group, the same pattern of body fatness was reported whereby those classified with disordered eating (30.2% BF) had significantly higher ($p < 0.05$) levels of body fat (24.1% BF) than those who were not classified with ordered eating even though the two eating pattern groups were similar in weight (57.6 and 57.2 kg, respectively). Unfortunately, no bone mineral density data were provided. Javed and associates (2013) identified athletes participating in the lean body or "aesthetic" sports such as gymnastics, ballet, and long-distance running as being at the greatest risk for developing female athlete triad. Although the majority of research on athletes with disordered eating identifies the problem to be one associated with the female athlete, it has also been reported in males. In their study of elite Swedish adolescent athletes (n = 611), Martinsen and Sundgot-Borgen (2013) confirmed that the prevalence of those with eating disorders was statistically ($p < 0.05$) higher in females (14%) compared to males (3.2%). Of note, they did not report any differences for prevalence of disordered eating for the female athletes based on the weight sensitivity of their respective sports. Martinsen and Sundgot-Borgen also reported that many of the athletes underreported their unhealthy behaviors on a questionnaire in comparison to a clinical interview. One of their concluding remarks was the suggestion that clinical interviews be used to assess disordered eating habits of young athletes (Martinsen and Sundgot-Borgen 2013).

Nichols and colleagues (2007) investigated the influence of sport type (high/odd impact vs. repetitive/nonimpact), menstrual status, and bone mineral density (DXA: GE Lunar DPX-NT) in 161 high school female athletes. Those with eumenhorreic status were placed in one group and everyone else was combined into the second group. As expected, for the eumenhorreic group, the high/odd-impact sport participants (soccer, volleyball, softball, lacrosse, tennis, sprinters, jumpers) had greater ($p < 0.05$) bone mineral density for the hip and trochanter than did their repetitive/no-impact sport participants (swimmers, cross-country, long-distance runners). The repetitive/no-impact sport athletes in the oligo/amenorrheic group had lower lumbar spine and trochanter bone mineral density values than did the eumenhorreic high/odd-impact athletes ($p < 0.05$). The repetitive/no-impact athletes had a greater ($p < 0.05$) prevalence (33.9%) of low bone mineral density (Z-score ≤ -1) in the spine than did the high/odd-impact athletes (11.8%) (Nichols et al. 2007). Nichols' work corroborates earlier findings of To et al. (2005) who compared bone mineral density values for adolescent female dancers to eumenhorreic sedentary controls. To et al. (2005) reported that the eumenhorreic dancers (18.3 ± 0.79 years, 18.8 ± 1.76 kg/m^2, 19.1 ± 4.01% BF) had significantly greater bone mineral density (DXA: Norland XR26 Mark II) at the lumbar spine, Ward's triangle, femoral neck, and trochanter than did the controls (18.3 ± 0.49 years, 20.4 ± 3.21 kg/m^2, 25.5 ± 6.01% BF); $p < 0.05$. These differences were no longer apparent when comparing the oligo/amenhorreic dancers (18.1 ± 0.69 years, 17.9 ± 0.93 kg/m^2, 18.1 ± 2.28% BF) to the eumenhorreic controls (To et al. 2005).

2.2.4 Recommendations Regarding Body Fatness of Child and Adolescent Athletes

It is tempting for athletes, parents, and coaches to evaluate child and adolescent athletes against standard values or recommendations. Key factors such as individual responses to training, nutrition, and maturation as well as an athlete's sport of choice can all impact the level of body fatness or FFM development exhibited by each athlete. For these reasons, it is difficult to identify a specific % BF for the male and female athlete that would be considered ideal for all athletes, regardless of their age. However, professional opinion regarding the minimal healthy level of % BF for adult men is 5%–7% BF; whereas, for adult women, the minimum % BF level for competitive sport is 12%–14% BF (Meyer et al. 2013). Although these values are deemed arbitrary and are intended to be employed for adult athletes who have reached biological maturation, they have been accepted by the majority of practitioners (Meyer et al. 2013). The National Athletic Training Association cites 14% BF as being the lowest value for an adolescent female athlete and 7% BF for adolescent males (Turocy et al. 2011). However, it is not uncommon for adolescent male athletes to fall within the 5%–12% BF range, while their female counterparts tend to range between 16% and 18% BF (Burke et al. 2012). In consideration of the many factors that create individualism, these ranges are offered as recommendations and should not be used to overtly classify an athlete's body composition as acceptable or unacceptable.

2.3 SUMMARY AND CONCLUSIONS

Optimal athletic performance is deeply intertwined with both athletic ability and skill; however, individualized nutritional needs and accurate body composition monitoring is critical to the athlete's health and ability to perform. Ensuring adequate caloric needs based on individual requirements of carbohydrates, proteins, and fats are vital in order to support the body as well as promote sports performance of an athlete.

While the athlete's support team (coaches, parents, nutritionists, etc.) are wise to appreciate the tendencies reported as mean and standard deviation values in the available research, understanding the interindividual variability of each athlete is key to the young athlete's ability to maintain normal development patterns and competitive aspirations as they enter and move through adulthood. Owing to the lack of research and the inherent differences that may exist and in many situations are very likely to exist between two athletes of the same gender with the exact same age, it is difficult to provide specific energy intake recommendations; however, professionals guiding the child or adolescent athlete must take their developmental stage and demands of physical exercise into account. Like adult athletes, examining the overall profile of the athlete in terms of how rested and recovered they feel, has their attitude or mood toward training or competing changed, how is their body composition changing, and how well they are performing are also key factors that provide indicators of the adequacy of the diet. In terms of body composition assessment, it is this interindividual variability that makes one assessment method or technique more accurate than another.

REFERENCES

American Academy of Pediatrics Committee on Sports Medicine and Fitness. 2005. Promotion of healthy weight-control practices in young athletes. *Pediatrics* 116(6): 1557–1564.

American Dietetic Association. 2014, May 30, 2014. *Pediatric Nutrition Care Manual*. https://www.nutritioncaremanual.org.

Behnke, A.R., Jr., Feen, B.G. and Welham, W.C. 1995. The specific gravity of healthy men. Body weight divided by volume as an index of obesity. 1942. *Obes Res* 3(3): 295–300.

Blaak, E.E., Westerterp, K.R., Bar-Or, O., Wouters, L.J. and Saris, W.H. 1992. Total energy expenditure and spontaneous activity in relation to training in obese boys. *Am J Clin Nutr* 55(4): 777–782.

Boisseau, N., Vermorel, M., Rance, M., Duche, P. and Patureau-Mirand, P. 2007. Protein requirements in male adolescent soccer players. *Eur J Appl Physiol* 100(1): 27–33.

Bolster, D.R., Pikosky, M.A., Mccarthy, L.M. and Rodriguez, N.R. 2001. Exercise affects protein utilization in healthy children. *J Nutr* 131(10): 2659–2663.

Bourgois, J., Claessens, A.L., Vrijens, J. et al. 2000. Anthropometric characteristics of elite male junior rowers. *Br J Sports Med* 34(3): 213–216; discussion 216–217.

Brozek, J., Grande, F., Anderson, J.T. and Keys, A. 1963. Densitometric analysis of body composition: Revision of some quantitative assumptions. *Ann N Y Acad Sci* 110: 113–140.

Burke, M., Smith, A.D. and Loud, K.J. 2012. Young athletes. *Team Physician Manual: International Federation of Sports Medicine*. L. J. Mitchell, F. Pigozzi, K. M. Chan et al. New York, Routledge: 195–205.

Centers for Disease Control. 2012. Physical Activity Guidelines for Americans. Retrieved July 18, 2014, http://www.cdc.gov/physicalactivity/data/facts.html.

Centers for Disease Control and Prevention. 2000, published May 2000, modified October 2000, retrieved July 19, 2014. Growth charts. http://www.cdc.gov/growthcharts.

Cheng, S., Nicholson, P.H., Kroger, H., Alen, M. and Tylavsky, F. 2005. Differences in estimates of change of bone accrual and body composition in children because of scan mode selection with the prodigy densitometer. *J Clin Densitom* 8(1): 65–73.

Claessens, A.L., Bourgois, J., Beunen, G. et al. 2003. Age at menarche in relation to anthropometric characteristics, competition level and boat category in elite junior rowers. *Ann Hum Biol* 30(2): 148–159.

Clarys, P., Geelan, B., Aerenouts, D., Deriemaeker, P. and Zinzen, E. 2011. Estimation of body composition in adolescent judo athletes. *J Combat Sports Martial Arts* 2: 73–77.

Coelho, G.M., De Farias, M.L., De Mendonca, L.M. et al. 2013. The prevalence of disordered eating and possible health consequences in adolescent female tennis players from Rio de Janeiro, Brazil. *Appetite* 64: 39–47.

Conroy, B.P., Kraemer, W.J., Maresh, C.M. et al. 1993. Bone mineral density in elite junior Olympic weightlifters. *Med Sci Sports Exerc* 25(10): 1103–1109.

Cunningham, E. 2010. Where can I find resources to assist in the determination of pediatric energy needs that account for physical activity of child and adolescent athletes? *J Am Diet Assoc* 110(8): 1264.

Delamarche, P., Monnier, M., Gratas-Delamarche, A. et al. 1992. Glucose and free fatty acid utilization during prolonged exercise in prepubertal boys in relation to catecholamine responses. *Eur J Appl Physiol Occup Physiol* 65(1): 66–72.

Ebine, N., Feng, J.Y., Homma, M., Saitoh, S. and Jones, P.J. 2000. Total energy expenditure of elite synchronized swimmers measured by the doubly labeled water method. *Eur J Appl Physiol* 83(1): 1–6.

Ellis, K.J. 2000. Human body composition: *In vivo* methods. *Physiol Rev* 80(2): 649–680.

Ellis, K.J., Shypailo, R.J., Abrams, S.A. and Wong, W.W. 2000. The reference child and adolescent models of body composition. A contemporary comparison. *Ann N Y Acad Sci* 904: 374–382.

Etchison, W.C., Bloodgood, E.A., Minton, C.P. et al. 2011. Body mass index and percentage of body fat as indicators for obesity in an adolescent athletic population. *Sports Health* 3(3): 249–252.

Fakhouri, T.H., Hughes, J.P., Burt, V.L. et al. 2014. Physical activity in U.S. youth aged 12–15 years, 2012. *NCHS Data Brief* 141: 1–8.

Feldmann, J.M., Belsha, J.P., Eissa, M.A. and Middleman, A.B. 2011. Female adolescent athletes' awareness of the connection between menstrual status and bone health. *J Pediatr Adolesc Gynecol* 24(5): 311–314.

Ferreira, J.E., De Souza, P.R., Jr., Da Costa, R.S., Sichieri, R. and Da Veiga, G.V. 2013. Disordered eating behaviors in adolescents and adults living in the same household in metropolitan area of Rio de Janeiro, Brazil. *Psychiatry Res* 210(2): 612–617.

Ferry, B., Lespessailles, E., Rochcongar, P., Duclos, M. and Courteix, D. 2013. Bone health during late adolescence: Effects of an 8-month training program on bone geometry in female athletes. *Joint Bone Spine* 80(1): 57–63.

Fornetti, W.D., Pivarnik, J.M., Foley, J.M. and Fiechtner, J.J. 1999. Reliability and validity of body composition measures in female athletes. *J Appl Physiol* 87(3): 1114–1122.

Forsythe, H.L. and Sinning, W.E. 1973. The anthropometric estimation of body density and lean body weight of male athletes. *Med Sci Sports Exerc* 5(3): 174–180.

Gabbett, T., Kelly, J., Ralph, S. and Driscoll, D. 2009. Physiological and anthropometric characteristics of junior elite and sub-elite rugby league players, with special reference to starters and non-starters. *J Sci Med Sport* 12(1): 215–222.

Going, S.B. and Farr, J.N. 2010. Exercise and bone macro-architecture: Is childhood a window of opportunity for osteoporosis prevention? *Int J Body Compos Res* 8: 1–9.

Hannan, W.J., Cowen, S.J., Freeman, C.P. and Wrate, R.M. 1993. Can bioelectrical impedance improve the prediction of body fat in patients with eating disorders? *Eur J Clin Nutr* 47(10): 741–746.

Heyward, V.H. and Wagner, D.R. 2004. *Applied Body Composition Assessment*. Champaign, IL, Human Kinetics.

Ibnziaten, A., Poblador, M.S., Leiva, A. et al. 2002. Body composition in 10 to 14-year-old handball players. *Eur J Anat* 6(3): 153–160.

Jackson, A.S. and Pollock, M.L. 1978. Generalized equations for predicting body density of men. *Brit J Nutr* 40: 487–504.

Jackson, A.S. and Pollock, M.L. 2004. Generalized equations for predicting body density of men. 1978. *Br J Nutr* 91(1): 161–168.

Jackson, A.S., Pollock, M.L. and Ward, A. 1980. Generalized equations for predicting body density of women. *Med Sci Sports Exerc* 12(3): 175–181.

Javed, A., Tebben, P.J., Fischer, P.R. and Lteif, A.N. 2013. Female athlete triad and its components: Toward improved screening and management. *Mayo Clin Proc* 88(9): 996–1009.

Keys, A. and Brozek, J. 1953. Body fat in adult man. *Physiol Rev* 33(3): 245–325.

Klungland Torstveit, M. and Sundgot-Borgen, J. 2012. Are under- and overweight female elite athletes thin and fat? A controlled study. *Med Sci Sports Exerc* 44(5): 949–957.

Lohman, T.G. 1981. Skinfolds and body density and their relation to body fatness: A review. *Hum Biol* 53(2): 181–225.

Lohman, T.G. 1986. Applicability of body composition techniques and constants for children and youths. *Exerc Sport Sci Rev* 14: 325–357.

Lohman, T.G., Slaughter, M.H., Boileau, R.A., Bunt, J. and Lussier, L. 1984. Bone mineral measurements and their relation to body density in children, youth and adults. *Hum Biol* 56(4): 667–679.

Loomba-Albrecht, L.A. and Styne, D.M. 2009. Effect of puberty on body composition. *Curr Opin Endocrinol Diabetes Obes* 16(1): 10–15.

Maimoun, L., Coste, O., Philibert, P. et al. 2013. Peripubertal female athletes in high-impact sports show improved bone mass acquisition and bone geometry. *Metabolism* 62(8): 1088–1098.

Malina, R.M. 2005. Variation in body composition associated with sex and ethnicity. *Human Body Composition*. S.B. Heymsfeld, T.G. Lohman, Z. Wang and S.B. Going. Champaign, IL, Human Kinetics: 271–298.

Martinez, L.R. and Haymes, E.M. 1992. Substrate utilization during treadmill running in prepubertal girls and women. *Med Sci Sports Exerc* 24(9): 975–983.

Martinsen, M. and Sundgot-Borgen, J. 2013. Higher prevalence of eating disorders among adolescent elite athletes than controls. *Med Sci Sports Exerc* 45(6): 1188–1197.

Maughan, R.J. and Burke, L.M. 2002. *Sports Nutrition*. Malden, MA, Blackwell Science.

Meyer, N.L., Sundgot-Borgen, J., Lohman, T.G. et al. 2013. Body composition for health and performance: A survey of body composition assessment practice carried out by the Ad Hoc Research Working Group on Body Composition, Health and Performance under the auspices of the IOC Medical Commission. *Br J Sports Med* 47(16): 1044–1053.

Moon, J.R. 2013. Body composition in athletes and sports nutrition: An examination of the bioimpedance analysis technique. *Eur J Clin Nutr* 67(Suppl 1): S54–S59.

Nichols, J.F., Rauh, M.J., Barrack, M.T. and Barkai, H.S. 2007. Bone mineral density in female high school athletes: Interactions of menstrual function and type of mechanical loading. *Bone* 41(3): 371–377.

Olmedillas, H., Gonzalez-Aguero, A., Moreno, L.A., Casajus, J.A. and Vicente-Rodriguez, G. 2011. Bone related health status in adolescent cyclists. *PLoS One* 6(9): e24841.

Petrie, H.J., Stover, E.A. and Horswill, C.A. 2004. Nutritional concerns for the child and adolescent competitor. *Nutrition* 20(7–8): 620–631.

Phillips, S.M. 2004. Protein requirements and supplementation in strength sports. *Nutrition* 20(7–8): 689–695.

Plank, L.D. 2005. Dual-energy x-ray absorptiometry and body composition. *Curr Opin Clin Nutr Metab Care* 8(3): 305–309.

Portal, S., Rabinowitz, J., Adler-Portal, D. et al. 2010. Body fat measurements in elite adolescent volleyball players: Correlation between skinfold thickness, bioelectrical impedance analysis, air-displacement plethysmography, and body mass index percentiles. *J Pediatr Endocrinol Metab* 23(4): 395–400.

Quiterio, A.L., Silva, A.M., Minderico, C.S. et al. 2009. Total body water measurements in adolescent athletes: A comparison of six field methods with deuterium dilution. *J Strength Cond Res* 23(4): 1225–1237.

Rakovac, M., Smoljanovic, T., Bojanic, I. et al. 2011. Body size changes in elite junior rowers: 1997 to 2007. *Coll Antropol* 35(1): 127–131.

Sanchez-Munoz, C., Sanz, D. and Zabala, M. 2007. Anthropometric characteristics, body composition and somatotype of elite junior tennis players. *Br J Sports Med* 41(11): 793–799.

Silva, A.M., Minderico, C.S., Teixeira, P.J., Pietrobelli, A. and Sardinha, L.B. 2006. Body fat measurement in adolescent athletes: Multicompartment molecular model comparison. *Eur J Clin Nutr* 60(8): 955–964.

Siri, W.E. 1961. Body composition from fluid space and density. *Techniques for Measuring Body Compostion*. J. Brezek and A. Henschel. Washington D.C., National Academy of Sciences: 223–224.

Slaughter, M.H., Lohman, T.G., Boileau, R.A. et al. 1984. Influence of maturation on relationship of skinfolds to body density: A cross-sectional study. *Hum Biol* 56(4): 681–689.

Slaughter, M.H., Lohman, T.G., Boileau, R.A. et al. 1988. Skinfold equations for estimation of body fatness in children and youth. *Hum Biol* 60(5): 709–723.

Sundgot-Borgen, J., Meyer, N.L., Lohman, T.G. et al. 2013. How to minimise the health risks to athletes who compete in weight-sensitive sports review and position statement on behalf of the Ad Hoc Research Working Group on Body Composition, Health and Performance, under the auspices of the IOC Medical Commission. *Br J Sports Med* 47(16): 1012–1022.

Tenforde, A.S. and Fredericson, M. 2011. Influence of sports participation on bone health in the young athlete: A review of the literature. *PM R* 3(9): 861–867.

Thorland, W.G., Tipton, C.M., Lohman, T.G. et al. 1991. Midwest wrestling study: Prediction of minimal weight for high school wrestlers. *Med Sci Sports Exerc* 23(9): 1102–1110.

To, W.W., Wong, M.W. and Lam, I.Y. 2005. Bone mineral density differences between adolescent dancers and non-exercising adolescent females. *J Pediatr Adolesc Gynecol* 18(5): 337–342.

Turocy, P.S., Depalma, B.F., Horswill, C.A. et al. 2011. National Athletic Trainers' Association position statement: Safe weight loss and maintenance practices in sport and exercise. *J Athl Train* 46(3): 322–336.

Van Loan, M.D., Boileau, R.A., Slaughter, M.H. et al. 1990. Association of bioelectrical resistance with estimates of fat-free mass determined by densitometry and hydrometry. *Amer J Hum Biol* 2(3): 219–226.

Wang, Z.M., Pierson, R.N., Jr. and Heymsfield, S.B. 1992. The five-level model: A new approach to organizing body-composition research. *Am J Clin Nutr* 56(1): 19–28.

Watts, P.B., Joubert, L.M., Lish, A.K., Mast, J.D. and Wilkins, B. 2003. Anthropometry of young competitive sport rock climbers. *Br J Sports Med* 37(5): 420–424.

3 Carbohydrate Needs of the Young Athlete

Julia K. Zakrzewski and Keith Tolfrey

CONTENTS

Abstract 35
3.1 Introduction 36
3.2 Recommended Values for Carbohydrate Intake for Young Athletes 36
3.3 Current Levels of Carbohydrate Intake in Young Athletes 37
3.4 Child–Adult Metabolic Differences 39
3.5 Carbohydrate Intake: Days and Hours before Endurance Exercise 40
3.6 Carbohydrate Intake: During Endurance Exercise 42
    3.6.1 Performance 42
    3.6.2 Substrate Oxidation 45
3.7 Carbohydrate Intake: Postexercise 47
3.8 Short-Duration High-Intensity Exercise and Skill Performance 49
3.9 Sports Drinks and Hydration 49
3.10 Health, Glycemic Index, and Insulin Sensitivity 50
3.11 Summary 52
References 53

ABSTRACT

Carbohydrate (CHO) typically provides the majority of energy in the athlete's diet and is essential to fuel high-intensity exercise. Ensuring adequate energy is available to meet the demands of high energy expenditure is important in the young athlete to ensure proper growth, development, and maturation. Physiological and metabolic changes that accompany the transition from childhood to adolescence and to adulthood, combined with the additional energy expenditure arising from exercise, mean that the dietary needs of young athletes require special consideration. However, in contrast to the well-documented literature in adults, little research attention has been given to child and adolescent populations. Thus, the development of specific recommendations for CHO intake in young athletes is difficult. Nevertheless, it is possible to make some general recommendations. Both the total daily CHO intake and the timing of CHO consumption in relation to exercise can determine whether adequate CHO substrate is available for muscles and the central nervous system, or whether CHO fuel sources might limit exercise performance. In terms of the overall diet, CHO should contribute to the majority of energy intake, which must be high enough to support growth and maturation while fueling the additional physical activity, and consequently elevated energy expenditure in young athletes. In particular, CHO is an important fuel for high-intensity exercise in young athletes. Decrements in exercise performance, fatigue, and changes in body composition may serve as useful indicators that CHO intake may not be adequate, particularly in female adolescent athletes. During exercise, drinks containing CHO could be considered for young athletes engaged in endurance exercise due to the preferential use of exogenous CHO in younger athletes in the pre- or early-pubertal stages. However, evidence on CHO loading and CHO for postexercise recovery does not appear to be available in children or adolescents. This chapter provides an overview of the available evidence that can be used to determine recommendations for CHO intake and timing in young athletes. Where no direct evidence in young athletes is available, we have relied on the relevant adult-based literature while emphasizing that the direct translation and application of these findings to children and adolescents must be viewed cautiously.

3.1 INTRODUCTION

Good nutritional practice is essential for both health and exercise performance in athletes. Although young people today are generally less active and heavier than recommended, numbers of young athletes involved in competitive sport and intense regular training with high energy expenditures have increased in recent years (Malina 2010). Ensuring adequate energy is available to meet the demands of high energy expenditures is important in the young athlete to ensure proper growth, development, and maturation (Malina 2010). Physiological and metabolic changes that accompany the transition from childhood to adolescence and to adulthood, combined with the additional energy expenditure arising from exercise, mean that the dietary needs of young athletes require special consideration.

Carbohydrate (CHO) intake provides the majority of energy in the diet and is also essential to fuel high-intensity exercise. Dietary CHO intake in young athletes may be evaluated in terms of both the total daily intake and the timing of consumption in relation to exercise; these factors can determine whether adequate CHO substrate is available for muscles and the central nervous system (CNS) or whether CHO fuel sources might limit exercise performance. Although the CHO needs of adults have been well documented, little research attention has been given to child and adolescent populations; this is surprising given the plethora of physical, physiological, and metabolic child–adult differences that are seen in the pediatric sport and exercise science literature. Therefore, there is no doubt that specific evidence focusing on young athletes is required to inform CHO recommendations tailored to this age group. This chapter provides an overview of the available evidence that can be used to determine recommendations for CHO intake and timing in young athletes. Where no direct evidence in young athletes is available, we have relied on the relevant adult-based literature while emphasizing that the direct translation and application of these findings to children and adolescents must be viewed cautiously.

3.2 RECOMMENDED VALUES FOR CARBOHYDRATE INTAKE FOR YOUNG ATHLETES

The Dietary Guidelines for Americans (USDA; U.S. Department of Health and Human Services and US Department of Agriculture 2010) provide estimated daily energy needs by age, sex, and physical activity level (Table 3.1). Rather than using kilojoules (kJ; the SI unit), the recommendations for energy intake are provided in kilocalories (kcal), which typically provide more meaningful values for the general public to interpret. The Institute of Medicine (2002) has established ranges for the percentage of energy (kcal) in the diet that should come from CHO, protein, and fat; these acceptable macronutrient distribution ranges (AMDR) take into account both chronic disease risk reduction and intake of essential nutrients. However, unlike daily total energy intake, recommendations for CHO intake have not been stratified by physical activity level, age, or sex; the AMDR is 45%–65% of total energy intake. Combining these details with the recommendations in Table 3.1, older and more active children should consume more CHO (g) due to the higher total energy intake that is recommended. Accordingly, perhaps it would be preferable for young athletes to aim to consume the amount of CHO (g) equal to 45%–65% of daily energy within the "active" energy intake category of Table 3.1. For example, a 12-year-old female athlete should consume 1800–2200 kcal day^{-1}, with 203–248 g (45% of total kcal) to 293–358 g (65% of total kcal) from CHO. However, the dietary reference intake (DRI) remains

TABLE 3.1
Estimated Daily Total Energy (kcal) Needs by Age, Sex, and Physical Activity Level

Sex	Age (Years)	Physical Activity Level		
		Sedentary	Moderately Active	Active
Female	4–8	1200–1400	1400–1600	1400–1800
	9–13	1400–1600	1600–2000	1800–2200
	14–18	1800	2000	2400
Male	4–8	1200–1400	1400–1600	1600–2000
	9–13	1600–2000	1800–2200	2000–2600
	14–18	2000–2400	2400–2800	2800–3200

Source: Adapted from U.S. Department of Agriculture and U.S. Department of Health and Human Services. *Dietary Guidelines for Americans, 2010.* 7th Edition, Washington, DC: U.S. Government Printing Office, December 2010.

Note: The values here may be used in conjunction with the AMDR for CHO (45%–65% of total energy intake) to estimate CHO needs specific to age, sex, and physical activity level.

at 100 g day^{-1} and recommended dietary allowance (RDA) at 130 g day^{-1} for all age and sex categories (children ≥1 year), which are not specific to physical activity level.

For young athletes, the RDAs appear to require further consideration due to the additional energy expenditures in this population. The American College of Sports Medicine (Rodriguez et al. 2009) recommends that adult athletes should consume 6–10 g CHO kg^{-1} body mass^{-1} each day, depending on the athlete's total daily energy expenditure, type of sport, sex, and environmental conditions, but excludes children and adolescents explicitly from these recommendations. Based on the combination of a higher reliance on fat as a fuel, lower glycogen stores, and limited glycolytic capacity in younger athletes, they may require less dietary CHO (% total energy intake) than adults (see Section 3.4). The Academy of Nutrition and Dietetics has provided some general guidance for adolescent athletes, recommending the consumption of a training diet that meets nutrition needs for physical activity and health with 55%–60% of total energy from CHO (Steen et al. 1996). They also emphasize the importance of a diet, including variety, balance, and moderation in food choices, as well as targeting athletes with an increased risk for developing eating disorders. However, no specific guidelines for prepubertal children were provided due to the lack of child-specific evidence.

3.3 CURRENT LEVELS OF CARBOHYDRATE INTAKE IN YOUNG ATHLETES

Nutritional surveys reporting CHO intakes of young athletes are important in identifying groups or individuals who may be at risk of inadequate dietary CHO consumption. The increased independence and peer pressure that often accompanies adolescence can influence food selections, which may lead to certain nutrient deficiencies and an increased risk of negative health consequences; for example, stunted growth, loss of lean body mass, reduced bone mineral content or density, fatigue, delayed injury recovery, menstrual dysfunction, and diminished performance (Malina 2010, Tamminen et al. 2012).

A number of small-scale studies have assessed daily absolute CHO intake in young athletes—examples are displayed in Table 3.2. Intakes are likely influenced by a number of factors, including age, sex, body composition, and specific event and/or sport. Even when considering only a single sport, assessments of CHO intakes have shown daily values ranging from 293 to 469 g,

TABLE 3.2
Examples of Reported CHO Intakes in Young Athletes

Sport/Event	Age (Years)	Sex	CHO Intake (g day^{-1})	References
Mixed endurance ($n = 93$)	17 (1)	F	352 (127)	Malczewska et al. (2000)
Gymnastics ($n = 29$)	7–10	F	219 (57)	Benardot et al. (1989)
Gymnastics ($n = 22$)	11–14	F	227 (64)	Benardot et al. (1989)
Figure skating ($n = 48$)	15 (2)	F	243 (111)	Ziegler et al. (2002)
Wrestling ($n = 18$)	16 (2)	M	367 (123) (BWL) 209 (136) (DWL)	Horswill et al. (1990)
U.S. football ($n = 46$)	12–14	M	302 (125)	Hickson et al. (1987)
U.S. football ($n = 88$)	15–18	M	366 (170)	Hickson et al. (1987)
Volleyball ($n = 65$)	14–19	F	195 (88)	Papadopoulou et al. (2002)
Association football ($n = 8$)	17 (2)	M	526 (62)	Rico-Sanz et al. (1998)

Note: Mean (SD); BWL = preseason before weight loss; DWL = during-season during weight loss.

corresponding to 41%–55% of daily energy intake, in adolescent association football players (Bar-Or and Unnithan 1994; Boisseau et al. 2002; Giovannini et al. 2000; Iglesias-Gutierrez et al. 2005; Rico-Sanz et al. 1998). For female adolescents, CHO represented 54% of total energy intake in athletes of various sports (Cupisti et al. 2002), but only 46% of total energy in volleyball players (Papadopoulou et al. 2002) were found. However, longitudinal nutrient intake assessments are needed to estimate any changes in CHO intake in relation to growth. In a 3-year follow-up study of 19 young French association football players, daily CHO intake increased from 320 g to 360 g from 13 to 14 years of age, and then to 396 g at 15 years, but did not increase when expressed per kilogram body mass (Leblanc et al. 2002). A 3-year longitudinal study in female runners reported an increased CHO intake relative to total energy intake, but decreased total absolute energy and CHO intakes (Wiita and Stombaugh 1996). Further longitudinal nutritional surveys that consider age, sex, puberty, body composition, and sport or specific event would provide valuable information on current CHO intakes in young athletes and changes with growth.

It is difficult to ascertain whether reported CHO intakes are adequate for health and performance due to the lack of specific CHO intake recommendations in young athletes that account for individual considerations, such as age, sex, body composition, and training load (see Section 3.2). However, it may be possible to identify certain groups susceptible to "low" CHO intakes, where sex appears to be an important factor. Intake of CHO is generally higher in boys (6 and 9 g kg^{-1}) (Chen et al. 1989; Leblanc et al. 2002; Montfort-Steiger et al. 2005) compared with girls (3–5.5 g kg^{-1}) (Cupisti et al. 2002; Papadopoulou et al. 2002; Wiita and Stombaugh 1996). The prevalence of eating disorders is also higher in adolescent female athletes compared to male athletes, and is higher in elite athletes compared with nonathletes (Martinsen and Sundgot-Borgen 2013). Disordered eating and low-energy intake associated with specific sports may also place certain individuals at risk of inadequate CHO intake. Events where it is seen as an advantage to remain lean, have an aesthetically appealing appearance, and make weight for sports all carry an increased risk of low energy and CHO intake. Thus, athletes, including distance runners, figure skaters, divers, synchronized swimmers, rhythmic dancers, gymnasts, and boxers may require special attention (Manore 2002). Restricted eating with the belief that it can delay puberty is a concern among young girls participating in aesthetic sports (Malina 2010), but is fairly simple to identify using specific questionnaires. For example, the children's Dutch Eating Behavior Questionnaire (DEBQ) for the measurement of restrained, emotional, and external eating (van Strien and Oosterveld 2008) may be a useful tool for coaches and parents to screen young athletes for restrictive eating and inadequate CHO intakes.

3.4 CHILD–ADULT METABOLIC DIFFERENCES

An insight into exercise substrate metabolism in children and adolescents underpins our understanding of young athletes' CHO needs. Differences in substrate metabolism between children and adults have been known for some time now. It was demonstrated more than 70 years ago that children have lower respiratory exchange ratio (RER) values during exercise compared with adults, indicating a higher reliance on fat and lower reliance on CHO oxidation (Robinson 1938). Subsequently, lower RER values have been observed in boys and girls compared with adults during submaximal exercise performed at similar absolute (Montoye 1982) and relative (Foricher et al. 2003; Martinez and Haymes 1992) exercise intensities. Prepubertal boys and girls also have low CHO oxidation rates compared with matched sex adolescents during exercise at the same relative intensity (Timmons et al. 2007a,b), suggesting puberty may modulate these changes in fat oxidation. Data are not entirely consistent in females; however, some studies indicate that girls and women exhibit similar contributions of fat oxidation to energy expenditure (Rowland and Rimany 1995). Discrepancies in the results of studies investigating females (Martinez and Haymes 1992; Rowland and Rimany 1995) may be due to inadequate control for the menstrual cycle (Oosthuyse and Bosch 2010).

Possible mechanisms that can explain the lower reliance on CHO and higher reliance on fat as fuels at rest and during exercise in children are unclear. The commonly held belief that children have an underdeveloped glycolytic system was based initially on a series of muscle biopsy studies with a small sample of boys by Eriksson and colleagues more than 40 years ago, reviewed by Eriksson (1980). In these studies, the glycogen content of muscle in 11- to 16-year-old boys was 50%–60% lower than reported in untrained adults (Eriksson et al. 1973) and increased with maturation (Eriksson and Saltin 1974). The activity of the rate-limiting enzyme for glycolysis in 11-year-old boys, phosphofructokinase (PFK), was only approximately 30% of that reported in published studies of untrained men (Eriksson et al. 1973). Although other researchers have not measured PFK, quantification of other glycolytic enzyme activities from muscle biopsies has proffered equivocal results. In a mixed sex comparison of 8 6-year-old children with 12 13-year-old mid-adolescents and 13 17-year-old young adults, lactate dehydrogenase (LDH) activity was highest in the adolescents (143% > children; 55% > young adults) (Berg et al. 1986). Although aldolase and pyruvate kinase were also greatest in the adolescent group, the enzyme activities were only significantly higher than the children, not the young adults (Berg et al. 1986).

In contrast, several oxidative enzymes, including succinate dehydrogenase (SDH), fumarase, and isocitrate dehydrogenase (ICDH), measured in young boys and adolescent girls were considerably higher when compared directly and indirectly with activities at physiological temperatures in men and women (Eriksson et al. 1973; Haralambie 1979, 1982). The young children in Berg's study (1986) had ~40% higher fumarase activity than the young adults; furthermore, when the data for the three age groups were pooled (n = 33; age range 3–19 years), fumarase was inversely related to chronological age ($r^2 = 0.23$). Comparing the ratio of PFK to ICDH (glycolytic: oxidative) activity in a mixed sex group of adults and 13- to 15-year-old adolescent girls, Haralambie (1982) found it doubled in adults (1.63 vs. 0.84). This strongly suggests that oxidation of tricarboxylic acid cycle intermediates is more prominent during adolescence than glycolysis. Some of the enzymes included in these studies were described as equilibrium or non-rate-limiting, which may diminish their influence on the flux through physiological pathways; more importantly, the comparisons between young people and adults were indirect in the Scandinavian studies, and all of the studies were with small sample sizes because of the ethical and logistical difficulties in obtaining tissue samples from this population. Nevertheless, there is evidence supporting the lower LDH activity (Kaczor et al. 2005) and blood lactate concentration during exercise (Macek et al. 1976; Mahon et al. 1997) in young people compared with adults. This is important, as lactate, an intermediate of CHO oxidation, is inversely related to fat oxidation (Achten and Jeukendrup 2004). Moreover, the lactate increase above baseline (LIAB) coincides with the intensity at which fat oxidation begins to decline in adolescents (Tolfrey et al. 2010) and adults (Achten and Jeukendrup 2004), and the increase in blood lactate with intensity is more pronounced in men than boys (Mahon et al. 1997). It is possible that a higher proportion of type I muscle fibers and intramuscular triacylglycerol (IMTAG) stores observed in children compared with adults may contribute to their increased ability to oxidize fat, but such data obtained from muscle biopsies in children are sparse and may also depend on training status (Bell et al. 1980; Fournier et al. 1982). Increased free fatty acid (FFA) availability and uptake during exercise in children compared with adults has also been reported (Delamarche et al. 1992), but not always confirmed (Boisseau and Delamarche 2000; Martinez and Haymes 1992). Although no age-related changes in carnitine palmitoyltransferase (CPT1) activity or major differences in enzyme activities of fat metabolism were observed in children compared with adults (Haralambie 1982; Kaczor et al. 2005), the CPT/2-oxoglutarate dehydrogenase ratio of enzyme activities in skeletal muscle may be higher in children (Kaczor et al. 2005), suggesting a preferential oxidation of fat over CHO.

More recent work using stable isotope techniques indicates that children do not have an underdeveloped glycolytic flux and it has been suggested that glycogen stores limit CHO oxidation. Indeed, younger, less mature boys rely more on exogenous CHO oxidation during exercise (Timmons et al. 2007b) (see Section 3.2). Although no difference in exogenous CHO oxidation was reported between 12- and 14-year-old girls, this may have been due to the small difference in puberty between the two groups (Tanner 3 and 4) (Timmons et al. 2007a). These findings should be considered in the context of exercise training, however, as the early work by Eriksson et al. (1973) showed that 4 months of training increased muscle glycogen concentration in 11- to 13-year-old boys and, after maximal work, blood and muscle lactate levels were higher and a greater reduction in muscle glycogen occurred. In a second experiment, 6 weeks of training increased SDH and PFK activities by 30% and 83%, respectively (Eriksson et al. 1973). Therefore, the capacity to store and use glycogen may increase with training in boys; there is no available direct evidence of this in girls.

3.5 CARBOHYDRATE INTAKE: DAYS AND HOURS BEFORE ENDURANCE EXERCISE

Manipulating CHO intake in the days ("CHO loading") and hours before an important exercise training session or competition allows adult athletes to commence exercise with glycogen stores sufficient to fuel the event. In adults, glycogen stores are an important source of blood glucose to provide energy for exercise and studies using invasive methods have shown that severe reductions in muscle glycogen (Bergstrom et al. 1967) and blood glucose derived from liver glycogen (Coyle and Coggan 1984) are associated with early onset of fatigue. Accordingly, elevating muscle glycogen content prior to exercise through the consumption of a high-CHO diet (CHO loading) postpones fatigue by approximately 20% in endurance events lasting more than 90 min, where exhaustion often coincides with critically low muscle glycogen content (Hawley et al. 1997). Carbohydrate loading and the associated glycogen supercompensation (i.e., increase above original baseline concentration) may also improve endurance performance by 2%–3% where a predetermined distance is covered as quickly as possible. Conversely, there is little or no effect of elevating preexercise muscle glycogen content above normal resting values on a single exhaustive bout of high-intensity exercise lasting less than 5 min or for moderate-intensity running or cycling lasting 60–90 min, where substantial quantities of glycogen remain in the working muscles at the end of exercise (Hawley et al. 1997). Adult endurance athletes can achieve glycogen supercompensation without the need for the "traditional" depletion phase (exhaustive exercise and low-CHO diet to achieve glycogen depletion) in the days before loading, and with as little as 24–36 h of high CHO intake and rest (Burke et al. 2011).

Based on dietary recommendations for adults, young athletes may be under the impression that consuming a high-CHO diet in the days and hours before exercise will improve performance, and consequently they might CHO load to some degree in preparation for major events. However, the effects of CHO loading on glycogen supercompensation and performance in children and adolescents remain unknown, partly due to ethical issues surrounding the use of invasive procedures with young people (e.g., muscle biopsies for the determination of muscle glycogen) and side effects associated with the glycogen depletion stage of the "traditional" CHO loading protocol (Bergstrom et al. 1967). In fact, the commonly held understanding that CHO loading can improve performance may not apply as readily to young people for various reasons. First, the relevance of CHO loading to youth athletes engaging in events lasting less than 90 min should be questioned, based on evidence from adults. Second, it appears that the physiological mechanism underpinning the effect of CHO loading on performance in adults may not translate to children due to their limited capacity to store glycogen (Eriksson et al. 1973) and utilize endogenous CHO during exercise (Timmons et al. 2007a, b). This suggests that children may not be able to "supercompensate" and, even if children did exhibit an ability to increase muscle glycogen through CHO loading, they are less likely to use endogenous CHO to provide energy for exercise (see Section 3.4). Indeed, there is evidence that adult women may not benefit from CHO loading and, like children, appear to rely to a greater extent on fat and exogenous CHO oxidation during exercise than adult men (Horton et al. 1998; Tarnopolsky 2008; Tarnopolsky et al. 1995). Although 6 days of a high-CHO diet can increase muscle glycogen and cycling time to fatigue in women, the magnitude of these changes was smaller than those observed previously in men (Walker et al. 2000), with further research revealing the increase in CHO availability and oxidation following CHO loading (plus CHO ingestion during exercise) did not translate to improved performance in women (Andrews et al. 2003). When comparing men and women directly, the increase in muscle glycogen concentration and time-trial performance in endurance-trained men following a 4-day CHO loading regimen did not occur in women of a similar training status (Tarnopolsky et al. 1995).

Evidence that the performance-enhancing effect of CHO loading in men may not be equally effective in women implies the applicability of CHO loading to young athletes is questionable. However, increasing muscle glycogen stores through CHO loading may benefit male adolescents during the later stages of puberty (Tanner stage 4 and 5) when the metabolic profile is similar to that of adult men (Riddell et al. 2008; Stephens et al. 2006; Timmons et al. 2007b). Furthermore, as noted in Section 3.4, training resulted in an increased capacity to store and use glycogen in boys (Eriksson et al. 1973); thus, young athletes who train regularly may exhibit an ability to increase their glycogen stores through CHO loading, with potential effects on performance. For these reasons, the interaction between training, CHO loading, and exercise performance in young people warrants examination. Since it is now known that the glycogen depletion phase of CHO loading is not required in adults, some ethical issues associated with this research in children may no longer exist and there may be scope to study whether the effects of CHO loading in adults translate to young athletes.

Similar to CHO loading, research over the past three decades has supported the recommendation that adults should consume an easily digestible high-CHO meal 2–4 h before endurance competition. This practice replenishes liver glycogen stores (which are reduced to low values after an overnight fast), increases muscle glycogen stores, and can extend endurance capacity (time to exhaustion), but does not necessarily improve time-trial performance (Chryssanthopoulos et al. 2004; Wee et al. 2005; Williams and Lamb 2008). Yet again, it is unclear whether the performance-enhancing effects of preexercise CHO consumption translate to young people. As with CHO loading, the potential for children to increase their glycogen stores needs to be examined systematically. Children do, however, have a higher capacity to use exogenous CHO (Timmons et al. 2003, 2007b), suggesting that provision of adequate preexercise CHO to maintain blood glucose concentration during exercise may be beneficial. In particular, consuming a meal rich in low glycemic index (LGI—see Section 3.10) CHO releases glucose gradually (Jenkins et al. 1981; Ludwig et al. 1999); the attenuated postprandial glucose and insulin response maintains blood glucose concentrations during exercise, can reduce the suppression of fat oxidation that normally accompanies CHO feeding, and may improve exercise performance in adults (Burke et al. 2011). Furthermore, the blunted glucose and insulin response to meals with LGI has been demonstrated in children and adolescents, but no effect on substrate oxidation during postprandial exercise was observed (Zakrzewski et al. 2012) and the effect on exercise performance has not been investigated. Although not all studies have supported the benefits of consuming LGI foods in the hours before exercise, this practice may be beneficial when it is difficult to consume CHO during exercise and in individuals who are sensitive to a hyperinsulinemic response to CHO feedings (e.g., those with low insulin sensitivity). From a general health and well-being perspective, it is also worth mentioning that regular breakfast consumption is associated with improved health, nutrition, and academic performance in young people (Rampersaud et al. 2005). In addition, exercise in the fasted state, often the alternative to consuming a high-CHO meal 2–4 h before exercise, may not be a practical option for young people. Consequently, fasted exercise involving "skipping breakfast" may not be a feasible or healthful behavior in young people.

There is no doubt that further research is required to provide specific recommendations for CHO consumption in the days and hours before exercise in young people. Importantly, the efficacy and safety of "CHO loading" has not been studied in children and should be considered. Rather than CHO loading to "supercompensate," it may be preferable for young athletes to ensure that CHO intake in the days and hours leading up to competition is sufficient to avoid depletion of glycogen stores and, perhaps more importantly, adequate CHO is available to meet daily requirements. Indeed, CHO provides an important source of energy for growth in children, who require more energy per kilogram of body weight during physical activity than adults (Bar-Or 2001). Inadequate energy intake in combination with high energy expenditures should be avoided due to the potential consequences of negative energy balance (see Section 3.3).

3.6 CARBOHYDRATE INTAKE: DURING ENDURANCE EXERCISE

The majority of experimental research on CHO intake in young athletes has involved the provision of different mono- and disaccharides during exercise (see Table 3.3). Since CHO oxidation increases with exercise intensity, increasing glucose availability should logically help sustain a higher exercise intensity and enhance performance. The available evidence in young people has generally supported these claims through examination of performance and substrate metabolism, as discussed below. Potential mechanisms explaining the enhanced performance with CHO intake during exercise in adults include provision of an additional fuel source when glycogen stores become depleted, muscle glycogen sparing, prevention of low blood glucose concentrations, and effects on the CNS, some of which may also apply to children and depend on the characteristics of the exercise.

3.6.1 Performance

A small number of studies have investigated the effects of exogenous CHO ingestion immediately before or during exercise on performance in young people, but have produced conflicting results. In contrast to much of the adult literature, one of the first studies in young people to examine the effects of CHO ingestion immediately before exercise reported no effect on performance (Hendelman et al. 1997). Three hours after a standardized breakfast, 15-year-old untrained adolescent boys consumed a candy bar, fat-free fig bars, or a sweetened drink (placebo) 10 min before exercise. Despite varying quantities of CHO, the preexercise CHO snacks did not affect blood glucose concentrations or substrate oxidation during 75 min cycling at 60% of VO_{2max} or subsequent time-trial performance (Hendelman et al. 1997). However, the performance trial may have been too short (5–6 min) to detect differences due to substrate availability. Furthermore, it is not possible to isolate the effects of CHO from total energy intake on performance as the snacks were not standardized for macronutrient or energy content, and participants were provided with absolute amounts of CHO, resulting in individual variation in amounts relative to body size. Notwithstanding the shortcomings of the study, it should be noted that performance times were faster in the CHO conditions (311.9 and

TABLE 3.3
Studies Investigating the Effect of CHO Intake during Exercise on Metabolism and Performance

Participants	Experimental Design	Contribution of CHO_{exo} Oxidation to Total EE	Metabolic Effect of CHO Ingestion	Performance Effect	References
13 ♂ 14.9(0.5) years	Candy bar (280 kcal, 36 g CHO), fat-free fig bars (200 kcal, 44 g CHO), or placebo consumed 10 min before 75 min CE at 60% VO_{2peak} + 2500 m CE time trial	Not assessed	No effect between conditions	No effect between conditions	Hendelman et al. (1997)
8 ♂ 13–17 years	Placebo or glucose drink (3 g glucose kg BM^{-1}) consumed during 120 min CE at 60% VO_{2peak}	~ 25%	↑ CHO oxidation ↓ Fat oxidation ↑ Blood glucose and plasma insulin ↓ CHO_{endo}	↓ RPE	Riddell et al. (2000b)
12 ♂ 10–14 years	Placebo, 6% glucose (G), or 3% fructose plus 3% glucose (FG) consumed during 90 min CE at 53% + VO_{2peak} TT_{ex} test at 90% PP	17% in G 16% in FG	↑ CHO oxidation in G and FG ↓ Fat oxidation in G and FG ↑ Lactate in G and FG ↑ Insulin and glucose in G	G↓ TT_{ex} 25% FG↓ TT_{ex} 40%	Riddell et al. (2001)
12 ♂ 9.8 years (PP and EP) 10 men 22.1 years	Placebo or 6% CHO drink (4% sucrose, 2% glucose) consumed during 60 min CE at 70% VO_{2peak}	22% boys 15% men	↑ CHO oxidation ↓ Fat oxidation ↑ Postexercise blood glucose and lactate ↓ CHO_{endo} (24% boys; 15% men) *Age-related effects* ↑ Fat and ↓ CHO oxidation in boys vs. men ↓ CHO_{endo} and ↑ CHO_{exo} oxidation in boys vs. men (CHO trial)	Not assessed	Timmons et al. (2003)

(Continued)

TABLE 3.3 (Continued)
Studies Investigating the Effect of CHO Intake during Exercise on Metabolism and Performance

Participants	Experimental Design	Contribution of CHO_{exo} Oxidation to Total EE	Metabolic Effect of CHO Ingestion	Performance Effect	References
20 ♂ 12 years (7 PP, 7 EP, 6 M-LP)	Placebo or 6% CHO drink (4% sucrose, 2% glucose) consumed during 60 min CE at 70% VO_{2peak}	30% in PP and EP 24% in M-LP and 14-year-old boys	↑ CHO oxidation ↓ Fat oxidation ↑ Postexercise blood glucose and lactate ↓ CHO_{endo} oxidation *Age- and puberty-related effects* ↑ Fat oxidation in younger vs. older boys ↓ CHO_{endo} oxidation in younger vs. older boys ↑ CHO_{exo} oxidation (% total EE) in younger vs. older boys and M-LP vs. PP and EP	Not assessed	Timmons et al. (2007b)
9 ♂ 14 years					
12 ♀ 12 years (YG) 10 ♀ 14 years (OG)	Placebo or 6% CHO drink (4% sucrose, 2% glucose) consumed during 60 min CE at 70% VO_{2peak}	~19% (similar in YG and OG)	↓ Fat oxidation in YG (not OG) ↓ CHO_{endo} oxidation in OG (not YG) *Age-related effects* ↓ CHO_{endo} oxidation in YG vs. OG. ↑ Fat oxidation in YG during placebo	Not assessed	Timmons et al. (2007a)
8 ♂ 15.7(0.7) years with IDDM 6 ♂ 14.9(0.6) years nondiabetic	Placebo or 8% glucose drink consumed during 60 min CE at 59% VO_{2peak}	9% IDDM 12% nondiabetic	Similar CHO oxidation ↓ Fat oxidation (tendency) ↓ CHO_{endo} *Between-group differences* ↑ Blood glucose and plasma insulin concentrations in IDDM vs. controls ↓ CHO_{exo} in IDDM vs. controls	Not assessed	Riddell et al. (2000a)
7 ♂ 11(1) years obese	Placebo or 6% glucose drink consumed during 60 min CE at Fatmax	23%	↑ CHO oxidation ↓ Fat oxidation	Not assessed	Chu et al. (2011)

Note: EE = energy expenditure; CHO_{exo} = exogenous carbohydrate oxidation; CHO_{endo} = endogenous carbohydrate oxidation; CE = cycle ergometry; TT_{ex} = time trial to exhaustion; PP = peak power; ♂ = boys, ♀ = girls; PP = prepubertal, EP = early pubertal, M-LP = mid-to-late pubertal.

316.2 s) compared with the placebo (328.1 s), a difference that was not statistically significant, but may be meaningful for young athletes competing against others of a similar standard.

Subsequent work has supported the benefits of CHO ingestion during exercise for endurance performance in young people and suggests that the composition of the ingested CHO can affect the extent of the improvement. Compared with a placebo (water), ingestion of a 6% glucose or 3% glucose plus 3% fructose solution during 90 min of moderate-intensity exercise delayed time to exhaustion at 90% of maximal power output in boys aged 10–14 years (Riddell et al. 2001). Indirect support for this finding comes from reports of reduced ratings of perceived exertion (RPE) during exercise with glucose ingestion in adolescent boys, indicating that the boys felt the exercise was "easier" (Riddell et al. 2000b). Interestingly, consuming the glucose–fructose mixed drink enhanced time to exhaustion more than glucose alone (40% and 25% delays, respectively) compared with water (Riddell et al. 2001). Although the authors speculated that the enhanced performance with the glucose–fructose mix may be related to the additional muscle glycogen-sparing effect of fructose, endogenous CHO oxidation (i.e., liver and muscle glycogen) did not differ between trials despite a reduced reliance on exogenous glucose sources with the fructose plus glucose drink. It is also possible that the improvement in performance with CHO intake could be due partly to a nonmetabolic mechanism. In adults, mouth rinsing can enhance performance when a high-power output is required over durations of 45–75 min via its effects on the CNS, with CHO-rich pre-event meals dampening this effect (Jeukendrup and Chambers 2010). It is interesting to note that the boys in the aforementioned Hendelman et al. (1997) study may have not benefited from the nonmetabolic effects of CHO ingestion during exercise, as CHO was provided 10 min before exercise.

The finding that performance only improved in 7 of 12 subjects in the glucose trial and 9 out of 12 in the glucose–fructose mix trial highlights the need for future research to consider individual variation. In particular, the inclusion of 10- to 14-year-olds in Tanner stages 2–4 (early to late pubertal) coupled with the known effects of age and puberty on metabolism is likely to have contributed to individual variation (Timmons et al. 2007b). Future studies should also consider the performance test used, which could contribute to some of the variability; the reliability of tests to volitional exhaustion in children is not known and prolonged tests to exhaustion have a high coefficient of variation in adults (Jeukendrup et al. 1996). Although the order of the trials was counterbalanced, the inclusion of a habituation session has been suggested to reduce the coefficient of variation in adolescents completing a cycling time trial (Montfort-Steiger et al. 2005).

Further research is required to clarify the potential benefits of CHO supplementation on performance in young people, including identification of the optimal CHO feeding regimen (dosage, composition, timing) for peak performance, taking into consideration individual factors such as age, puberty, sex, training status, and previous diet. Studies investigating reasons for between-subject variability could pave the way to a more individualized approach to CHO prescription. In particular, although an improvement in performance with glucose ingestion throughout exercise has been documented in women (Campbell et al. 2001), this finding requires investigation in prepubertal and adolescent girls to determine sex-specific dietary recommendations for athletic performance.

3.6.2 Substrate Oxidation

The improved endurance performance with CHO intake in adults is attributed largely to increased CHO oxidation and maintenance of euglycemia during exercise, particularly as exercise duration increases and endogenous CHO stores become depleted. Although the invasive nature of the techniques employed to quantify glycogen stores has posed ethical restrictions when considering similar research with children, stable isotope tracer techniques used in conjunction with indirect calorimetry represents a promising noninvasive method of estimating endogenous and exogenous substrate oxidation in younger age groups and has been used to examine the effects of CHO ingestion during exercise (Riddell et al. 2000b; Timmons et al. 2003, 2007b).

In young people, CHO ingestion during exercise increases total CHO oxidation and lowers total fat oxidation when compared with a placebo, often flavored water (Table 3.3). These findings have been demonstrated mainly in healthy boys aged 10–17 years (Riddell et al. 2000b; Timmons et al. 2007b) and may also apply to girls (Timmons et al. 2007a) and obese boys (Chu et al. 2011), although the evidence is sparse. The mechanisms responsible for the reduction in fat oxidation following CHO ingestion relate to the rise in insulin that inhibits lipolysis and FFA availability (Horowitz et al. 1997) and the increase in blood glucose uptake and, therefore, CHO oxidation, which inhibits the rate of FFA entry into the mitochondria (Coyle et al. 1997; Sidossis et al. 1996). During exercise, glucose supplementation increases glucose and insulin concentrations, increases CHO oxidation, and suppresses fat oxidation in boys (Riddell et al. 2001; Timmons et al. 2007b). Separate examination of exogenous and endogenous substrate stores has revealed that the reduction in fat oxidation and increased exogenous CHO oxidation during exercise with CHO ingestion is accompanied by a sparing of endogenous CHO in boys (Timmons et al. 2007b). Thus, it appears that CHO is preferable over fat as a fuel when exogenous CHO is provided at a sufficient rate during exercise in young people.

Consideration of age and pubertal status is crucial when evaluating the effects of CHO ingestion during exercise in young people. Whether exercise is performed with or without CHO ingestion, boys and girls oxidize a proportionally higher amount of fat and lower amount of CHO than adults (Riddell et al. 2008; Timmons et al. 2007a,b). When CHO is ingested during exercise, pre- and early-pubertal boys exhibit a higher rate of exogenous CHO oxidation, which provides a greater relative proportion of total energy, compared with adult men (Timmons et al. 2003). Interestingly, the rate of exogenous CHO oxidation in boys (Timmons et al. 2003) is similar to trained adults, who also have increased rates of fat oxidation during exercise (Burelle et al. 1999; Jeukendrup et al. 1997), highlighting the need to consider training status when comparing young people and adults. Independent of chronological age, advanced pubertal status reduces the contribution of exogenous CHO oxidation to total energy expenditure, and testosterone concentration is inversely related to exogenous CHO oxidation in males (Timmons et al. 2007b). Therefore, the age-related effects of CHO intake on exercise metabolism are likely attributed to puberty.

The higher exogenous CHO oxidation in younger and less mature boys when CHO is ingested during exercise is accompanied by a greater conservation of endogenous glycogen stores compared with more mature boys and adult men (Timmons et al. 2003, 2007b). Since it is unlikely that a blunted ability to oxidize CHO can explain the lower total CHO and higher fat oxidation in these boys due to their well-developed capacity to oxidize exogenous CHO, the greater "sparing" of endogenous CHO stores could indicate a reduced capacity to store muscle glycogen in younger, less mature boys. Moreover, the decrease in blood glucose during the onset of exercise suggests reduced glycogen stores in boys (Riddell et al. 2000b) and girls (Delamarche et al. 1994). Children may compensate for the limited glycogen stores by increasing their reliance on exogenous fuels, such as consumption of CHO snacks and beverages, when available. It has been suggested that the greater reliance on exogenous CHO in younger, less mature boys may be important in protecting endogenous substrates for growth and development of the musculoskeletal system and CNS. Overall, consuming exogenous CHO during exercise may be of particular benefit to young and less mature boys.

Dietary recommendations for young athletes should consider these findings by advocating the consumption of orally consumed CHO during or immediately before exercise to ensure sufficient exogenous CHO is available to fuel exercise in younger, less mature children, perhaps more so than adults. Ideally, CHO recommendations should be specific to pubertal status rather than chronological age, with a reduced need to provide exogenous CHO as maturation progresses. Since rates of exogenous CHO oxidation in more mature 12-year-old boys were similar to those of 14-year-old pubertal boys, it may be sufficient to distinguish between young people in pre- and early puberty and those in mid-late puberty, rather than each of the five Tanner stages (Timmons et al. 2007b). Importantly, exogenous CHO oxidation increases with exercise duration (Timmons et al. 2003), meaning that boys competing in endurance events, in particular, could benefit from CHO ingestion during exercise. However, the direct application of this recommendation for young athletes who exercise less than 60–120 min, as used in the supporting evidence, is questionable.

Whether from the pediatric or adult literature, the majority of research on exercise metabolism has been conducted in males. Similar to boys, there is some evidence that younger, less mature girls have higher fat and lower endogenous CHO oxidation rates during exercise compared with older adolescents (Timmons et al. 2007a). However, CHO supplementation only reduced fat oxidation in those aged 12 years, not those aged 14 years, and the balance between exogenous and endogenous CHO oxidation during exercise was not different between 12- and 14-year-old girls. Consequently, it is possible the reported age- and maturation-related differences in exogenous CHO oxidation in males and the potential implications for performance may not apply to girls. Alternatively, the similarity in exogenous CHO oxidation reported between 12- and 14-year-old girls may have been due to the small, albeit statistically significant, difference in puberty between the two groups (Tanner 3 and 4) (Timmons et al. 2007a). This is complicated further by issues related to menstrual cycle stage; all 14-year-old girls were tested in the early follicular phase, but only four of the 12-year-olds had experienced their first menstrual period and were not tested at a standardized time due to the sporadic nature of their menstruation. It is advisable to control for menstrual cycle stage, as variations in ovarian hormone levels throughout the menstrual cycle alter exercise metabolism in women (Oosthuyse and Bosch 2010). Interestingly, ingestion of glucose minimizes these effects and there is evidence that the performance-enhancing effects of glucose ingestion during exercise are more pronounced in the luteal compared with the follicular stage (26% vs. 19% improvement) (Campbell et al. 2001).

Unfortunately, studies that replicate the reported findings in girls are not available, making it impossible to draw any firm conclusions based on the available evidence. Owing to some of the data inconsistencies between studies including boys and girls, studies directly examining between-sex differences in the response to CHO supplementation in young people are needed. In adults, there is evidence that women may derive a greater benefit from CHO ingestion than men; women oxidize a greater relative proportion of exogenous CHO during endurance exercise, which spares more endogenous fuel (Campbell et al. 2001; Riddell et al. 2003). Moreover, glucose ingestion improved time-trial performance by 19%–26% in trained women (Campbell et al. 2001), but only 7% in trained men (Angus et al. 2000), although differences in study design mean these values cannot be compared directly. A direct comparison of trained men and women, however, reported remarkably similar metabolic responses to CHO supplementation, with both groups experiencing an increased plasma glucose turnover and oxidation, which suppressed fat and endogenous CHO oxidation (Wallis et al. 2006). Future studies with children and adolescents, controlling for training status and puberty, should include both boys and girls to determine possible sex-related differences to CHO supplementation during exercise to determine nutritional recommendations for athletic performance in young male and female athletes.

3.7 CARBOHYDRATE INTAKE: POSTEXERCISE

Timing of food consumption based on competition or exercise event time is important to not only enhance exercise performance, but also improve recovery time. Consuming the correct nutrients during the period after exercise is essential for initiating the rebuilding of damaged muscle tissue and the restoration of energy reserves. Since a fundamental goal of traditional postexercise nutrient timing is to replenish glycogen stores, CHO intake after exercise is critical when glycogen is depleted. Although the postexercise period is widely considered the most important part of nutrient timing in adults (Burke et al. 2004, 2011), very few studies have examined postexercise CHO intake in young people. Consequently, the evidence discussed within this section is based on studies with adults and it is important to highlight from the beginning that the findings may not apply to young people, particularly pre- and early-pubertal children.

Consumption of CHO (or CHO plus protein) within 30 min of an exercise session results in higher glycogen levels than when ingestion is delayed for 2 h (Ivy et al. 1988, 2002). When postexercise CHO intake is proportional to body mass, men and women are able to benefit to a similar extent from faster glycogen resynthesis compared with placebo ingestion (Tarnopolsky et al. 1997). This enhanced capacity to replenish glycogen stores may allow performance to be maintained during periods of training, with postexercise CHO consumption over a 7-day training period improving subsequent performance (increased time to exhaustion) compared with a placebo (Roy et al. 2002). The composition of the snack and type of CHO consumed after exercise affects the extent of glycogen synthesis. Carbohydrates with a high glycemic index (HGI) supply energy quickly for glycogen resynthesis during recovery and result in higher muscle glycogen levels 24 h after a glycogen-depleting exercise bout when compared with LGI CHO (Burke et al. 1993). Accordingly, when comparing simple sugars, it appears that glucose and sucrose are equally effective, whereas fructose alone (which has a lower GI) is less effective (Blom et al. 1987). Therefore, consumption of HGI CHO snacks after exercise rather than LGI CHO and fructose-containing snacks are recommended for adults. When considering meal composition, it is often recommended that adults should consume a mixed CHO and protein meal following exercise, ideally in a 3:1 CHO-to-protein ratio (Kerksick et al. 2008). Although glycogen synthesis rates may not necessarily be improved with the coingestion of protein and CHO compared with isoenergetic CHO ingestion (Millard-Stafford et al. 2008), the provision of protein and amino acids for muscle protein repair and promoting a more anabolic hormonal profile (Rodriguez et al. 2007) may be particularly important for growing young people. Milk may, therefore, be a convenient source of protein and CHO when it is not possible to consume a meal after exercise. Indeed, glycogen repletion is similar when CHO is consumed in the form of solids and liquids (Burke et al. 2004) and liquids are sometimes preferred by athletes immediately after exercise for practical reasons. However, caution should be taken when translating such findings to young people, as the efficacy of postexercise fluid "supplements" has not been studied in children and adolescents. This practice might be best avoided in younger populations, who can gain the same benefits from consuming postexercise CHO and protein as part of a well-balanced diet.

Based on the available evidence in adults, the joint position stand of the American College of Sports Medicine and American Dietetic Association (2009) recommends the consumption of approximately 1.0–1.5 g per kg body weight of CHO during the first 30 min after exercise and again every 2 h for 4–6 h to replace glycogen stores (Rodriguez et al. 2009). These recommendations are particularly important when the time between two training sessions is less than 8 h or sessions are very prolonged (Berardi et al. 2006; Ivy et al. 2002). It is unnecessary for athletes who rest one or more days between intense training sessions to practice nutrient timing provided sufficient CHO is consumed during the 24-h period after the exercise bout (Burke et al. 1996). For instance, glycogen stores would be depleted to a large extent following a marathon, but these athletes are not likely to perform another race or exercise session the same day; CHO intake after exercise would be more important for triathletes training for durations of around 60–90 min twice a day. When considering whether the benefits of postexercise CHO intake apply to children and adolescents, age- and maturation-related changes in metabolism must be considered. As discussed in Sections 3.4 and 3.5, the lower muscle CHO stores in younger, less mature children may indicate that "supercompensation" of muscle glycogen is not possible. Alternatively, the effects of postexercise CHO intake may actually be enhanced in this population if glycogen levels can be increased to some degree; boys may be able to raise muscle glycogen concentration and use more muscle glycogen during maximal exercise in response to training (Eriksson et al. 1973). Nevertheless, consuming a meal or snack after exercise may be important for all athletes, regardless of age, to meet daily CHO and energy balance goals. Although child and adolescent athletes do not typically engage in more than one intense training session per day, there may be occasions where they participate in multiple events in one day (e.g., track and field meetings) and it may be preferable for endurance athletes training every day (e.g., distance runners, swimmers, cyclists) to consume CHO within 30 min of training to aid recovery. Indeed, CHO supplementation during exercise in boys can diminish postexercise physiological stress and attenuate the immediate exercise-induced increase in immune counts in boys, indicating improved immune function (Timmons et al. 2004). Research investigating the effect of postexercise CHO intake on recovery, fuel stores, and subsequent performance in young people is much needed.

3.8 SHORT-DURATION HIGH-INTENSITY EXERCISE AND SKILL PERFORMANCE

Children typically engage in very short bursts of intense physical activity interspersed with varying intervals of low and moderate intensity during both habitual free-play (Bailey et al. 1995) and various team sports, rather than continuous bouts of 1–2 h that have been studied in much of the research discussed. Since CHO oxidation provides the majority of adenosine triphosphate (ATP) during higher-intensity exercise when the glycolytic energy pathway predominates, logic suggests that low CHO availability might limit high-intensity exercise performance, as reported in adults (Maughan et al. 1997). Carbohydrate ingestion during exercise can improve performance when the exercise is of high intensity (75% VO_{2max}) and relatively short duration (<1 h), and it has become clear that the underlying mechanism for this is not metabolic, but may reside in the CNS. Indeed, undigested CHO mouth rinses have been shown to result in similar performance improvements (Jeukendrup and Chambers 2010).

Again, data in young people are confined to only a few studies with inconsistent findings. When boys ingested CHO 30 min before repeated Wingate anaerobic tests (WAnT), peak power and mean power were not different compared with placebo ingestion, indicating no improvement in performance. Postexercise glucose concentration and blood lactate concentration were also unaffected, despite higher preexercise glucose concentration in the CHO trial (Marjerrison et al. 2007). Similarly, CHO ingestion immediately before and during exercise did not affect sprint times during a modified version of the Loughborough Intermittent Shuttle Test in team game players aged 12–14 years (Phillips et al. 2010), with follow-up studies showing no effect of the concentration of CHO consumed (Phillips et al. 2012a) or a CHO (maltodextrin) compared with a placebo gel (Phillips et al. 2012b) on 15 s sprint time. Likewise, during a 90-min basketball-specific training session in 14- to 15-year-old male basketball players, sprint performance was not influenced by *ad libitum* consumption of an 8% carbohydrate solution compared with no fluid ingestion (Carvalho et al. 2011). However, it may be noteworthy that the 6% CHO-electrolyte drink improved time to exhaustion by 24% (Phillips et al. 2010). In a separate study, the same group found a 6% CHO-electrolyte solution improved time to exhaustion during intermittent exercise by 34% compared with a 10% solution (Phillips et al. 2012a). Furthermore, a CHO (maltodextrin) gel increased intermittent endurance capacity by 21% (Phillips et al. 2012b). This indicates that supplementation benefitted at least some of the players, with the greatest benefits from consuming a 6% solution. Overall, the limited evidence suggests that preexercise CHO ingestion may improve intermittent endurance capacity, but not sprint performance in adolescent boys. Again, it is not possible to make firm conclusions based on the available evidence, which is limited to a few studies that have not typically included girls.

3.9 SPORTS DRINKS AND HYDRATION

Despite the paucity of literature on exogenous CHO ingestion during exercise and performance in young athletes, evidence does suggest that adding CHO to sports drinks may be beneficial for maintaining hydration. The topic of fluid and hydration is discussed in greater detail in Chapter 7. Adding flavor, CHO, and sodium chloride (NaCl) to drinks has been used as a strategy to improve the palatability of sports drinks, increase voluntary fluid intake, and help maintain hydration during exercise. Compared with unflavored water, voluntary fluid intake increased by 45% when it was flavored and almost doubled with a 6% CHO and 18 mmol L^{-1} NaCl drink in boys (Wilk and Bar-Or 1996). Consequently, while flavoring water reduced voluntary dehydration, the further addition of

CHO and NaCl prevented it altogether. Similar findings were observed in trained, heat-acclimatized boys who experienced higher sweating rates during prolonged exercise (Rivera-Brown et al. 1999). These studies have focused on exercise in hot, humid conditions and have typically used 3-h exercise protocols consisting of four 20-min cycling bouts at 50%–60% maximal oxygen uptake (interspersed with 25-min rest periods). When using a different exercise protocol more closely reflecting real-life situations (a time-trial run followed the steady-state exercise bouts), voluntarily fluid consumption, hydration, and time to exhaustion were similar regardless of whether unflavored water, flavored water, or flavored water with CHO and NaCl was provided to heat-acclimatized adolescent male runners (Wilk et al. 2010). Furthermore, in nonacclimatized girls exercising in the heat, voluntary drinking was enhanced with flavored compared with unflavored water regardless of combination with CHO and NaCl, but hydration was promoted to a greater extent with the drink containing CHO and NaCl (Wilk et al. 2007). Similarly, there was a tendency toward improved hydration and greater fluid retention with the consumption of a CHO plus NaCl drink in trained, heat-acclimatized girls with high sweating rates, although voluntary dehydration was not prevented completely (Rivera-Brown et al. 2008). Based on these studies, it would appear that voluntary dehydration may be reduced to some extent by drinking a CHO-electrolyte drink in both girls and boys, but it is not possible to determine the independent effects of CHO and NaCl. Caution is recommended when interpreting these findings, based on prolonged exercise (4 × 20-min bouts with 25-min rest periods) in hot, humid conditions. For many young people training for shorter periods (<90 min) in temperate conditions, the promotion of these drinks may lead to unnecessary overconsumption of sugary drinks (see Section 3.10).

3.10 HEALTH, GLYCEMIC INDEX, AND INSULIN SENSITIVITY

Maintenance of good health is essential for disease prevention, to promote continued wellness throughout life, and for normal growth and development. Since habitual diet has a considerable impact on health, it is important to consider CHO intake recommendations for exercise performance alongside any potential health consequences of the practices advocated. This is particularly important for children and adolescents as they progress through puberty and develop lifestyle behaviors that can affect future health. Specifically, recommendations for CHO intake in young people may require special consideration, as insulin is a key hormone stimulating glucose uptake and regulating glycogen metabolism during rest and exercise, and the pubertal transition from Tanner stage 1–3 is associated with a 32% reduction in insulin sensitivity with concomitant increases in fasting glucose, insulin, and the acute response to glucose, which recovers by Tanner stage 5 (Goran and Gower 2001). Consequently, caution should be exercised when prescribing high-CHO diets or "CHO loading" and HGI foods to young people in the pre- to mid-stages of puberty.

Despite potential health concerns of prescribing specific diets to young people, the available evidence suggests that dramatic changes in CHO and fat intakes do not affect glucose and lipid metabolism adversely in the short term; most participants have been healthy, nonobese young people, meaning the findings are likely to apply to many young athletes. During a 7-day high-CHO diet (60% CHO, 25% fat) and low-CHO diet (30% CHO, 55% fat), prepubertal children (Tanner stage 1) and adolescents (Tanner stage 4 and 5) adapted rapidly by adjusting CHO and fat oxidation to macronutrient intake, with only minor changes in parameters of glucose metabolism (Sunehag et al. 2002). Interestingly, acute consumption of a high-CHO diet did not affect insulin sensitivity adversely in these children and adolescents, whereas insulin sensitivity actually improved when the adolescents changed from a low-CHO to high-CHO diet. Similar findings were observed when energy intake was adjusted for the maintenance of energy balance (estimated from individual basal metabolic rate), with healthy nonobese children and adolescents increasing their CHO oxidation during a high-CHO diet and fat oxidation during a high-fat diet (Treuth et al. 2003). However, the boys exhibited more pronounced changes in substrate oxidation than the girls, indicating boys may adapt more readily to changes in diet composition (Treuth et al. 2003). Unlike lean adolescents, obese adolescents failed to increase insulin sensitivity during the high-CHO diet, resulting in increased insulin secretion to maintain normal blood glucose levels (Sunehag et al. 2005). Consequently, high-CHO diets may not be suitable for certain populations, including overweight children and possibly girls.

When considering CHO ingestion during exercise, the presence of certain health conditions must be considered, particularly insulin-dependent diabetes mellitus (IDDM) and obesity. Although no difference in substrate oxidation between boys with and without IDDM occurred when a placebo was given during exercise, exogenous glucose oxidation was impaired in boys with IDDM when glucose was ingested despite two- to threefold higher blood glucose and plasma insulin concentrations than the healthy controls. Glucose ingestion did, however, spare endogenous glycogen stores to a similar extent in both groups (Riddell et al. 2000a). Moreover, glucose ingestion equivalent to total CHO utilization attenuated the drop in blood glucose, reducing the likelihood of hypoglycemia during moderate-intensity exercise in boys with IDDM (Riddell et al. 2000a). Overweight young people may also have specific nutritional needs due to their altered metabolism, including a greater reliance on CHO oxidation during exercise (McMurray and Hosick 2011). The suppression of whole body fat oxidation during exercise with CHO ingestion (vs. placebo) is likely to be counterproductive for obese children trying to maximize fat oxidation and weight management through regular physical activity (Chu et al. 2011). Moreover, consumption of sugar-sweetened beverages, including sports drinks, energy drinks, lemonade, and other fruit drinks, has been linked to excess weight gain in children and adults (Malik et al. 2006). Indeed, it would not be advisable to recommend CHO supplementation during exercise in overweight children if this adds to their total daily energy intake. It is also crucial that young people are aware of the difference between sports and energy drinks and do not consume these drinks on a regular basis as part of their diet. Sports drinks may be recommended for fuel and hydration before, during, and after prolonged exercise in hot humid conditions (see Section 3.9), but are categorized as "sugar-sweetened beverages." Thus, regular consumption of sports drinks for most young athletes is likely to be unwarranted and could result in the overconsumption of sugar. Energy drinks specifically are not recommended due to the health risks associated with many of the ingredients, related to cardiovascular disease and bone mineralization (Seifert et al. 2011), although limited empirical evidence exists at this point in time to confirm these potential concerns.

Rather than the total amount of CHO in the diet, the "quality" or GI of the CHO may have greater relevance for health. The concept of GI was introduced as a method of classifying different CHO-rich foods according to their effect on postprandial glycemia and is defined as the incremental area under the 2-h blood glucose curve following ingestion of 50 g available CHO as a percentage of the corresponding area following an equivalent amount of CHO from a standard reference product (glucose or white bread) (Jenkins et al. 1981). Foods classified as HGI include refined grain products, white bread, and potatoes, whereas LGI foods include whole-grain products, legumes, and fruits. There is now a large body of evidence providing robust support for LGI diets in the prevention of obesity, diabetes, and cardiovascular disease in adults (Brand-Miller et al. 2009) with similar findings emerging in young people (Fajcsak et al. 2008; Rouhani et al. 2013; Rovner et al. 2009). Therefore, although HGI snacks may be recommended after exercise to promote the replenishment of muscle glycogen stores in adults, caution should be exercised when promoting the regular consumption of HGI foods in young people. This is particularly pertinent in adolescents within the mid-pubertal stages who are characterized by a reduction in insulin sensitivity.

Finally, it should be highlighted that many of the reviewed studies within the pediatric literature refer to "CHO supplementation" rather than meals or snacks. In general, the use of dietary supplements is not advocated for children or adolescents. Young athletes who consume sports drinks and energy drinks for their perceived physiological benefits may not be aware of the potential risks (e.g., high sugar content) and, in many cases, specific health benefits from nutritional supplements and drinks may be better achieved through appropriate consumption of a nutritious diet. Regarding

CHO supplementation specifically, glucose drinks consumed during prolonged exercise when it is not possible to consume food may be beneficial. However, pre- and postexercise CHO needs can be met by consuming food and drink as part of a healthy balanced diet. In particular, the benefits and efficacy of "recovery drinks" for young people have not been studied, perhaps partly due to the concerns linked with promoting this practice in children.

3.11 SUMMARY

Nutrition, including adequate CHO intake, is essential for the health and performance of young athletes. Since young athletes have physiological and metabolic characteristics that distinguish them from adults, nutritional recommendations must be tailored to the age and pubertal stage of the athlete. Unfortunately, most of the knowledge on the CHO needs of athletes is informed by evidence from adult-based research. The development of specific recommendations for young athletes is difficult due to the lack of child-specific evidence, which is further complicated by the dietary intake required for growth and development in conjunction with that required for training and competition. Although many unanswered questions remain concerning CHO needs of the young athlete, it is possible to make some general recommendations.

In terms of the overall diet, CHO should contribute to the majority of energy intake, which must be high enough to support growth and maturation while also fueling the additional physical activity in young athletes. For child and adolescent athletes, CHO is also an important fuel for high-intensity exercise. The Dietary Guidelines for Americans (USDA, U.S. Department of Health and Human Services and US Department of Agriculture 2010) for energy intake and the AMDR values for CHO intake may provide useful guidance in calculating age-specific CHO needs in relation to physical activity level. Based on the current evidence, some authors have also attempted to make general recommendations for CHO intake in young athletes; for example, at least 50% of total daily energy intake (Petrie et al. 2004). Decrements in exercise performance, fatigue, and changes in body composition may serve as useful indicators that CHO intake may not be adequate. Given the tendency of adolescent girls to limit their daily energy intake, attention should be directed to female adolescent athletes to ensure that CHO needs are met daily and energy balance is maintained.

Timing of CHO consumption in relation to training and competition requires examination in young athletes. Currently, evidence on CHO loading in young athletes is not available. During exercise, drinks containing CHO could be considered for young athletes engaged in endurance exercise due to the preferential use of exogenous CHO in younger athletes in the pre- or early-pubertal stages. Although CHO-electrolyte drinks can minimize voluntary dehydration, there are health concerns associated with excessive consumption of such sugary beverages. Therefore, a healthy, balanced diet in line with the AMDR for total and CHO-derived energy would be sufficient to fuel exercise for most young athletes. More research with young athletes is needed to determine specific recommendations for CHO intake and timing in relation to exercise, including dosage and composition, and the efficacy of exogenous CHO intake in sport-specific situations (e.g., cycling, running, team sports). In adults, the restoration of muscle and liver glycogen is a fundamental goal of recovery between training sessions or competitive events; this requires examination in children and adolescents. Most dietary CHO should be from LGI sources (e.g., unsweetened porridge, whole-grain bread, whole-grain pasta, brown rice, lentils), with limited quantities of simple sugars and HGI CHO, but easily digestible, HGI foods may provide a useful source of CHO in the hours before and immediately after exercise, another area warranting examination in young athletes. Undoubtedly, research that can address such issues is crucial to inform CHO recommendations for young athletes in terms of both total daily intakes and in relation to exercise timing (before, during, and after exercise). Providing evidence-based recommendations for young athletes would be valuable in ensuring the maintenance of overall health and to enhance exercise performance during these important years of growth and maturation.

REFERENCES

Achten, J. and A. E. Jeukendrup. 2004. Relation between plasma lactate concentration and fat oxidation rates over a wide range of exercise intensities. *Int J Sports Med* 25 (1): 32–7. doi: 10.1055/s-2003-45231.

Andrews, J. L., D. A. Sedlock, M. G. Flynn, J. W. Navalta, and H. Ji. 2003. Carbohydrate loading and supplementation in endurance-trained women runners. *J Appl Physiol (1985)* 95 (2): 584–90. doi: 10.1152/japplphysiol.00855.2002.

Angus, D. J., M. Hargreaves, J. Dancey, and M. A. Febbraio. 2000. Effect of carbohydrate or carbohydrate plus medium-chain triglyceride ingestion on cycling time trial performance. *J Appl Physiol (1985)* 88 (1): 113–9.

Bailey, R. C., J. Olson, S. L. Pepper, J. Porszasz, T. J. Barstow, and D. M. Cooper. 1995. The level and tempo of children's physical activities: An observational study. *Med Sci Sports Exerc* 27 (7): 1033–41.

Bar-Or, O. 2001. Nutritional considerations for the child athlete. *Can J Appl Physiol* 26 (Suppl): S186–91.

Bar-Or, O., and V. B. Unnithan. 1994. Nutritional requirements of young soccer players. *J Sports Sci* 12 (Spec No): S39–42.

Bell, R. D., J. D. MacDougall, R. Billeter, and H. Howald. 1980. Muscle fiber types and morphometric analysis of skeletal muscle in six-year-old children. *Med Sci Sports Exerc* 12 (1): 28–31.

Benardot, D., M. Schwarz, and D. W. Heller. 1989. Nutrient intake in young, highly competitive gymnasts. *J Am Diet Assoc* 89 (3): 401–3.

Berardi, J. M., T. B. Price, E. E. Noreen, and P. W. Lemon. 2006. Postexercise muscle glycogen recovery enhanced with a carbohydrate-protein supplement. *Med Sci Sports Exerc* 38 (6): 1106–13. doi: 10.1249/01.mss.0000222826.49358.f3.

Berg, A., S. S. Kim, and J. Keul. 1986. Skeletal muscle enzyme activities in healthy young subjects. *Int J Sports Med* 7 (4): 236–9. doi: 10.1055/s-2008–1025766.

Bergstrom, J., L. Hermansen, E. Hultman, and B. Saltin. 1967. Diet, muscle glycogen and physical performance. *Acta Physiol Scand* 71 (2): 140–50. doi: 10.1111/j.1748-1716.1967.tb03720.x.

Blom, P. C., A. T. Hostmark, O. Vaage, K. R. Kardel, and S. Maehlum. 1987. Effect of different post-exercise sugar diets on the rate of muscle glycogen synthesis. *Med Sci Sports Exerc* 19 (5): 491–6.

Boisseau, N., and P. Delamarche. 2000. Metabolic and hormonal responses to exercise in children and adolescents. *Sports Med* 30 (6): 405–22.

Boisseau, N., C. Le Creff, M. Loyens, and J. R. Poortmans. 2002. Protein intake and nitrogen balance in male non-active adolescents and soccer players. *Eur J Appl Physiol* 88 (3): 288–93. doi: 10.1007/s00421-002-0726-x.

Brand-Miller, J., J. McMillan-Price, K. Steinbeck, and I. Caterson. 2009. Dietary glycemic index: Health implications. *J Am Coll Nutr* 28 (Suppl): 446S–9S.

Burelle, Y., F. Peronnet, S. Charpentier, C. Lavoie, C. Hillaire-Marcel, and D. Massicotte. 1999. Oxidation of an oral [13C]glucose load at rest and prolonged exercise in trained and sedentary subjects. *J Appl Physiol (1985)* 86 (1): 52–60.

Burke, L. M., G. R. Collier, P. G. Davis, P. A. Fricker, A. J. Sanigorski, and M. Hargreaves. 1996. Muscle glycogen storage after prolonged exercise: Effect of the frequency of carbohydrate feedings. *Am J Clin Nutr* 64 (1): 115–9.

Burke, L. M., G. R. Collier, and M. Hargreaves. 1993. Muscle glycogen storage after prolonged exercise: Effect of the glycemic index of carbohydrate feedings. *J Appl Physiol (1985)* 75 (2): 1019–23.

Burke, L. M., J. A. Hawley, S. H. Wong, and A. E. Jeukendrup. 2011. Carbohydrates for training and competition. *J Sports Sci* 29 (Suppl) 1: S17–27. doi: 10.1080/02640414.2011.585473.

Burke, L. M., B. Kiens, and J. L. Ivy. 2004. Carbohydrates and fat for training and recovery. *J Sports Sci* 22 (1): 15–30. doi: 10.1080/0264041031000140527.

Campbell, S. E., D. J. Angus, and M. A. Febbraio. 2001. Glucose kinetics and exercise performance during phases of the menstrual cycle: Effect of glucose ingestion. *Am J Physiol: Endocrinol Metab* 281 (4): E817–25.

Carvalho, P., B. Oliveira, R. Barros, P. Padrao, P. Moreira, and V. H. Teixeira. 2011. Impact of fluid restriction and *ad libitum* water intake or an 8% carbohydrate-electrolyte beverage on skill performance of elite adolescent basketball players. *Int J Sport Nutr Exerc Metab* 21 (3): 214–21.

Chen, J. D., J. F. Wang, K. J. Li, Y. W. Zhao, S. W. Wang, Y. Jiao, and X. Y. Hou. 1989. Nutritional problems and measures in elite and amateur athletes. *Am J Clin Nutr* 49 (5 Suppl): 1084–9.

Chryssanthopoulos, C., C. Williams, A. Nowitz, and G. Bogdanis. 2004. Skeletal muscle glycogen concentration and metabolic responses following a high glycaemic carbohydrate breakfast. *J Sports Sci* 22 (11–12): 1065–71. doi: 10.1080/02640410410001730007.

Chu, L., M. C. Riddell, T. Takken, and B. W. Timmons. 2011. Carbohydrate intake reduces fat oxidation during exercise in obese boys. *Eur J Appl Physiol* 111 (12): 3135–41. doi: 10.1007/s00421-011-1940-1.

Coyle, E. F. and A. R. Coggan. 1984. Effectiveness of carbohydrate feeding in delaying fatigue during prolonged exercise. *Sports Med* 1 (6): 446–58.

Coyle, E. F., A. E. Jeukendrup, A. J. Wagenmakers, and W. H. Saris. 1997. Fatty acid oxidation is directly regulated by carbohydrate metabolism during exercise. *Am J Physiol* 273 (2 Pt 1): E268–75.

Cupisti, A., C. D'Alessandro, S. Castrogiovanni, A. Barale, and E. Morelli. 2002. Nutrition knowledge and dietary composition in Italian adolescent female athletes and non-athletes. *Int J Sport Nutr Exerc Metab* 12 (2): 207–19.

Delamarche, P., A. Gratas-Delamarche, M. Monnier, M. H. Mayet, H. E. Koubi, and R. Favier. 1994. Glucoregulation and hormonal changes during prolonged exercise in boys and girls. *Eur J Appl Physiol Occup Physiol* 68 (1): 3–8.

Delamarche, P., M. Monnier, A. Gratas-Delamarche, H. E. Koubi, M. H. Mayet, and R. Favier. 1992. Glucose and free fatty acid utilization during prolonged exercise in prepubertal boys in relation to catecholamine responses. *Eur J Appl Physiol Occup Physiol* 65 (1): 66–72.

Eriksson, B. O. 1980. Muscle metabolism in children—A review. *Acta Paediatr Scand Suppl* 283: 20–8.

Eriksson, B. O., P. D. Gollnick, and B. Saltin. 1973. Muscle metabolism and enzyme activities after training in boys 11–13 years old. *Acta Physiol Scand* 87 (4): 485–97. doi: 10.1111/j.1748-1716.1973.tb05415.x.

Eriksson, O. and B. Saltin. 1974. Muscle metabolism during exercise in boys aged 11 to 16 years compared to adults. *Acta Paediatr Belg* 28 (Suppl): 257–65.

Fajcsak, Z., A. Gabor, V. Kovacs, and E. Martos. 2008. The effects of 6-week low glycemic load diet based on low glycemic index foods in overweight/obese children—Pilot study. *J Am Coll Nutr* 27 (1): 12–21.

Foricher, J. M., N. Ville, A. Gratas-Delamarche, and P. Delamarche. 2003. Effects of submaximal intensity cycle ergometry for one hour on substrate utilisation in trained prepubertal boys versus trained adults. *J Sports Med Phys Fitness* 43 (1): 36–43.

Fournier, M., J. Ricci, A. W. Taylor, R. J. Ferguson, R. R. Montpetit, and B. R. Chaitman. 1982. Skeletal muscle adaptation in adolescent boys: Sprint and endurance training and detraining. *Med Sci Sports Exerc* 14 (6): 453–6.

Giovannini, M., C. Agostoni, M. Gianni, L. Bernardo, and E. Riva. 2000. Adolescence: Macronutrient needs. *Eur J Clin Nutr* 54 (Suppl) 1: S7–10.

Goran, M. I. and B. A. Gower. 2001. Longitudinal study on pubertal insulin resistance. *Diabetes* 50 (11): 2444–50.

Haralambie, G. 1979. Skeletal muscle enzyme activities in female subjects of various ages. *Bull Eur Physiopathol Respir* 15 (2): 259–68.

Haralambie, G. 1982. Enzyme activities in skeletal muscle of 13–15 years old adolescents. *Bull Eur Physiopathol Respir* 18 (1): 65–74.

Hawley, J. A., E. J. Schabort, T. D. Noakes, and S. C. Dennis. 1997. Carbohydrate-loading and exercise performance. An update. *Sports Med* 24 (2): 73–81.

Hendelman, D. L., K. Ornstein, E. P. Debold, S. L. Volpe, and P. S. Freedson. 1997. Preexercise feeding in untrained adolescent boys does not affect responses to endurance exercise or performance. *Int J Sport Nutr* 7 (3): 207–18.

Hickson, J. F., Jr., M. A. Duke, W. L. Risser, C. W. Johnson, R. Palmer, and J. E. Stockton. 1987. Nutritional intake from food sources of high school football athletes. *J Am Diet Assoc* 87 (12): 1656–9.

Horowitz, J. F., R. Mora-Rodriguez, L. O. Byerley, and E. F. Coyle. 1997. Lipolytic suppression following carbohydrate ingestion limits fat oxidation during exercise. *Am J Physiol* 273 (4 Pt 1): E768–75.

Horswill, C. A., S. H. Park, and J. N. Roemmich. 1990. Changes in the protein nutritional status of adolescent wrestlers. *Med Sci Sports Exerc* 22 (5): 599–604.

Horton, T. J., M. J. Pagliassotti, K. Hobbs, and J. O. Hill. 1998. Fuel metabolism in men and women during and after long-duration exercise. *J Appl Physiol* (*1985*) 85 (5): 1823–32.

Iglesias-Gutierrez, E., P. M. Garcia-Roves, C. Rodriguez, S. Braga, P. Garcia-Zapico, and A. M. Patterson. 2005. Food habits and nutritional status assessment of adolescent soccer players. A necessary and accurate approach. *Can J Appl Physiol* 30 (1): 18–32.

Ivy, J. L., H. W. Goforth, Jr., B. M. Damon, T. R. McCauley, E. C. Parsons, and T. B. Price. 2002. Early postexercise muscle glycogen recovery is enhanced with a carbohydrate-protein supplement. *J Appl Physiol* (*1985*) 93 (4): 1337–44. doi: 10.1152/japplphysiol.00394.2002.

Ivy, J. L., A. L. Katz, C. L. Cutler, W. M. Sherman, and E. F. Coyle. 1988. Muscle glycogen synthesis after exercise: Effect of time of carbohydrate ingestion. *J Appl Physiol* (*1985*) 64 (4): 1480–5.

Jenkins, D. J., T. M. Wolever, R. H. Taylor, H. Barker, H. Fielden, J. M. Baldwin, A. C. Bowling, H. C. Newman, A. L. Jenkins, and D. V. Goff. 1981. Glycemic index of foods: A physiological basis for carbohydrate exchange. *Am J Clin Nutr* 34 (3): 362–6.

Jeukendrup, A. E. and E. S. Chambers. 2010. Oral carbohydrate sensing and exercise performance. *Curr Opin Clin Nutr Metab Care* 13 (4): 447–51. doi: 10.1097/MCO.0b013e328339de83.

Jeukendrup, A. E., M. Mensink, W. H. Saris, and A. J. Wagenmakers. 1997. Exogenous glucose oxidation during exercise in endurance-trained and untrained subjects. *J Appl Physiol (1985)* 82 (3): 835–40.

Jeukendrup, A., W. H. M. Saris, F. Brouns, and A. D. M. Kester. 1996. A new validated endurance performance test. *Med Sci Sports Exerc* 28 (2): 266–70. doi: 10.1097/00005768-199602000-00017.

Kaczor, J. J., W. Ziolkowski, J. Popinigis, and M. A. Tarnopolsky. 2005. Anaerobic and aerobic enzyme activities in human skeletal muscle from children and adults. *Pediatr Res* 57 (3): 331–5. doi: 10.1203/01.Pdr.0000150799.77094.De.

Kerksick, C., T. Harvey, J. Stout, B. Campbell, C. Wilborn, R. Kreider et al. 2008. International Society of Sports Nutrition position stand: Nutrient timing. *J Int Soc Sport Nutr* 5. doi: Artn 17 Doi 10.1186/1550-2783-5-17.

Leblanc, J. C., F. Le Gall, V. Grandjean, and P. Verger. 2002. Nutritional intake of French soccer players at the Clairefontaine Training Center. *Int J Sport Nutr Exerc Metab* 12 (3): 268–80.

Ludwig, D. S., J. A. Majzoub, A. Al-Zahrani, G. E. Dallal, I. Blanco, and S. B. Roberts. 1999. High glycemic index foods, overeating, and obesity. *Pediatrics* 103 (3). doi: Artn e26 DOI 10.1542/peds.103.3.e26.

Macek, M., J. Vavra, and J. Novosadova. 1976. Prolonged exercise in prepubertal boys.1. Cardiovascular and metabolic adjustment. *Eur J Appl Physiol Occup Physiol* 35 (4): 291–8. doi: 10.1007/Bf00423289.

Mahon, A. D., G. E. Duncan, C. A. Howe, and P. Del Corral. 1997. Blood lactate and perceived exertion relative to ventilatory threshold: Boys versus men. *Med Sci Sports Exerc* 29 (10): 1332–7.

Malczewska, J., G. Raczynski, and R. Stupnicki. 2000. Iron status in female endurance athletes and in non-athletes. *Int J Sport Nutr Exerc Metab* 10 (3): 260–76.

Malik, V. S., M. B. Schulze, and F. B. Hu. 2006. Intake of sugar-sweetened beverages and weight gain: A systematic review. *Am J Clin Nutr* 84 (2): 274–88.

Malina, R. M. 2010. Early sport specialization: Roots, effectiveness, risks. *Curr Sports Med Rep* 9 (6): 364–71. doi: 10.1249/JSR.0b013e3181fe3166.

Manore, M. M. 2002. Dietary recommendations and athletic menstrual dysfunction. *Sports Med* 32 (14): 887–901.

Marjerrison, A. D., J. D. Lee, and A. D. Mahon. 2007. Preexercise carbohydrate consumption and repeated anaerobic performance in pre- and early-pubertal boys. *Int J Sport Nutr Exerc Metab* 17 (2): 140–51.

Martinez, L. R. and E. M. Haymes. 1992. Substrate utilization during treadmill running in prepubertal girls and women. *Med Sci Sports Exerc* 24 (9): 975–83.

Martinsen, M. and J. Sundgot-Borgen. 2013. Higher prevalence of eating disorders among adolescent elite athletes than controls. *Med Sci Sports Exerc* 45 (6): 1188–97. doi: 10.1249/MSS.0b013e318281a939.

Maughan, R. J., P. L. Greenhaff, J. B. Leiper, D. Ball, C. P. Lambert, and M. Gleeson. 1997. Diet composition and the performance of high-intensity exercise. *J Sports Sci* 15 (3): 265–75. doi: 10.1080/026404197367272.

McMurray, R. G. and P. A. Hosick. 2011. The interaction of obesity and puberty on substrate utilization during exercise: A gender comparison. *Pediatr Exerc Sci* 23 (3): 411–31.

Millard-Stafford, M., W. L. Childers, S. A. Conger, A. J. Kampfer, and J. A. Rahnert. 2008. Recovery nutrition: Timing and composition after endurance exercise. *Curr Sports Med Rep* 7 (4): 193–201. doi: 10.1249/JSR.0b013e31817fc0fd.

Montfort-Steiger, V., C. A. Williams, and N. Armstrong. 2005. The reproducibility of an endurance performance test in adolescent cyclists. *Eur J Appl Physiol* 94 (5–6): 618–25. doi: 10.1007/s00421-005-1352-1.

Montoye, H. J. 1982. Age and oxygen utilization during submaximal treadmill exercise in males. *J Gerontol* 37 (4): 396–402.

Oosthuyse, T. and A. N. Bosch. 2010. The effect of the menstrual cycle on exercise metabolism: Implications for exercise performance in eumenorrhoeic women. *Sports Med* 40 (3): 207–27. doi: 10.2165/11317090-000000000-00000.

Papadopoulou, S. K., S. D. Papadopoulou, and G. K. Gallos. 2002. Macro- and micro-nutrient intake of adolescent Greek female volleyball players. *Int J Sport Nutr Exerc Metab* 12: 73–80.

Petrie, H. J., E. A. Stover, and C. A. Horswill. 2004. Nutritional concerns for the child and adolescent competitor. *Nutrition* 20 (7–8): 620–31. doi: 10.1016/j.nut.2004.04.002.

Phillips, S. M., A. P. Turner, S. Gray, M. F. Sanderson, and J. Sproule. 2010. Ingesting a 6% carbohydrate-electrolyte solution improves endurance capacity, but not sprint performance, during intermittent, high-intensity shuttle running in adolescent team games players aged 12–14 years. *Eur J Appl Physiol* 109 (5): 811–21. doi: 10.1007/s00421-010-1404-z.

Phillips, S. M., A. P. Turner, M. F. Sanderson, and J. Sproule. 2012a. Beverage carbohydrate concentration influences the intermittent endurance capacity of adolescent team games players during prolonged intermittent running. *Eur J Appl Physiol* 112 (3): 1107–16. doi: 10.1007/s00421-011-2065-2.

Phillips, S. M., A. P. Turner, M. F. Sanderson, and J. Sproule. 2012b. Carbohydrate gel ingestion significantly improves the intermittent endurance capacity, but not sprint performance, of adolescent team games players during a simulated team games protocol. *Eur J Appl Physiol* 112 (3): 1133–41. doi: 10.1007/s00421-011-2067-0.

Rampersaud, G. C., M. A. Pereira, B. L. Girard, J. Adams, and J. D. Metzl. 2005. Review—Breakfast habits, nutritional status, body weight, and academic performance in children and adolescents. *J Am Diet Assoc* 105 (5): 743–60. doi: 10.1016/j.jada.2005.02.007.

Rico-Sanz, J., W. R. Frontera, P. A. Mole, M. A. Rivera, A. Rivera-Brown, and C. N. Meredith. 1998. Dietary and performance assessment of elite soccer players during a period of intense training. *Int J Sport Nutr* 8 (3): 230–40.

Riddell, M. C., O. Bar-Or, M. Hollidge-Horvat, H. P. Schwarcz, and G. J. F. Heigenhauser. 2000a. Glucose ingestion and substrate utilization during exercise in boys with IDDM. *J Appl Physiol* 88 (4): 1239–46.

Riddell, M. C., O. Bar-Or, H. P. Schwarcz, and G. J. F. Heigenhauser. 2000b. Substrate utilization in boys during exercise with [C-13]-glucose ingestion. *Eur J Appl Physiol* 83 (4–5): 441–8. doi: 10.1007/s004210000259.

Riddell, M. C., O. Bar-Or, B. Wilk, M. L. Parolin, and G. J. F. Heigenhauser. 2001. Substrate utilization during exercise with glucose and glucose plus fructose ingestion in boys ages 10–14 yr. *J Appl Physiol* 90 (3): 903–11.

Riddell, M. C., V. K. Jamnik, K. E. Iscoe, B. W. Timmons, and N. Gledhill. 2008. Fat oxidation rate and the exercise intensity that elicits maximal fat oxidation decreases with pubertal status in young male subjects. *J Appl Physiol* 105 (2): 742–8. doi: 10.1152/japplphysiol.01256.2007.

Riddell, M. C., S. L. Partington, N. Stupka, D. Armstrong, C. Rennie, and M. A. Tarnopolsky. 2003. Substrate utilization during exercise performed with and without glucose ingestion in female and male endurance-trained athletes. *Int J Sport Nutr Exerc Metabol* 13 (4): 407–21.

Rivera-Brown, A. M., R. Gutierrez, J. C. Gutierrez, W. R. Frontera, and O. Bar-Or. 1999. Drink composition, voluntary drinking, and fluid balance in exercising, trained, heat-acclimatized boys. *J Appl Physiol* 86 (1): 78–84.

Rivera-Brown, A. M., F. A. Ramirez-Marrero, B. Wilk, and O. Bar-Or. 2008. Voluntary drinking and hydration in trained, heat-acclimatized girls exercising in a hot and humid climate. *Eur J Appl Physiol* 103 (1): 109–16. doi: 10.1007/s00421-008-0682-1.

Robinson, S. 1938. Experimental studies of physical fitness in relation to age. *Arbeitphysiologie* 10: 251–323.

Rodriguez, N. R., N. M. DiMarco, S. Langley, American Dietetic Association, Dietitians of Canada, American College of Sports Medicine, Nutrition and Performance Athletic. 2009. Position of the American Dietetic Association, Dietitians of Canada, and the American College of Sports Medicine: Nutrition and athletic performance. *J Am Diet Assoc* 109 (3): 509–27.

Rodriguez, N. R., L. M. Vislocky, and R. C. Gaine. 2007. Dietary protein, endurance exercise, and human skeletal-muscle protein turnover. *Curr Opin Clin Nutr Metab Care* 10 (1): 40–5. doi: 10.1097/Mco.0b013e3280115e3b.

Rouhani, M. H., A. Salehi-Abargouei, and L. Azadbakht. 2013. Effect of glycemic index and glycemic load on energy intake in children. *Nutrition* 29 (9): 1100–5. doi: 10.1016/j.nut.2013.02.004.

Rovner, A. J., T. R. Nansel, and L. Gellar. 2009. The effect of a low-glycemic diet vs a standard diet on blood glucose levels and macronutrient intake in children with type 1 diabetes. *J Am Diet Assoc* 109 (2): 303–7. doi: 10.1016/j.jada.2008.10.047.

Rowland, T. W. and T. A. Rimany. 1995. Physiological responses to prolonged exercise in premenarcheal and adult females. *Pediatr Exerc Sci* 7: 183–91.

Roy, B. D., K. Luttmer, M. J. Bosman, and M. A. Tarnopolsky. 2002. The influence of post-exercise macronutrient intake on energy balance and protein metabolism in active females participating in endurance training. *Int J Sport Nutr Exerc Metab* 12 (2): 172–88.

Seifert, S. M., J. L. Schaechter, E. R. Hershorin, and S. E. Lipshultz. 2011. Health effects of energy drinks on children, adolescents, and young adults. *Pediatrics* 127 (3): 511–28. doi: 10.1542/peds.2009-3592.

Sidossis, L. S., C. A. Stuart, G. I. Shulman, G. D. Lopaschuk, and R. R. Wolfe. 1996. Glucose plus insulin regulate fat oxidation by controlling the rate of fatty acid entry into the mitochondria. *J Clin Invest* 98 (10): 2244–50. doi: 10.1172/Jci119034.

Steen, S. N., C. Bildsten, R. Johnson, B. Spears, B. B. Day, and D. Bernardot. 1996. Timely statement of the American Dietetic Association: Nutrition guidance for adolescent athletes in organized sports. *J Am Diet Assoc* 96 (6): 611–2. doi: 10.1016/S0002-8223(96)00170-8.

Stephens, B. R., A. S. Cole, and A. D. Mahon. 2006. The influence of biological maturation on fat and carbohydrate metabolism during exercise in males. *Int J Sport Nutr Exerc Metab* 16 (2): 166–79.

Sunehag, A. L., G. Toffolo, M. Campioni, D. M. Bier, and M. W. Haymond. 2005. Effects of dietary macronutrient intake on insulin sensitivity and secretion and glucose and lipid metabolism in healthy, obese adolescents. *J Clin Endocrinol Metab* 90 (8): 4496–502. doi: 10.1210/Jc.2005-0626.

Sunehag, A. L., G. Toffolo, M. S. Treuth, N. F. Butte, C. Cobelli, D. M. Bier, and M. W. Haymond. 2002. Effects of dietary macronutrient content on glucose metabolism in children. *J Clin Endocrinol Metab* 87 (11): 5168–78. doi: 10.1210/jc.2002-020674.

Tamminen, K. A., N. L. Holt, and P. R. E. Crocker. 2012. Adolescent athletes: Psychosocial challenges and clinical concerns. *Curr Opin Psychiatry* 25 (4): 293–300. doi: 10.1097/Yco.0b013e3283541248.

Tarnopolsky, M. A. 2008. Sex differences in exercise metabolism and the role of 17-beta estradiol. *Med Sci Sport Exerc* 40 (4): 648–54. doi: 10.1249/Mss.0b013e31816212ff.

Tarnopolsky, M. A., S. A. Atkinson, S. M. Phillips, and J. D. MacDougall. 1995. Carbohydrate loading and metabolism during exercise in men and women. *J Appl Physiol (1985)* 78 (4): 1360–8.

Tarnopolsky, M. A., M. Bosman, J. R. MacDonald, D. Vandeputte, J. Martin, and B. D. Roy. 1997. Postexercise protein-carbohydrate and carbohydrate supplements increase muscle glycogen in men and women. *J Appl Physiol* 83 (6): 1877–83.

Timmons, B. W., O. Bar-Or, and M. C. Riddell. 2003. Oxidation rate of exogenous carbohydrate during exercise is higher in boys than in men. *J Appl Physiol (1985)* 94 (1): 278–84. doi: 10.1152/japplphysiol.00140.2002.

Timmons, B. W., O. Bar-Or, and M. C. Riddell. 2007a. Energy substrate utilization during prolonged exercise with and without carbohydrate intake in preadolescent and adolescent girls. *J Appl Physiol (1985)* 103 (3): 995–1000. doi: 10.1152/japplphysiol.00018.2007.

Timmons, B. W., O. Bar-Or, and M. C. Riddell. 2007b. Influence of age and pubertal status on substrate utilization during exercise with and without carbohydrate intake in healthy boys. *Appl Physiol Nutr Metab* 32 (3): 416–25. doi: 10.1139/H07-004.

Timmons, B. W., M. A. Tarnopolsky, and O. Bar-Or. 2004. Immune responses to strenuous exercise and carbohydrate intake in boys and men. *Pediatr Res* 56 (2): 227–34. doi: 10.1203/01.PDR.0000132852.29770.C5.

Tolfrey, K., A. E. Jeukendrup, and A. M. Batterham. 2010. Group- and individual-level coincidence of the "Fatmax" and lactate accumulation in adolescents. *Eur J Appl Physiol* 109 (6): 1145–53. doi: 10.1007/s00421-010-1453-3.

Treuth, M. S., A. L. Sunehag, L. M. Trautwein, D. M. Bier, M. W. Haymond, and N. F. Butte. 2003. Metabolic adaptation to high-fat and high-carbohydrate diets in children and adolescents. *Am J Clin Nutr* 77 (2): 479–89.

U.S. Department of Agriculture and U.S. Department of Health and Human Services. *Dietary Guidelines for Americans, 2010*. 7th Edition, Washington, DC: U.S. Government Printing Office, December 2010.

van Strien, T. and P. Oosterveld. 2008. The children's DEBQ for assessment of restrained, emotional, and external eating in 7- to 12-year-old children. *Int J Eat Disord* 41 (1): 72–81. doi: 10.1002/eat.20424.

Walker, J. L., G. J. Heigenhauser, E. Hultman, and L. L. Spriet. 2000. Dietary carbohydrate, muscle glycogen content, and endurance performance in well-trained women. *J Appl Physiol (1985)* 88 (6): 2151–8.

Wallis, G. A., R. Dawson, J. Achten, J. Webber, and A. E. Jeukendrup. 2006. Metabolic response to carbohydrate ingestion during exercise in males and females. *Am J Physiol Endocrinol Metab* 290 (4): E708–15. doi: 10.1152/ajpendo.00357.2005.

Wee, S. L., C. Williams, K. Tsintzas, and L. Boobis. 2005. Ingestion of a high-glycemic index meal increases muscle glycogen storage at rest but augments its utilization during subsequent exercise. *J Appl Physiol (1985)* 99 (2): 707–14. doi: 10.1152/japplphysiol.01261.2004.

Wiita, B. G. and I. A. Stombaugh. 1996. Nutrition knowledge, eating practices, and health of adolescent female runners: A 3-year longitudinal study. *Int J Sport Nutr* 6 (4): 414–25.

Wilk, B. and O. Bar-Or. 1996. Effect of drink flavor and NaCl on voluntary drinking and hydration in boys exercising in the heat. *J Appl Physiol (1985)* 80 (4): 1112–7.

Wilk, B., A. M. Rivera-Brown, and O. Bar-Or. 2007. Voluntary drinking and hydration in non-acclimatized girls exercising in the heat. *Eur J Appl Physiol* 101(6): 727–34. doi: 10.1007/s00421-007-0539-z.

Wilk, B., B. W. Timmons, and O. Bar-Or. 2010. Voluntary fluid intake, hydration status, and aerobic performance of adolescent athletes in the heat. *Appl Physiol Nutr Metab* 35(6): 834–41. doi: 10.1139/H10-084.

Williams, C. and D. Lamb. 2008. Does a high-carbohydrate breakfast improve performance? *Gatorade Sports Sci Exch* 21: 88–95.

Zakrzewski, J. K., E. J. Stevenson, and K. Tolfrey. 2012. Effect of breakfast glycemic index on metabolic responses during rest and exercise in overweight and non-overweight adolescent girls. *Eur J Clin Nutr* 66(4): 436–42. doi: 10.1038/ejcn.2011.175.

Ziegler, P. J., S. S. Jonnalagadda, J. A. Nelson, C. Lawrence, and B. Baciak. 2002. Contribution of meals and snacks to nutrient intake of male and female elite figure skaters during peak competitive season. *J Am Coll Nutr* 21 (2): 114–9.

4 Protein Needs of Young Athletes

Kurt A. Escobar, Trisha A. McLain, and Chad M. Kerksick

CONTENTS

Abstract 59
4.1 An Action Compound 60
4.2 Protein Digestion 61
4.3 Many Physiological Roles of Protein 61
4.4 Building Up and Breaking Down: Protein Metabolism 62
4.5 On a Need-to-Eat Basis 64
4.6 Not All Proteins Are Created Equal 67
4.7 The Highs and Lows of Protein Quality and Understanding Protein Sources 69
4.8 Safety of Protein Intake 71
4.9 Conclusion 71
References 72

ABSTRACT

Protein is a key nutrient responsible for an array of biological functions including the repair and building of cellular structures such as skeletal muscle tissue. However, its reach extends far beyond tissue remodeling and growth. Dietary protein supplies the necessary amino acids required for gene activity, transport of biological molecules, energy production, synthesis of hormones, enzymes, and neurotransmitters. Protein metabolism is a dynamic process whereby proteins are constantly synthesized from and degraded into amino acids, dependent on the demand and their availability, which is reliant on dietary intake. For growth, repair, and synthesis of biologically active proteins, a positive protein balance must be achieved and the rate of protein synthesis must exceed the rate of degradation. For these reasons, adequate protein intake in children is critical for growth, development, and normal physiological function. The unique demands of growth and development experienced by children and adolescents call for a greater daily protein intake than that of adults. The recommended daily allowance for protein is 0.95 grams/kg/day for children of 4–13 years of age and 0.85 grams/kg/day for adolescents of 14–18 years of age. However, if a young individual engages in regular exercise or sport, 1.5 grams/kg/day may be necessary while a daily intake of 1.2–1.4 grams/kg/day may be required for those participating in exhaustive endurance performance. Additionally, the body can only endogenously synthesize some amino acids, and others must be consumed in the diet; these are called essential amino acids. The essential amino acids are found in high-quality proteins such as meat, poultry, fish, eggs, and milk-based foods. Lesser-quality proteins, such as plant-based proteins, must be strategically combined to provide a child with the necessary amino acids for growth and development. And finally, though historically it has been promoted in popular press that protein consumption above what is recommended leads to adverse renal and bone effects, studies have repeatedly shown that an elevated protein intake does not result in such effects in healthy individuals. Adequate and appropriate dietary protein should be ensured by parents and coaches concerned with not only athletic performance, but also with proper growth and development.

4.1 AN ACTION COMPOUND

From the microscopic level of gene activity all the way up to the incredible complexity of each system within our body, proteins are responsible for each action, signal, and response initiated and received by various parts of our body. It is important to fully appreciate that even though protein and amino acids garner exceptional focus for their involvement in skeletal muscle growth, development, and athletic performance, the roles and functions of proteins (and their constituent amino acids) exceed far beyond topics solely centered on health and fitness. Proteins, similar to fats and carbohydrates, contain carbon, hydrogen, and oxygen; however, unlike the other macronutrients, protein is unique in that it contains nitrogen. Proteins comprise amino acids and chemical structures that feature an amino or amine group ($-NH_2$). From there, amino acids combine together in a highly regulated process that eventually results in them folding and taking on intricate three-dimensional structures that ultimately create functional proteins.

Proteins support a vast number of processes including gene expression, transport of biological molecules, tissue remodeling and repair, energy production, synthesis of hormones, enzymes, and neurotransmitters. Specifically regarding children and adolescents, the functions of proteins are critical for growth, development, and physiological function, thus creating the need for adequate intake through diet. In the face of inadequate protein intake, children and adolescents may experience reductions in linear growth, delays in sexual maturation, as well as decreased lean body mass accumulation (Story and Stang 2005). Further, certain amino acids known as the essential amino acids cannot be readily produced within the body and for this reason their consumption in the diet is paramount. Alternatively, a group of amino acids used for protein development are able to be produced by the body in adequate amounts to meet physiological demands; these amino acids are nonessential amino acids. Finally, some scientists classify certain amino acids as conditionally essential meaning that only under certain conditions is the body not able to synthesize adequate

TABLE 4.1
Essential, Nonessential, and Conditionally Essential Amino Acids

Essential Amino Acids

Isoleucine	Phenylalanine
Leucine	Threonine
Lysine	Tryptophan
Methionine	Valine

Nonessential

Alanine[a]	Glutamic acid
Asparagine	Glycine
Aspartic acid	Serine
Citruline	

Conditionally Essential

Arginine	Proline
Cysteine[b]	Taurine
Glutamine	Tyrosine[c]
Histidine[d]	

[a] Children have reduced capacity to produce arginine.
[b] Cysteine is produced from methionine.
[c] Tyrosine is produced from phenyalanine.
[d] Infants cannot produce histidine.

amounts of them. As an example and from a growth and development perspective, it is known that children are unable to produce adequate amounts of arginine. Examples of essential, nonessential, and conditionally essential amino acids are provided in Table 4.1. It is important that coaches and practitioners understand the importance of dietary protein and the metabolic and physiological roles protein plays in regard to children and adolescent populations, while also recognizing dietary protein requirements, the wide variety of protein sources, and acknowledging safety concerns.

4.2 PROTEIN DIGESTION

Digestion of protein begins in the stomach, excluding, of course, the physical chewing and grinding that occurs in the mouth. The highly acidic environment of the stomach (pH of 1–3.5), initiates the denaturation and unfolding of protein. Pepsin, a key protein enzyme, works to cleave peptide bonds within the protein, dismantling the proteins into smaller subunits called proteoses, peptones, and polypeptides. Pepsin activity accounts for 10%–20% of total protein digestion, while the majority of digestion occurs in the intestines. Upon entering the small intestines, pancreatic secretions raise the pH of the digestive contents, paving the way for additional proteolytic enzymes to continue the digestive process. Endopeptidases (trypsin, chymotrypsin, and elastase) break apart peptide bonds within the protein molecule, generating many smaller peptides in the intestinal lumen while exopeptidases (carboxypeptidases) produce individual amino acids by cleaving peptide bonds at the carboxy-terminal ends of the peptides and proteins. Approximately 70% of protein digestion occurs via endopeptidases or exopeptidases, creating oligopeptides ranging in length from 2 to 5 amino acids, while 30% are found as free amino acids. The final phase of protein breakdown occurs when these peptide chains come in contact with thousands of peptidase enzymes found within the microvilli of the small intestine cells. Here, the oligopeptides are broken down into dipeptide and tripeptide chains that may be easily transported inside the intestinal cell and out of the digestive tract. Once inside the intestinal cell, peptidases, which are specific to a wide array of amino acids, complete the breakdown of the di- and tripeptides into individual amino acids. More than 99% of the final protein products are absorbed as individual amino acids and passed into the bloodstream, where they can be used for protein formation in the various tissues throughout the body.

4.3 MANY PHYSIOLOGICAL ROLES OF PROTEIN

The human body uses 20 amino acids to produce proteins resulting in a staggering number of possible combinations that result in a final protein product that is both structurally and functionally unique. Different estimates suggest that the human body may comprise anywhere from 60 to 100 trillion cells; each cell contains thousands of different proteins within them, and as expected, they come in an array of shapes and sizes, with distinct functions based on the one-by-one sequence of amino acids contained within it. As an example, proteins are known to function as cellular receptor molecules, transport vehicles of biological materials, aid the immune system fight against foreign substances, or act as enzymes that catalyze chemical reactions. Additionally, proteins are found in structural tissues such as bones, ligaments, tendons, and, of course, skeletal muscle. Skeletal muscle is an incredibly unique conglomerate of proteins; its complex organization of proteins can contract and generate force, allowing us to interact with our environment. Additionally, skeletal muscle is exceptionally plastic, responding to various types of stimuli and becoming more resilient to stress including those imposed from exercise and training. It is the plastic properties of skeletal muscle that lay the foundation for training adaptations to occur. A number of different protein types and their representative functions are listed in Table 4.2.

Body proteins arise from three predominant sources: blood or plasma, visceral tissue (organs), and skeletal muscle. More specifically, visceral proteins are looked upon as nonskeletal proteins found in various tissues and organs, and some even consider plasma proteins to be visceral proteins (Reeds 2000). The major types of protein found in the blood are albumins, globulins, and fibrinogens.

TABLE 4.2
Physiological Roles of Proteins in the Body

Proteins	Examples	Physiological Role
Albumin	Serum albumin	Capillary fluid movement
Cell surface antigens	Major histocompatibility complex (MHC) proteins	Antigen presentation
Cytokines	Interleukin 6, tumor necrosis factor-α	Immune response signaling
Enzymes	Lysosomes	Hydrolyzes polysaccharides
	Polymerases	Synthesis of nucleic acids
	Proteases	Degrades proteins
Globins	Cytochromes	Electron transport for energy production in mitochondria
	Hemoglobin	O_2 and CO_2 in transport in blood
	Myoglobin	O_2 and CO_2 in transport in muscle
Hormones	Testosterone	Male secondary sex characteristic modulation
	Thyroxine	Cellular metabolism
Ion binding	Calmodulin	Binding of calcium ions
	Ferritin	Storage of ions
Immunoglobulins	Antibodies	Recognizes and neutralizes foreign substances (antigens)
Muscle	Actin	Responsible for muscle contraction
	Myosin	Responsible for muscle contraction
Repressors	*Lac* repressor	Gene transcription
Transporters	Proton pump	Establishes membrane excitability
	Sodium–potassium pump	Mitochondrial energy production

Albumin is found in the highest concentration in the blood and works to provide osmotic pressure in the plasma and transport of fatty-based substances such as lipids and steroid hormones in the bloodstream. Globulins assist with transporting ions, perform a number of enzymatic functions in the plasma, and are primarily involved in supporting the immune system. Fibrinogen primarily works to build fibrin, a primary constituent of blood clots, making fibrinogen's primary role that is blood coagulation (Guyton and Hall 2006).

The nitrogen found in amino acids also plays a role in human function. For example, the nitrogen atom is incorporated into the primary energy system molecules nicotinamide dinucleotide (NAD+) and flavin dinucleotide (FAD). These compounds primarily operate to deliver electrons to drive energy production. In addition, nitrogen is used in the oxygen-carrying molecules in blood (hemoglobin) and muscle (myoglobin) and may also be found in many hormones, vitamins, minerals, and organic compounds critical to anabolic processes. In particular to the general theme of this book, in this chapter, protein's role in biological growth and development is paramount in addition to its place in anabolic deposition of lean body mass. In summary, the reach of protein function across our entire physiological system is vast. However, protein's role takes on an even greater level when the discussion is focused on children and adolescents who are growing and developing, but also have a strong desire to physically perform at their highest levels (Coleman and Rosenbloom 2012).

4.4 BUILDING UP AND BREAKING DOWN: PROTEIN METABOLISM

The primary function of protein in the diet is to provide amino acids to enable the production of necessary proteins for cell function across the body. Though proteins can contribute toward energy production, their preferential role is that of protein anabolism. At rest, protein contributes a modest 2%–5% of the body's energy needs, a value that may increase to 15% during prolonged exercise bouts with less-than-adequate energy and/or carbohydrate intake.

Protein use for energy increases when the body's ability to use carbohydrate is compromised, such as during periods when carbohydrate intake is inadequate (McArdle et al. 2001). To generate energy from amino acids, the nitrogen group found on each amino acid must be removed. This energy-expensive process is known as deamination. Owing to the process being energetically costly, the body works to avoid activating this mechanism. Once deaminated, the "carbon skeleton" may directly contribute toward energy production by entering various parts of the Krebs cycle, a key energy production process that is also known as the citric acid cycle (Figure 4.1). Additionally, other pathways exist where certain amino acids (alanine) or products of anaerobic metabolism (lactate), upon transportation to the liver, may be converted into glucose where it can then be used by the skeletal muscle for energy. Finally, many amino acids can have their amino group transferred in a process known as transamination that also works to regulate the pool of amino acids available to the cells.

The human body does not store protein like it stores carbohydrate (muscle and liver glycogen) and fat (triglycerides primarily stored in muscle, adipose tissue, and surrounding organs). This lack of storage is compensated by the dynamic nature of protein metabolism, whereby proteins are continuously being synthesized and degraded. Protein throughout the body exists as pools of amino acids, which are subsisted by a constant ebb and flow of amino acids into and out of these pools based on the current supply and demand of amino acids (Wolfe 2005, 2006). When dietary intake of protein provides necessary amino acids to replenish the free amino acid pools, the body's reliance on endogenous protein degradation (i.e., skeletal muscle breakdown) to build a new protein is reduced. Alternatively, if dietary supply is inadequate, rates of protein degradation must increase to supply the necessary amino acids required for the building of new cellular proteins. This dynamic balance of synthesis and degradation is called net protein balance, where a positive net protein balance is achieved when the rate of protein synthesis exceeds the rate of protein degradation, and vice versa during a negative net protein balance. This process, again, is dictated by amino

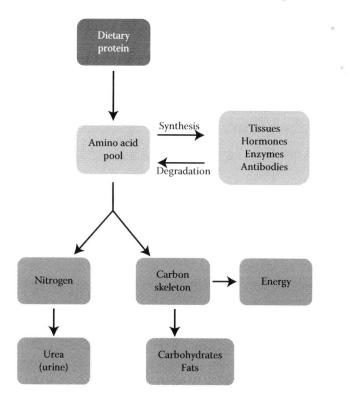

FIGURE 4.1 Simplified schematic of protein metabolism.

acid availability and need. Protein balance is often assessed via measurement of nitrogen balance, where the total intake of nitrogen is compared against the total excretion of nitrogen. Put simply, for appropriate muscle deposition and other tissue growth to occur in developing children, adolescents, or any other population, there must be adequate availability of amino acids to synthesize protein.

Continual protein turnover also provides the foundation for skeletal muscle plasticity in response to training, leading to increases in strength, a better ability to handle physical stresses, and an increase or accumulation of muscle tissue throughout periods of growth and development (Phillips 2004). During periods of exercise and training, protein intake must increase to offset the demands of training while also ensuring that adequate amino acids are available to maintain a positive protein balance. A positive protein balance is required to facilitate training adaptations and to optimize the repair and recovery processes of skeletal muscle. Given the impact of amino acid availability for child and adolescent athletes, it is important to consider the consequences of exercise on protein metabolism. Exercise, both aerobic and resistance training, have been shown to facilitate positive nitrogen balance (Bolster et al. 2001; Pikosky et al. 2002), which sets the stage for tissue growth and repair. However, this trend is dependent on protein intake in the diet, with inadequate daily protein intake failing to promote an increase in the body's nitrogen balance (Boisseau et al. 2005). Interestingly, it has been observed that with high levels of protein intake, whole-body protein metabolism may be altered during periods of exercise to facilitate growth, even in the face of negative energy balance due to inadequate calorie intake or increased energy expenditure (Bolster et al. 2001; Pikosky et al. 2002).

"Nutrient partitioning" is a concept that recognizes the body's ability to preferentially metabolize certain fuels during certain conditions. Using protein as an example, previous reports indicate that available protein may be prioritized toward growth and development functions (Beermann 1994). Of note and of a similar note, nutrition partitioning involving protein is well documented to occur during two other important physiological states: pregnancy and lactation (Bauman et al. 1982). Beyond nutrient partitioning, evidence in healthy men has consistently shown that as an individual becomes more adapted to a training program and/or has a higher level of training background, that protein usage or requirements go down, suggesting that protein demands changed due to an increased efficiency of the body to use protein. All such phenomena help to highlight the body's remarkable physiological orchestration to take precedence of growth and development. Additionally, it also highlights the need for adequate daily protein intake.

4.5 ON A NEED-TO-EAT BASIS

The stress of rapid growth and development experienced by children and adolescents requires an increased demand for nutrients, including protein. Adequate protein intake through diet is not only necessary for maintaining protein turnover and the synthesis of physiologically important amino acid products, but also for the deposition of a new tissue (Institute of Medicine 2005). Children and adolescents have a slightly higher recommended daily allowance (RDA) of protein when compared to adults to ensure that amino acids are available in adequate amounts to facilitate growth, accumulation of lean body mass, and sexual maturation (Story and Stang 2005). To illustrate, a 2009 study collected body composition data on 364 third graders and again when the same cohort was in ninth grade, it was found that dietary protein intake may play a significant role in body composition development during puberty for girls. Moreover, higher protein intakes were associated with less fat mass gain over the 6-year time period. These fat mass changes were accompanied by the largest increase in fat-free mass index in girls with a body mass index (BMI) in the fifth quintile (van Vught et al. 2009). This trend was also seen in boys; however, the associations did not reach significance that is likely attributed to the gender differences in body composition development among pubertal children (van Vught et al. 2009).

The RDA for protein is 0.95 grams/kg/day for children of 4–13 years of age and 0.85 grams/kg/day for adolescents of 14–18 years of age (Institute of Medicine 2005). For example, an 84-pound (38.2 kg) 12-year-old child would need 36.3 grams of protein per day, while a 110-pound (50 kg) 17-year-old teen would need 42.5 grams/day. When looking at protein need as a percent of total daily energy intake, the acceptable range of this macronutrient is 10%–35% (Institute of Medicine 2005).

When engaging in exercise, protein intake may need to be elevated above the RDA to ensure adequate repair and recovery. It has often been erroneously reported that protein intakes greater than RDA are unhealthy and may lead to a negative effect on renal function and bone health; however, recent published literature consistently indicates that both these concerns are unfounded in that there is little substantive evidence to indicate that protein intakes above the aforementioned ranges have adverse effects in healthy human beings (Campbell et al. 2007; Phillips 2014). To this point, there are insufficient data to recommend an upper limit (UL) for daily protein intake in children as well as an upper boundary for an acceptable macronutrient distribution range (AMDR) for protein (Institute of Medicine 2005; National Academies Press 2006). Such points are made to lay the foundation of and dismiss the concerns that may be associated with an elevated protein intake (both will be discussed further in subsequent sections), as scientific studies continue to indicate that protein is central to growth and development in children and adolescents, while also being important during periods of exercise and recovery.

Participation in sport and exercise has a tremendous amount of positive health outcomes for children and adolescents, including cardiorespiratory and muscular fitness, reduced body fat levels, decreased risk for cardiovascular and metabolic diseases, enhanced bone health, and a reduction of the symptoms associated with depression and anxiety (Coleman and Rosenbloom 2012). However, it is worth noting that training and sport participation places additional physiological stress on a young person's body, which is already undergoing the demands of growth and development. Therefore, additional attention should be focused toward a young athlete's nutrition. It is important that lost nutrients (i.e., carbohydrate and water) are replaced acutely (i.e., following physical activity), as well as adequately maintained through daily intake. Adequate daily protein intake is key to recovery, repair, facilitation of exercise adaptations, skill development, as well as to help prevent overtraining. All these aspects of training should be of primary concern for parents and coaches. Protein plays a critical role in all these processes and thus, adequate daily intake should be ensured to promote the gains elicited from training and sport practice while keeping the young athlete healthy and able to train, practice, and play.

While most of the literature pertaining to protein need and exercise is based on the adult population, where it is suggested that individuals participating in training should eat more protein than the RDA (Campbell et al. 2007; Rodriguez et al. 2009), it is reasonable that young athletes should also increase protein intake during periods of training (Petrie et al. 2004). The substantial demands of body growth and development already warrant a daily protein intake greater than what is needed by adults (0.8 grams/kg/day) (Table 4.3). When combined with the stresses elicited by training, the concern regarding adequacy becomes evident (Fink et al. 2012). Though the training demands experienced by young athletes may certainly be less than those accommodated by adults, it is important to give the body the nutrients it needs to repair from exercise, as well as reap the benefits from protein to ultimately improve performance outcomes. Indeed, young athletes beginning a training program should consume 1.0–1.5 grams/kg/day of protein (in addition to adequate calories), to reduce the associated protein loss from increased amino acid turnover and nitrogen loss (Spear 2005). Additionally, a young endurance athlete may need between 1.2 and 1.4 grams/kg/day of protein (Spear 2005). In light of this recommendation, caution is urged to parents, coaches, or athletes attempting to implement these approaches so as to ensure that adequate intake of other macronutrients (carbohydrates and fats) are also achieved. Growth and development as well as the increased demand from practice and training increases the nutrient needs of all macronutrients, not just protein. More information is available regarding carbohydrate and fat considerations in Chapters 3 and 5, respectively while Chapters 15 and 16 offer many practical tips and considerations to help recommended intakes to be met by athletes.

TABLE 4.3
Recommended Daily Intake of Protein

Age (Years)	Recommended Amount (g/kg/day)
4–8	0.95
9–13	0.95
14–18	0.85

Source: Adapted from DRIs. Dietary reference intakes for energy, carbohydrate, fiber, fat, fatty acids, cholesterol, protein, and amino acids, 2005. Institute of Medicine. 2005. Dietary Reference Intakes for Energy, Carbohydrate, Fiber, Fat, Fatty Acids, Cholesterol, Protein, and Amino Acids. 1-1357; National Academies Press. 2006. *Dietary Reference Intakes: The Essential Guide to Nutrient Requirements.* Washington, DC: National Academies Press.

Overall training load (i.e., intensity, volume, duration, and frequency) should influence where in the recommended range a young athlete's dietary intake should fall. In addition, paying attention to recovery factors such as readiness, energy levels, and desire to practice should also be considered as all these can be monitored and evaluated against changes in fitness and body composition to assess the adequacy of the young athlete's diet. Time periods that may warrant an intake toward the upper end of the range are the off-season and preseason, where it is not uncommon for practice and training volumes to be high; this may particularly be the case in middle-school and high-school athletics. For example, a 65-kg middle-school basketball player engaging in an off-season strength and conditioning program, daily practice, and weekly summer league games may benefit from a daily intake upward of 97.5 grams/kg/day (1.5 grams/kg/day). The same recommendation may be appropriate for a high-school football player during periods of heavy practice (i.e., twice a day) and an intense resistance-training program, where a daily intake of 1.5 grams/kg/day for a 75-kg teen would result in an intake of 112.5 grams/day. However, it is important for these recommendations to also be dialed back during periods or phases of training where training intensity and especially volume is lower.

It is well noted that resistance-training outcomes, such as increases in strength and fat-free mass may be enhanced by ingesting protein in amounts above the RDA (Cermak et al. 2012; Kerksick et al. 2006, 2007; Kreider 1999; Rodriguez et al. 2009). Protein ingestion increases amino acid availability and helps to promote a positive net protein balance, which effectively paves the way for muscle anabolism. Acute responses to a single bout of resistance training stimulate increases in muscle protein synthesis and also increase muscle protein breakdown. In the absence of feeding and amino acid availability, an overall negative nitrogen balance results after an acute strength-training bout (Biolo et al. 1995; Phillips et al. 1997). With youth strength and conditioning programs becoming more prevalent, particularly those with a resistance-training component, protein intake is an important dietary consideration as training outcomes achieved from a strength and conditioning program may be enhanced with adequate protein intake. Given that adaptations from chronic resistance training result from the provision of amino acids that leads to a robust increase in net protein balance (Kerksick and Kulovitz 2013), timely feeding of protein is the potent way to optimize training. The gains resulting from resistance training amidst successive periods of positive muscle protein balance from appropriate protein intake will likely translate into greater athletic performance, due to enhancements in strength, functional movement capability, and potentially kinesthetic awareness. Therefore, a common recommendation for young athletes participating in a resistance-training program is a daily protein intake of 1.0–1.5 grams/kg/day. It is worth mentioning that while adequate protein intake can promote optimal blood levels of amino acids for tissue growth, the circulating hormone levels of sexually immature males are insufficient to lead to the significant development of muscle mass; however, as mentioned earlier, improvements in strength and functional movement are well documented (Spear 2005). Additionally, excessive protein intake, as is the case of any other macronutrient, may lead to a caloric excess and body fat gain if the increased dietary intake is not matched with increased levels of physical training.

Though less discussed and an area that is somewhat surprising to parents, coaches, and uninformed health-care practitioners, endurance performance may also warrant a protein intake greater than the RDA. Prolonged and sustained aerobic performance such as cross-country, cycling, and perhaps soccer, may demand an increased need for amino acids to help repair tissues, prevent lean body mass breakdown, and maintain a healthy bodyweight. While protein's overall contribution to energy production is accepted to be relatively low, prolonged bouts of exercise, particularly if combined with substandard dietary practices, can increase the utilization of protein as an energy source. Therefore, adequate daily carbohydrate intake is an extremely important consideration, not only to deliver an efficient fuel source for the sporting activity, but also to spare amino acids for anabolic processes. For young athletes engaging in regular and/or exhaustive endurance training, a daily protein intake of 1.2–1.4 grams/kg/day may be required (Desbrow et al. 2014; Petrie et al. 2004; Spear 2005) to combat the potential of incurring a negative protein balance during periods of such strenuous endurance activity. Parents and coaches of young athletes should ensure that adequate daily protein intake (and carbohydrate intake) is achieved to allow for the sparing of amino acids for growth and development, as well as to maximize recovery and promote adaptations from endurance training and practice.

As stated previously, carbohydrate availability plays a role in protein metabolism and moderates protein need. Moreover, carbohydrate operates as the muscle's most-preferred source of fuel. Uniquely, carbohydrate is used as a fuel source in both anaerobic (higher intensity) and aerobic (lower-to-moderate intensity) exercising conditions. Throughout periods of intense exercise, glycogen (the body's stored form of carbohydrate) in the muscle and liver may become depleted and eventually reduces blood glucose levels. Since amino acids can be used to manufacture glucose (the constituent of carbohydrate) by a process known as gluconeogenesis, protein breakdown increases to maintain blood glucose levels when glycogen stores are depleted. Therefore, carbohydrate status is known to influence the metabolic fate of protein.

Finally, it is also important to note that while science has yet to identify a link between increased protein intake and negative health implications (Campbell et al. 2007; Martin et al. 2005), overconsumption of protein should not be construed as any more effective than what is required (i.e., >2.0 grams/kg/day in adults) (Campbell et al. 2007; Kreider 1999; Rodriguez et al. 2009). Excessive consumption of protein (like any other macronutrient) may lead to an excessive caloric intake, and potentially results in unwanted body mass gain and unfavorable shifts in one's body composition. Additionally, though protein intake above the RDA may serve as a beneficial nutritional strategy during periods of training or sport performance, it should not come at the cost of other nutrients (i.e., carbohydrate and fat) as an inadequate intake of carbohydrate can negatively impact exercise performance and inadequate fat intake can impact the absorption of key vitamins and production of necessary hormones.

4.6 NOT ALL PROTEINS ARE CREATED EQUAL

As we discussed previously, unlike fat and carbohydrate, there are no reservoirs of protein in the human body. In exchange, protein metabolism is known to be a dynamic process where amino acids are recycled in and out of a pool of amino acids. The amino acid pool is maintained through a continual ebb and flow of amino acids from endogenous (i.e., skeletal muscle) and/or exogenous (i.e., dietary protein) sources. Skeletal muscle is rich in protein, second only to water in its composition. For this reason, skeletal muscle is considered as the physiological location of which the body may depend on for amino acid donation when there is a demand. Historically, individual rates of protein synthesis and breakdown have been collectively measured using the nitrogen balance technique where the intake of nitrogen is compared relative to the amount of nitrogen that is excreted from the body. Both processes (muscle protein synthesis and muscle protein breakdown) are highly regulated and ultimately are predicated on the availability of amino acids. When dietary protein intake is sufficient enough to replenish the free amino acid pool, the body's reliance on endogenous stores (i.e., skeletal muscle) to synthesize new proteins is reduced. Conversely, if the dietary supply is inadequate, the rate of protein breakdown is increased to provide the necessary amino acids required to build new proteins. However, protein metabolism is not only influenced by the overall amount of amino acids available, but also what types of amino acids are available.

The human body requires 20 amino acids to build protein. However, the body cannot synthesize a group of them resulting in their classification as indispensable or, more commonly referred to as, essential amino acids. Therefore, these amino acids must be provided through the diet to facilitate optimal rates of protein synthesis and maintenance of normal bodily function. The remaining dispensable or nonessential amino acids should not be thought of as unnecessary amino acids, as these amino acids are of great importance for other aspects of protein as well as cellular metabolism. The term "nonessential" only suggests that these amino acids do not have to be consumed in the diet and that the body can endogenously manufacture them at a sufficient rate. Interestingly, while other types of body proteins may require their availability for synthesis, the nonessential amino acids have clearly been shown to have no measurable involvement with the growth and building of muscle proteins (Tipton et al. 1999; Volpi et al. 2003). Thus, the stresses of growth and development compounded with those of sport, practice, and training place a premium on essential amino acid availability to support the production of new proteins. To synthesize the vast number of proteins that the body needs, all the required amino acids must be available. If a protein requires an essential amino acid for its production, it cannot be produced if the particular amino acid has not been consumed through the diet.

Of the essential amino acids, three are widely reported to exert a unique influence on muscle protein metabolism: leucine, isoleucine, and valine (Drummond et al. 2009; Katsanos et al. 2006; Rennie et al. 2006). These three essential amino acids are known as the branched-chain amino acids (BCAAs) and are unique in that they are primarily metabolized in skeletal muscle. All other amino acids are metabolized in the liver; however, the liver lacks the enzyme branched-chain aminotransferase, which is needed to catabolize BCAAs. Luckily, this enzyme is found in skeletal muscle. Another interesting point regarding the BCAAs is that they are typically the most abundant essential amino acids in many dietary proteins making them easy to consume. One BCAA, in particular, leucine, has been a recent topic of much scientific inquiry due to its ability to enhance muscle protein balance. Leucine has been shown to be the most potent stimulator of muscle protein synthesis of *all* the amino acids (Norton et al. 2009, 2012) and accordingly ingestion of leucine-rich protein sources robustly stimulates muscle protein synthesis (Pasiakos et al. 2011; Rieu et al. 2006). While optimizing leucine content is an important consideration relative to the stimulation of protein synthesis, leucine intake must also be balanced against the ingestion of the other amino acids to maximally stimulate muscle protein synthesis (Norton et al. 2009, 2012). Protein foods are commonly classified by their "completeness," meaning that a complete protein source is any food that contains all the essential amino acids in amounts that support life and growth. Alternatively, incomplete proteins are foods that do not contain the full profile of essential amino acids in sufficient amounts. A diet consisting of incomplete protein sources will challenge cellular and metabolic function, and ultimately over time, can lead to protein malnutrition. This may occur even if the overall protein intake is being provided. In this respect, optimal delivery of the essential amino acids is needed to facilitate the synthesis of tissue, hormones, transport vesicles, antibodies, and enzymes. Consequently, the suboptimal delivery of the essential amino acids will negatively impact cellular function and other bodily functions while lean body mass will be leached in an attempt to compensate for the lack of sufficiency in the amino acid pool. In the simplest terms, all animal-based protein sources (i.e., eggs, milk, meat, fish, poultry, etc.) are complete protein sources while plant-based protein sources typically lack one or more of the essential amino acids rendering them complete protein sources. For example, grains lack the essential amino acid lysine, while legumes lack methionine. Interestingly, both these common food sources contain high amounts of the amino acid the other lacks; therefore, the combination of the two foods would result in a complete protein profile. It has been found that vegetarians, especially those participating in training or sports, have slightly higher protein needs to compensate for the high intake of incomplete protein sources (Fink et al. 2012). This point is of importance in that if a child does not receive sufficient amounts of essential amino acids due to high intake of low-quality protein, not only may sport and training performance suffer, but also these adolescents may run the risk of impaired growth, delayed sexual maturation, and decreased lean body mass deposition (Story and Stang 2005). Another key point of emphasis is that the same amino acid from an animal or plant source is fundamentally the same and if an athlete chooses to refrain or limit their consumption of animal-based proteins, they must become educated upon what amino acids are provided by various plant sources to ensure that a balance and optimal delivery of the essential amino acids occurs.

While the overall daily protein intake for young athletes is dependent on age, activity level, and mode of training, it is important to recognize that the essential amino acids are the primary effectors of muscle protein balance (Borsheim et al. 2002; Tipton et al. 1999; Volpi et al. 2003); therefore, these amino acids must be found in the protein consumed in the diet. Again, this does not require the consumption of meat, milk, and eggs, foods that are typically associated with protein (though these sources do indeed have a full essential amino acid profile), but may be acquired through thoughtful complementing of incomplete proteins.

4.7 THE HIGHS AND LOWS OF PROTEIN QUALITY AND UNDERSTANDING PROTEIN SOURCES

The quality of a protein has a tremendous effect on its ability to meet the nitrogen and amino acid requirements during growth and training. For a growing young athlete, a diet rich in high-quality protein is an effective way to ensure that amino acid requirements are indeed being met. A parent or coach may be curious as to what constitutes a high-quality protein and how that is determined. Of course, food sources such as beef, eggs, poultry, and milk products are rich in protein, but nonanimal foods contain protein as well. Indeed, many foods contain some amount of protein; however, as we discussed earlier, all proteins are not created equal. A number of means have been used to assess the quality of different sources of dietary protein. Biological value (BV), chemical score, protein efficiency ratio (PER), net protein utilization, and the protein digestibility-corrected amino acid score (PDCAAS) are the most commonly used. Chemical score compares the amino acid content, most particularly the essential amino acid content, of any given protein source to that of a reference protein (e.g., egg protein). For example, if chicken breast is found to contain 80% of the limiting amino acid level as that is found in egg protein, a chemical score of 80 would be assigned to chicken. Proteins with higher chemical scores are considered to be of higher quality and proteins with lower chemical scores are of lower quality. A similar concept is utilized for BV and PER with one key difference: BV and PER account for how much of the protein is actually utilized by the test protein in comparison to the standard egg protein. The higher the BV and PER value, the better the protein will be at meeting bodily demands of a young athlete. Finally, another commonly used method compares the amino acid profile of a protein to the essential amino acid requirements in humans established by The Food and Agriculture Organization. This method, known as the PDCAAS, is currently recognized as the best method of comparing proteins for humans (Schaafsma 2005). A protein with a PDCAAS of 1.0 indicates that the protein exceeds the essential amino acid requirements of the body and is therefore an excellent source of protein. One notable shortcoming with PDCAAS, however, is that all values are truncated at a value of 1.0 leading one to believe that all protein sources with a value of 1.0 are equal where in fact some protein sources (e.g., milk solids,

TABLE 4.4
PDCAASs and PERs for Common and Supplemented Protein Sources

Protein	PDCAAS	PER
Whey	1.00	3.0–3.2
Bovine colostrum	1.00	3.0
Casein	1.00	2.9
Milk protein	1.00	2.8
Ovalbumin (egg)	1.00	2.8
Soy	1.00	1.8–2.3
Beef/Poultry/Fish	0.8–0.92	2.0–2.3
Wheat	0.43	1.5
Gelatin (collagen)	0.08	–

whey, casein, and soy) would have PDCAA values greater than 1.0 (Phillips et al. 2009). Table 4.4 highlights several types of protein along with their estimated PER and PDCAA scores.

It is not uncommon for a parent to be concerned with fat content of certain protein sources (meats, dairy products), and therefore, limit their children's intake. Indeed, some protein sources do contain considerable amounts of fat, particularly saturated fats, which may be found in red meats, eggs, and whole-fat dairy products. However, there is an emerging literature suggesting that the association between total fat, saturated fat, and cardiovascular disease may not be as strong as previously thought (Carrera-Bastos et al. 2011; Forsythe et al. 2008; Mente et al. 2009; Volek et al. 2008). In a meta-analysis by Siri-Tarino and colleagues (2010), using 21 studies and a total of 347,747 participants, no significant evidence was found suggesting that dietary saturated fat is associated with an increased risk of coronary heart disease (Siri-Tarino et al. 2010). Moreover, a study by Forsythe and colleagues reported that a low-carbohydrate/high-fat/high-protein diet resulted in greater positive effects on blood lipids (serum fatty acid composition) and inflammation compared to a high-carbohydrate/low-fat/moderate-protein diet despite consuming 3 times the amount of saturated fat than the low-fat diet (Forsythe et al. 2008). It is important to note that participants in these studies were adults and this is still a highly debated topic; however, these findings lead to questions regarding previously held assumptions about fat intake and health. Moreover, it is important to note that not only proteins, but also fats, play a major role in the growth and maturation of adolescents.

A large number of protein supplements are available and marketed to the active/athletic population as a superior means to enhance body composition, build muscle, and increase sport performance. Limited evidence is available to indicate that protein supplements are no more effective than high-quality protein from standard dietary sources alone at promoting exercise-training adaptations (Phillips 2004). However, this point takes away from the potential benefits derived from (1) optimal timing of protein as a nutrient, (2) the convenience offered by a protein supplement, and (3) the favorable appetite and metabolic impact of high-quality protein ingestion. Moreover and as highlighted throughout this chapter, biological growth and development demands energy and the combination of regular exercise and training further stresses the importance of optimal energy and macronutrient intake. For this reason alone, protein supplementation can be considered to allow for adequate fueling in scenarios where poor planning may result in no feeding at all or consumption of quick, convenient foods that are typically void of healthful nutrients. In this respect, controlled investigations using protein supplements and a recent meta-analysis indicate that protein supplementation may indeed promote favorable exercise-training adaptations (Cermak et al. 2012; Kerksick et al. 2006, 2007).

In summary, the source of protein is an important consideration with the consumption of animal-based foods being the simplest way to ensure that optimal intake and distribution of the essential amino acids is provided. While many plant-based protein sources are available and encouraged, athletic children (and adults), particularly those who regularly exercise and train while choosing to restrict their intake of animal-based proteins to any degree are encouraged to closely monitor their diet to ensure that optimal delivery of the amino acids takes place.

4.8 SAFETY OF PROTEIN INTAKE

Habitual protein consumption in excess of the RDA has been reported to promote chronic renal disease through increased glomerular pressure and hyperfiltration (Brenner et al. 1982; Metges and Barth 2000). However, these reports often fail to highlight the fact that the majority of this scientific evidence was generated either from animal models or patients with a coexisting renal disease (Brenner et al. 1982); a generalization to healthy humans is not appropriate (Martin et al. 2005). When well-designed prospective cohort study designs have been used, high protein intakes have not been associated with renal function impairment in normal-operating kidneys (in adults) (Knight et al. 2003). Furthermore, when nonvegetarians and vegetarians were compared, no statistically significant differences in kidney function were found (Blum et al. 1989). While dietary protein intakes above the RDA are not deleterious for healthy, exercising individuals, those individuals with mild renal insufficiency or a family history of renal disease should closely monitor their protein intake to accurately observe their progression of renal disease (Lentine and Wrone 2004; Martin et al. 2005). Indeed, this caution extends to children with preexisting kidney health issues (National Institute of Diabetes and Digestive and Kidney Diseases 2014). It is important to highlight as well that insufficient data are available to suggest a UL for protein in children or an upper boundary for an AMDR (National Academies Press 2006). As a final point, comments made by both the World Health Organization and a panel setting the Nutrient Reference Values for Australia and New Zealand indicate that no evidence is available linking a higher protein diet to renal disease (Nutrient Reference Values for Australia and New Zealand 2014; Phillips 2014; World Health Organization 2007).

In addition to renal function, dietary protein intake and bone metabolism has been an area of concern and controversy. This concern primarily revolves around the leaching of calcium from bones secondary to an elevated protein intake, which may lead to osteopenia and predispose some individuals to osteoporosis. Studies reporting this effect were limited by small sample sizes, methodological errors, and the use of high doses of purified forms of protein (Ginty 2003). Furthermore, data from stable calcium isotope studies have emerged and instead point toward dietary calcium sources, not from bone resorption, as being the origin of the increased urinary calcium (Kerstetter et al. 2005). Overall, there is a lack of scientific evidence linking higher dietary protein intakes to adverse outcomes in healthy, exercising individuals. Again, it is important to note that there is no evidence of a UL or upper boundary of AMDR for protein in children (National Academies Press 2006), but there is, as we have learned, a minimum need that must be met to avoid negative health effects such as impairments in linear growth, sexual maturation, and lean mass deposition (Story and Stang 2005).

4.9 CONCLUSION

Protein is a vital nutrient responsible for many crucial bodily functions, including growth and development of children and adolescents. Protein is digested primarily in the small intestines and upon absorption is transported through the blood to build new proteins. Proteins are composed of individual amino acids arranged in highly specific sequences and folded into intricate three-dimensional structures; their function in the body is determined by the three-dimensional conformation. At rest, proteins make a small contribution to energy production; however, during starvation, carbohydrate depletion, or during prolonged exercise, body proteins, such as skeletal muscle, may be degraded into amino acids to serve as a fuel source. Protein metabolism is a dynamic process where proteins are constantly synthesized and degraded and amino acids flow in and out of an amino acid pool. Overall protein balance is determined by the amino acid supply and demand. When dietary intake of amino acids is sufficient, the body's reliance on endogenous protein degradation (i.e., skeletal muscle breakdown) to build a new protein is reduced and a positive protein balance is achieved.

The unique demands of growth and development experienced by children and adolescents call for a greater daily protein requirement than that of adults. It is essential that they receive adequate protein on a daily basis to promote normal development including the deposition of lean body mass. Insufficient dietary protein may result in reductions in linear growth, delays in sexual maturation, as well as decreased lean body mass accumulation (Story and Stang 2005). The RDA for protein is 0.95 grams/kg/day for children of 4–13 years of age and 0.85 grams/kg/day for adolescents of 14–18 years of age (Institute of Medicine 2005). Regular exercise and sport participation further elevate protein need to account for increased muscle protein turnover. Adequate protein intake is important for repair, recovery, and facilitation of training adaptations and skill acquisition. For young athletes beginning a training program, 1.5 grams/kg/day may be necessary while a daily intake of 1.2–1.4 grams/kg/day may be required for those participating in exhaustive endurance performance (Spear 2005). The body uses 20 different amino acids to build proteins, some of which are readily synthesized in the body while others must be consumed from the diet. High-quality protein sources are those that contain a broad and plentiful spectrum of the essential amino acids, including BCAAs and leucine. These sources are the most efficient way to meet amino acid and nitrogen needs. Insufficient data are currently available to suggest a UL for protein in children or an upper boundary for an AMDR (National Academies Press 2006). Finally, increased intakes of protein by healthy individuals are well tolerated and have not been shown to result in impaired renal function or bone health but positively influence body composition in growing children (Nutrient Reference Values for Australia and New Zealand 2014; Phillips 2014; Story and Stang 2005; World Health Organization 2007).

REFERENCES

Bauman, D. E., J. H. Eisemann, and W. B. Currie. 1982. Hormonal effects on partitioning of nutrients for tissue growth: Role of growth hormone and prolactin. *Fed Proc* 41 (9):2538–44.

Beermann, D. H. 1994. Coordination of nutrient use by peripheral and visceral tissues. *J Nutr* 124 (8 Suppl):1392S.

Biolo, G., S. P. Maggi, B. D. Williams, K. D. Tipton, and R. R. Wolfe. 1995. Increased rates of muscle protein turnover and amino acid transport after resistance exercise in humans. *Am J Physiol* 268 (3 Pt 1):E514–20.

Blum, M., M. Averbuch, Y. Wolman, and A. Aviram. 1989. Protein intake and kidney function in humans: Its effect on "normal aging." *Arch Intern Med* 149 (1):211–2.

Boisseau, N., C. Persaud, A. A. Jackson, and J. R. Poortmans. 2005. Training does not affect protein turnover in pre- and early pubertal female gymnasts. *Eur J Appl Physiol* 94 (3):262–7. doi: 10.1007/s00421-004-1264-5.

Bolster, D. R., M. A. Pikosky, L. M. McCarthy, and N. R. Rodriguez. 2001. Exercise affects protein utilization in healthy children. *J Nutr* 131 (10):2659–63.

Borsheim, E., K. D. Tipton, S. E. Wolf, and R. R. Wolfe. 2002. Essential amino acids and muscle protein recovery from resistance exercise. *Am J Physiol Endocrinol Metab* 283 (4):E648–57. doi: 10.1152/ajpendo.00466.2001.

Brenner, B. M., T. W. Meyer, and T. H. Hostetter. 1982. Dietary protein intake and the progressive nature of kidney disease: The role of hemodynamically mediated glomerular injury in the pathogenesis of progressive glomerular sclerosis in aging, renal ablation, and intrinsic renal disease. *N Engl J Med* 307 (11):652–9. doi: 10.1056/NEJM198209093071104.

Campbell, B., R. Kreider, T. Ziegenfuss, P. La Bounty, M. Roberts, D. G. Burke, J. Landis, H. L. Lopez, and J. Antonio. 2007. International Society of Sports Nutrition position stand: Protein and exercise. *J Int Soc Sports Nutr* 4 (1):8.

Carrera-Bastos, P., M. Fontes-Villalba, J. H. O'Keefe, S. Lindeberg, and L. Cordain. 2011. The western diet and lifestyle and diseases of civilization. *Res Rep Clin Cardiol* 2:15–35.

Cermak, N. M., P. T. Res, L. C. de Groot, W. H. Saris, and L. J. van Loon. 2012. Protein supplementation augments the adaptive response of skeletal muscle to resistance-type exercise training: A meta-analysis. *Am J Clin Nutr* 96 (6):1454–64. doi: 10.3945/ajcn.112.037556.

Coleman, E. and C. Rosenbloom. 2012. *Sports Nutrition: A Practice Manual for Professionals*. Chicago, IL: Academy of Nutrition and Dietetics.

Desbrow, B., J. McCormack, L. M. Burke, G. R. Cox, K. Fallon, M. Hislop, R. Logan et al. 2014. Sports dietitians Australia position statement: Sports nutrition for the adolescent athlete. *Int J Sport Nutr Exerc Metab* 24 (5):570–84. doi: 10.1123/ijsnem.2014-0031.

Drummond, M. J., H. C. Dreyer, C. S. Fry, E. L. Glynn, and B. B. Rasmussen. 2009. Nutritional and contractile regulation of human skeletal muscle protein synthesis and mTORC1 signaling. *J Appl Physiol (1985)* 106 (4):1374–84. doi: 10.1152/japplphysiol.91397.2008.

Fink, H. F., A. E. Mikesky, and L. A. Burgoon. 2012. *Practical Applications in Sports Nutrition*. 3rd ed. Burlington, MA: Jones & Bartlett Learning.

Forsythe, C. E., S. D. Phinney, M. L. Fernandez, E. E. Quann, R. J. Wood, D. M. Bibus, W. J. Kraemer, R. D. Feinman, and J. S. Volek. 2008. Comparison of low fat and low carbohydrate diets on circulating fatty acid composition and markers of inflammation. *Lipids* 43 (1):65–77. doi: 10.1007/s11745-007-3132-7.

Ginty, F. 2003. Dietary protein and bone health. *Proc Nutr Soc* 62 (4):867–76. doi: 10.1079/PNS2003307.

Guyton, A. C. and J. E. Hall. 2006. *Textbook of Medical Physiology*. 11th ed. Philadelphia, PA: Elsevier Saunders.

Institute of Medicine. 2005. Dietary Reference Intakes for Energy, Carbohydrate, Fiber, Fat, Fatty Acids, Cholesterol, Protein, and Amino Acids. 1-1357.

Katsanos, C. S., H. Kobayashi, M. Sheffield-Moore, A. Aarsland, and R. R. Wolfe. 2006. A high proportion of leucine is required for optimal stimulation of the rate of muscle protein synthesis by essential amino acids in the elderly. *Am J Physiol Endocrinol Metab* 291 (2):E381–7. doi: 10.1152/ajpendo.00488.2005.

Kerksick, C. M. and M. G. Kulovitz. 2013. Requirements of energy, carbohydrates, proteins, and fats for athletes. In *Nutrition and Enhance Sports Performance: Muscle Building, Endurance, and Strength*. Eds. D. Bagchi, S. Nair, and C. K. Sen. Salt Lake City, UT: Academies Press.

Kerksick, C. M., C. J. Rasmussen, S. L. Lancaster, B. Magu, P. Smith, C. Melton, M. Greenwood, A. L. Almada, C. P. Earnest, and R. B. Kreider. 2006. The effects of protein and amino acid supplementation on performance and training adaptations during ten weeks of resistance training. *J Strength Cond Res* 20 (3):643–53. doi: 10.1519/R-17695.1.

Kerksick, C. M., C. Rasmussen, S. Lancaster, M. Starks, P. Smith, C. Melton, M. Greenwood, A. Almada, and R. Kreider. 2007. Impact of differing protein sources and a creatine containing nutritional formula after 12 weeks of resistance training. *Nutrition* 23 (9):647–56. doi: 10.1016/j.nut.2007.06.015.

Kerstetter, J. E., K. O. O'Brien, D. M. Caseria, D. E. Wall, and K. L. Insogna. 2005. The impact of dietary protein on calcium absorption and kinetic measures of bone turnover in women. *J Clin Endocrinol Metab* 90 (1):26–31. doi: 10.1210/jc.2004-0179.

Knight, E. L., M. J. Stampfer, S. E. Hankinson, D. Spiegelman, and G. C. Curhan. 2003. The impact of protein intake on renal function decline in women with normal renal function or mild renal insufficiency. *Ann Intern Med* 138 (6):460–7.

Kreider, R. B. 1999. Dietary supplements and the promotion of muscle growth with resistance exercise. *Sports Med* 27 (2):97–110.

Lentine, K. and E. M. Wrone. 2004. New insights into protein intake and progression of renal disease. *Curr Opin Nephrol Hypertens* 13 (3):333–6.

Martin, W. F., L. E. Armstrong, and N. R. Rodriguez. 2005. Dietary protein intake and renal function. *Nutr Metab (Lond)* 2:25. doi: 10.1186/1743-7075-2-25.

McArdle, W. D., F. I. Katch, and V. L. Katch. 2001. *Exercise Physiology: Energy, Nutrition and Human Performance*. Baltimore, MD: Lippincott Williams and Wilkins.

Mente, A., L. de Koning, H. S. Shannon, and S. S. Anand. 2009. A systematic review of the evidence supporting a causal link between dietary factors and coronary heart disease. *Arch Intern Med* 169 (7):659–69. doi: 10.1001/archinternmed.2009.38.

Metges, C. C. and C. A. Barth. 2000. Metabolic consequences of a high dietary-protein intake in adulthood: Assessment of the available evidence. *J Nutr* 130 (4):886–9.

National Academies Press. 2006. *Dietary Reference Intakes: The Essential Guide to Nutrient Requirements*. Washington, DC: National Academies Press.

National Institute of Diabetes and Digestive and Kidney Diseases. 2014. Nutrition for chronic kidney disease in children. Retrieved from http://www.niddk.nih.gov/health-information/health-topics/kidney-disease/nutrition-for-chronic-kidney-disease-in-children/Pages/facts.aspx.

Norton, L. E., D. K. Layman, P. Bunpo, T. G. Anthony, D. V. Brana, and P. J. Garlick. 2009. The leucine content of a complete meal directs peak activation but not duration of skeletal muscle protein synthesis and mammalian target of rapamycin signaling in rats. *J Nutr* 139 (6):1103–9. doi: 10.3945/jn.108.103853.

Norton, L. E., G. J. Wilson, D. K. Layman, C. J. Moulton, and P. J. Garlick. 2012. Leucine content of dietary proteins is a determinant of postprandial skeletal muscle protein synthesis in adult rats. *Nutr Metab (Lond)* 9 (1):67. doi: 10.1186/1743-7075-9-67.

Nutrient Reference Values for Australia and New Zealand. 2014. Macronutrient balance. Retrieved from https://www.nrv.gov.au/chronic-disease/macronutrient-balance.

Pasiakos, S. M., H. L. McClung, J. P. McClung, L. M. Margolis, N. E. Andersen, G. J. Cloutier, M. A. Pikosky, J. C. Rood, R. A. Fielding, and A. J. Young. 2011. Leucine-enriched essential amino acid supplementation during moderate steady state exercise enhances postexercise muscle protein synthesis. *Am J Clin Nutr* 94 (3):809–18. doi: 10.3945/ajcn.111.017061.

Petrie, H. J., E. A. Stover, and C. A. Horswill. 2004. Nutritional concerns for the child and adolescent competitor. *Nutrition* 20 (7–8):620–31. doi: 10.1016/j.nut.2004.04.002.

Phillips, S. M. 2004. Protein requirements and supplementation in strength sports. *Nutrition* 20 (7–8):689–95. doi: 10.1016/j.nut.2004.04.009.

Phillips, S. M. 2014. A brief review of higher dietary protein diets in weight loss: A focus on athletes. *Sports Med* 44 (Suppl 2):S149–53. doi: 10.1007/s40279-014-0254-y.

Phillips, S. M., J. E. Tang, and D. R. Moore. 2009. The role of milk- and soy-based protein in support of muscle protein synthesis and muscle protein accretion in young and elderly persons. *J Am Coll Nutr* 28 (4):343–54.

Phillips, S. M., K. D. Tipton, A. Aarsland, S. E. Wolf, and R. R. Wolfe. 1997. Mixed muscle protein synthesis and breakdown after resistance exercise in humans. *Am J Physiol* 273 (1 Pt 1):E99–107.

Pikosky, M., A. Faigenbaum, W. Westcott, and N. Rodriguez. 2002. Effects of resistance training on protein utilization in healthy children. *Med Sci Sports Exerc* 34 (5):820–7.

Reeds, P. J. 2000. Dispensable and indispensable amino acids for humans. *J Nutr* 130 (7):1835S–40S.

Rennie, M. J., J. Bohe, K. Smith, H. Wackerhage, and P. Greenhaff. 2006. Branched-chain amino acids as fuels and anabolic signals in human muscle. *J Nutr* 136 (1 Suppl):264S–8S.

Rieu, I., M. Balage, C. Sornet, C. Giraudet, E. Pujos, J. Grizard, L. Mosoni, and D. Dardevet. 2006. Leucine supplementation improves muscle protein synthesis in elderly men independently of hyperaminoacidaemia. *J Physiol* 575 (Pt 1):305–15. doi: 10.1113/jphysiol.2006.110742.

Rodriguez, N. R., N. M. Di Marco, and S. Langley. 2009. American College of Sports Medicine position stand. Nutrition and athletic performance. *Med Sci Sports Exerc* 41 (3):709–31. doi: 10.1249/MSS.0b013e31890eb8600005768-200903000-00027 [pii].

Schaafsma, G. 2005. The protein digestibility—Corrected amino acid score (PDCAAS)—A concept for describing protein quality in foods and food ingredients: A critical review. *J AOAC Int* 88 (3):988–94.

Siri-Tarino, P. W., Q. Sun, F. B. Hu, and R. M. Krauss. 2010. Meta-analysis of prospective cohort studies evaluating the association of saturated fat with cardiovascular disease. *Am J Clin Nutr* 91 (3):535–46. doi: 10.3945/ajcn.2009.27725.

Spear, B. 2005. Sports nutrition. In *Guidelines for Adolescent Nutrition Services*, Stang, J. and Story, M. (Eds). 199–208. Minneapolis, MN: Center for Leadership, Education and Training in Maternal and Child Nutrition, Division of Epidemiology and Community Health, School of Public Health, University of Minnesota.

Story, M. and J. Stang. 2005. Nutrition needs of adolescents. In *Guidelines for Adolescent Nutrition Services*, Stang, J. and Story, M. (Eds). 21–34. Minneapolis, MN: Center for Leadership, Education and Training in Maternal and Child Nutrition, Division of Epidemiology and Community Health, School of Public Health, University of Minnesota.

Tipton, K. D., B. E. Gurkin, S. Matin, and R. R. Wolfe. 1999. Nonessential amino acids are not necessary to stimulate net muscle protein synthesis in healthy volunteers. *J Nutr Biochem* 10 (2):89–95.

van Vught, A. J., B. L. Heitmann, A. G. Nieuwenhuizen, M. A. Veldhorst, R. J. Brummer, and M. S. Westerterp-Plantenga. 2009. Association between dietary protein and change in body composition among children (EYHS). *Clin Nutr* 28 (6):684–8. doi: 10.1016/j.clnu.2009.05.001.

Volek, J. S., M. L. Fernandez, R. D. Feinman, and S. D. Phinney. 2008. Dietary carbohydrate restriction induces a unique metabolic state positively affecting atherogenic dyslipidemia, fatty acid partitioning, and metabolic syndrome. *Prog Lipid Res* 47 (5):307–18. doi: 10.1016/j.plipres.2008.02.003.

Volpi, E., H. Kobayashi, M. Sheffield-Moore, B. Mittendorfer, and R. R. Wolfe. 2003. Essential amino acids are primarily responsible for the amino acid stimulation of muscle protein anabolism in healthy elderly adults. *Am J Clin Nutr* 78 (2):250–8.

Wolfe, R. R. 2005. Regulation of skeletal muscle protein metabolism in catabolic states. *Curr Opin Clin Nutr Metab Care* 8 (1):61–5.

Wolfe, R. R. 2006. The underappreciated role of muscle in health and disease. *Am J Clin Nutr* 84 (3):475–82.

World Health Organization. 2007. Protein and amino acid requirements in human nutrition: Report of a joint FAO/WHO/UNU expert consultation. Retrieved from http://apps.who.int/iris/bitstream/10665/43411/1/WHO_TRS_935_eng.pdf?ua=1.

5 Fat Needs

Trisha A. McLain and Carole A. Conn

CONTENTS

Abstract 78
5.1 Fats, Fats, Fats 78
    5.1.1 Introducing the "Lipid" Lineup 78
    5.1.2 Favorable Functions of Fats 78
    5.1.3 Are All Fats Created Equally? 79
        5.1.3.1 Saturated Fats 79
        5.1.3.2 Unsaturated Fats 79
        5.1.3.3 Trans Fats 79
    5.1.4 Omega-3 and Omega-6 Fatty Acid Teams 80
    5.1.5 Linoleic Acid and the Omega-6 Team 80
    5.1.6 Alpha-Linolenic Acid and the Omega-3 Team 81
    5.1.7 Fat as Fuel: Basic Fat Utilization 81
    5.1.8 Dietary Reference Intake for Fats 81
5.2 Fueling the Young Athlete: How Do Fats Play a Role? 82
    5.2.1 Differences between Adults and Children 83
    5.2.2 Fats: The Quarterback of Children's Metabolic Playing Field 83
5.3 Fat Supplements and Human Performance 84
    5.3.1 Medium-Chain Triglycerides 84
    5.3.2 Long-Chain Triglycerides 86
    5.3.3 Fish Oils 86
        5.3.3.1 RBC Deformability and VO_2 Max 87
        5.3.3.2 Muscle Damage, Inflammation, and Immune Function 88
        5.3.3.3 Asthma and Exercise-Induced Asthma 88
    5.3.4 Conjugated Linoleic Acids 88
    5.3.5 Fats and Testosterone 89
5.4 Finding the Right Fats and Oils for the Child Athlete 89
    5.4.1 Fats Young Athletes Should Avoid and Ways to Avoid Them 89
    5.4.2 Reading Food Labels for Fat 90
        5.4.2.1 Find Out How Much Energy from Fat is in Food 90
        5.4.2.2 How Much Fat Should the Child Athlete Consume? 90
        5.4.2.3 The Facts about Zero Trans Fat 90
        5.4.2.4 Trans Fats are Everywhere Though! 91
        5.4.2.5 Natural Trans Fats 91
        5.4.2.6 Find and Avoid Those Artificial Trans Fats! 92
    5.4.3 Snacks and Meal Recommendations for the Child Athlete 93
    5.4.4 Special Considerations 94
        5.4.4.1 Fats for Vegetarian Athletes 94
        5.4.4.2 Fats for Female Athletes 94
5.5 Guidelines for Young Athletes for Daily Consumption of Fats 95
References 95

ABSTRACT

Fats are a subcategory of fat-soluble substances known as lipids, consisting of carbon, hydrogen, and oxygen molecules. Dietary fat is a dense fuel source that is essential for both normal physiological processes and for providing energy to children during physical activity. Though fat has a bad reputation in today's society, fat plays a multitude of important roles for active children. Fats are especially important when considering the higher basal metabolic rates and overall differences in daily physical activity of children when compared to adults. Fat allows for proper nutrient transport, hormone production, protection of internal organs, and serves as one of the primary fuel sources both at rest and during exercise. Free fatty acids are the primary source for fat metabolism, which provide energy for aerobic events such as running and swimming. Fats consumed through the diet may be classified as saturated, unsaturated, monounsaturated, polyunsaturated, and/or trans fats. It is important that coaches, parents, and athletes understand that not all dietary sources of fat are beneficial. It is crucial that these individuals have the knowledge and ability to differentiate between those fats that could be beneficial versus hinder their child's development, health, and performance. Determining the optimal fat intake is largely dependent on the child; however, if the child's type and level of physical activity is taken under consideration, a healthy balance of dietary fat intake and calorie expenditure can be achieved. Balancing dietary fat intake should be the goal of any coach or parent in order to maximize the developmental potential as well as athletic ability. Although it is highly recommended to meet with a trained professional to develop and implement a tailored diet, the recommended dietary intake for fat is currently 25%–35% of a child's overall energy intake.

5.1 FATS, FATS, FATS

Every time you turn on the television or walk into the grocery store, foods low in fats are being advertised and advocated as the ideal, healthy foods. Food companies are continuously releasing "fat free" or "low-fat versions" of their products. To put it simply, fat in foods has a bad reputation. The question is, how important is the macronutrient fat? Do we need fat at all, or can we remove it from our diet? The word fat provokes a knee-jerk reaction for most people; however, fat is essential for all of us, especially young, active children who participate in sports. The truth is, we all need fat, but young children need it the most. Fat plays important roles in the human body, especially the bodies of growing and active children.

5.1.1 Introducing the "Lipid" Lineup

Fats are a subcategory of fat-soluble substances known as lipids, and are compounds consisting of carbon, hydrogen, and oxygen molecules. Their function depends primarily on their physical arrangement of carbon, hydrogen, and oxygen, which subsequently impacts the molecule's chemical properties. Like the other two macronutrients, carbohydrates and proteins, lipids can provide energy for our bodies. Lipids are insoluble and subsequently, do not dissolve in water. Lipids include fats, oils, and cholesterol. Approximately 95% of the lipids found in the human body and in foods are classified as triglycerides. Table 5.1 summarizes some of the major functions of lipids.

When people mention fat, they most commonly refer to triglycerides. Triglycerides are fats where a glycerol molecule is attached to three fatty acids. Triglycerides are the predominant type of fat in foods and they operate as the predominant storage depot of fatty acids inside the body. For the purposes of this discussion we will use the term *fat* instead of lipids or triglyceride, due to its familiarity and common usage in everyday language.

5.1.2 Favorable Functions of Fats

Fats serve many useful roles in the human body. Fats are not only an important source of energy, but are necessary for absorption of fat-soluble vitamins, including vitamins A, D, E, and K, while

Fat Needs

TABLE 5.1
Functions of Lipids
- Provide a concentrated source of energy and serve as an energy reserve (fat stores)
- Absorb and carry fat-soluble vitamins
- Increase the flavor and palatability of foods
- Provide relief from hunger
- Serve as structural components of cell membranes
- Production of sex hormones, including estrogen and testosterone
- Health and development of brain and eyes
- Production of signaling molecules especially important for immune function

also protecting vital organs such as the heart, lungs, and reproductive organs, providing insulation, and aiding in proper immune function. Moreover, fats are important sources of essential fatty acids (EFA), such as omega-6 and omega-3 fatty acids, which are important for brain development and eye health [56].

5.1.3 Are All Fats Created Equally?

Although fats are needed in our diets, there are different types of fats, some better for you than others. Fats can be saturated or unsaturated. "Saturation" is related to the chemical structure of the fat molecule; specifically, whether or not a fat is holding all of the hydrogen atoms it can hold. If every available bond of the carbons making up a fatty acid in the triglyceride molecule is holding a hydrogen ion, the chain forms a saturated fatty acid. Triglycerides containing mostly saturated fatty acids are called "saturated fats."

However, sometimes the fatty acid chain has a place where a hydrogen is missing (and a double bond between carbons is subsequently formed), forming an unoccupied spot or point of "unsaturation." Fatty acid chains containing one or more unoccupied spots are termed unsaturated fatty acids. Unsaturated fatty acids can be broken down even further. If a fatty acid chain contains one point of unsaturation, the fatty acid is termed a monounsaturated fatty acid, abbreviated MUFA. If there are two or more points of unsaturation, the fatty acid is termed polyunsaturated fatty acid, abbreviated PUFA. Collectively, when a triglyceride contains at least one unsaturated fatty acid it is termed an "unsaturated" fat.

5.1.3.1 Saturated Fats
Saturated fats are usually hard or solid at room temperature. Foods high in saturated fat include fatty meats, such as a non-lean ($\geq 30\%$ fat) steak, lamb chops, coconut oil, lard, and high-fat dairy products, including cheese, whole-milk, butter, and ice cream.

5.1.3.2 Unsaturated Fats
Alternatively, unsaturated fats tend to be liquid at room temperature, so foods that contain mainly unsaturated fats are typically vegetable oils such as corn oil, peanut oil, safflower oil, and fish oils. Unsaturated fats include both monounsaturated (one double bond or point of unsaturation) and polyunsaturated (two or more double bonds or points of unsaturation) fatty acids. Popular foods that have relatively high amounts of monounsaturated fatty acids (MUFAs) include olive oil, avocados, and some margarines, while fish oil, corn oil, soybean oil, and nut oils are rich in polyunsaturated fatty acids (PUFAs).

5.1.3.3 Trans Fats
The process of hydrogenation adds hydrogen molecules to an unsaturated fatty acid causing unsaturated fatty acids to change their shape. This change in chemical structure creates unusual

SIDEBAR 5.1   TYPES OF FATS

Saturated fats: Lipid molecules comprising fatty acids whose adjacent carbons are linked by single bonds. The carbons are "saturated" with hydrogens, having the maximal possible number of hydrogens attached. Saturated fats tend to be solid at room temperature.

Examples: Animal products and coconut oils.

Unsaturated fats: Lipid molecules comprising fatty acids whose adjacent carbons are linked by one or more double bonds. The carbons are "unsaturated" or not saturated with hydrogens. This means these molecules have fewer than the maximum possible number of hydrogens attached to them. Unsaturated fats tend to be liquid at room temperature.

Examples: Found in plants, fish, vegetable oils, and soft margarines.

Monounsaturated fats: Fats that contain predominantly fatty acids in which one carbon–carbon bond is not saturated with hydrogen.

Polyunsaturated fats: Fats that contain predominantly fatty acids in which two or more carbon–carbon bonds are not saturated with hydrogen. All essential fatty acids are polyunsaturated.

Trans fats: Fatty acids with unusual shapes due to hydrogenation creating fatty acids with bonds in the trans form. Also known as trans fatty acids. This type of fat is thought to be particularly unhealthy.

---

unsaturated fatty acids, which are similar in shape to saturated fatty acids, but have distinct physical and chemical properties as well as their detrimental effects on one's health. During hydrogenation some bonds become saturated, but others remain unsaturated, but transform to the unusual unsaturated trans bonds. These fatty acids are termed trans fatty acids, often referred to as *trans fats*. When unsaturated fatty acids are converted into trans fats, the body will not benefit from any of the potential health benefits of the original unsaturated fatty acid. A summary of the different types of fats may be seen in Sidebar 5.1.

5.1.4   OMEGA-3 AND OMEGA-6 FATTY ACID TEAMS

The human body can synthesize the fatty acids it needs from carbohydrates and proteins, except two, "linoleic acid" and "alpha-linolenic acid." The fatty acids linoleic acid and alpha (α)-linolenic acid are called EFA because they must be consumed in the diet. They are members of the fatty acid team of omega-6 fatty acids, commonly referred to as n-6 fatty acids, and omega-3 fatty acids, commonly referred to as n-3 fatty acids. Both n-6 and n-3 are PUFAs and are excellent sources of energy. They are important to the body for many reasons. Let us explore each of these teams individually.

5.1.5   LINOLEIC ACID AND THE OMEGA-6 TEAM

Linoleic acid serves as the "parent" to the "players" of the omega-6 fatty acid team. When consumed, linoleic acid produces the necessary players of the omega-6 team. Arachidonic acid (AA) is one of many notable omega-6 fatty acids, aiding in the production of eicosanoids, which are signaling molecules that play a major role in our body's many functions, particularly inflammatory immune responses important for defense against bacteria and viruses.

A component of all cell membranes in the body, omega-6 fatty acids are essential and may be consumed through sunflower, corn, and soybean oils. The molecules created in the body from omega-6 fatty acids play a major role in the central nervous system (CNS), particularly in the nerves and brain. They are required for growth and maintenance of healthy skin, as well as maintaining a normal functioning reproduction system. Evidence indicates that they play a major role in forming substrates and substances that regulate blood pressure, aid in blood clotting, and assure robust immune responses.

5.1.6 Alpha-Linolenic Acid and the Omega-3 Team

Alpha-linolenic acid serves as the "parent" to the "players" of the omega-3 fatty acid team. When consumed, linolenic acid can be used by the body to produce the necessary players of the omega-3 team. The two most important omega-3 fatty acids include eicosapentaenoic acid (e-co-sah-pent-tahee-no-ick) usually abbreviated to EPA and docosahexaenoic acid (dough-co-sah-hex-ah-ee-no-ick) usually called DHA. The body makes limited amounts of these omega-3 fatty acids from linolenic acid, but luckily, both EPA and DHA are found abundantly in oils of fish.

Omega-3 fatty acids are needed in high quantities in the brain and nervous system tissues. They are particularly important in visual development of infants. They also play a major role in the maintenance of blood pressure and blood clotting, and in helping control inflammation and pain. Recognition of the importance of omega-3 fatty acids originated when researchers found and reported a low prevalence of heart disease in Eskimos, who consume diets very high in fat from fish. The Eskimos did well using fish for food, benefiting from the omega-3 containing oils, and since the original observation, numerous studies have documented other health benefits of increasing consumption of omega-3s, or fish oil, including a reduction in blood triglyceride levels [23,75].

5.1.7 Fat as Fuel: Basic Fat Utilization

This chapter will later discuss the differences between children and adults in how fats and carbohydrates are used to produce energy. However, it holds true that fats primarily supply energy and dominate during prolonged, low-intensity exercises such as the Presidential 1-mile run test or a 1600-m swim. The storage capacity of fat, and therefore potential energy, is substantially larger than the reserves for carbohydrate storage. Approximately 70,000–75,000 kcal of fat are stored in the subcutaneous and visceral stores, while another 1,500 kcal are stored in the muscles of persons who weigh around 70 kg, representative of 14–18-year-old athletes [73]. However, fat takes longer than carbohydrate to breakdown due to its complex form of long-carbon chains. When broken down, substantially more energy is derived from a gram of fat (9.4 kcal/g) than from the same amount of carbohydrate (4.1 kcal/g).

As previously mentioned, many different compounds are classified as fats, with triglycerides providing the majority of fat energy. We store triglycerides in adipose tissue or "groups of fat cells" and inside muscle cells. Both storage areas provide an important endogenous source of fuel for a child at play. Triglycerides are broken down into one molecule of glycerol and three free fatty acid (FFA) molecules. This process is referred to as lipolysis. The free fatty acids (FFAs) derived from triglycerides are the primary source for fat metabolism, which produces energy for use in events such as running and swimming, as well as other fuel needs.

Before FFAs can be used for energy production, they must be broken down into a small molecule known as acetyl-CoA, using a process called beta-oxidation (β-oxidation). β-Oxidation is a series of steps in which two carbon "acetyl" units are cleaved off the longer carbon chain of the FFA. The number of steps is dependent on the number of carbons making up the FFA. For example, if the FFA chain consists of 18 carbons, 8 sequential passes through β-oxidation will yield 9 molecules of acetyl-CoA. Alternatively, if an FFA chain spans 12 carbons, the process of β-oxidation will yield 6 acetyl-CoA. The acetyl-CoA can then enter several sequential metabolic pathways ending in the formation of energy, or adenosine triphosphate (ATP), the energy currency of the body. Due to the high numbers of steps involved, producing energy from fats takes time, but because fat is easily stored in higher quantities than carbohydrates, it is the preferred fuel for long-term activities.

5.1.8 Dietary Reference Intake for Fats

It has been difficult to establish a dietary reference intake (DRI) for the overall energy requirements of young athletes, making it even more difficult to establish a dietary guideline for fat needs

TABLE 5.2
DRIs: Acceptable Fat Distribution Ranges for Children, 4–18 Years[a]

Macronutrient	Range (% of Energy Intake)
Fat	25–35
n-6 polyunsaturated fatty acids (linoleic acid)	5–10
n-3 polyunsaturated fatty acids (α-linolenic acid)	0.6–1.2

Source: Adapted from Bass S and Inge K. Nutrition for special populations: Children and young athletes, in: *Clinical Sports Nutrition.* V Deakin, LM Burke, eds. Sydney, NSW: McGraw-Hill, 2006.

[a] Published by the Food and Nutrition Board, Institute of Medicine, National Academy of Science.

TABLE 5.3
Recommended Dietary Allowances and Adequate Intakes of n-3 and n-6 Polyunsaturated Fatty Acids for Male and Female Children[a]

Males		Females	
9–13 Years	14–18 Years	9–13 Years	14–18 Years
n-6 Polyunsaturated Fatty Acids (Linoleic Acid) (g/day)			
12	16	10	11
n-3 Polyunsaturated Fatty Acids (α-Linolenic Acid) (g/day)			
1.2	1.6	1.0	1.1

Source: Adapted from Bass S and Inge K. Nutrition for special populations: Children and young athletes, in: *Clinical Sports Nutrition.* V Deakin, LM Burke, eds. Sydney, NSW: McGraw-Hill, 2006.

[a] Published by the Food and Nutrition Board, Institute of Medicine, National Academy of Science.

in children, especially active children. Most guidelines regarding DRI accommodate sedentary to active individuals (i.e., active, extremely active) for specific ages and genders; however, these categories are vague and do not consider the variation often observed between maturation level and chronological age. Below are the current fat distribution ranges and recommended dietary allowances for both male and female children aged 4–18 years (Tables 5.2 and 5.3).

5.2 FUELING THE YOUNG ATHLETE: HOW DO FATS PLAY A ROLE?

Athletes who pursue large training volumes, spending hours and hours training, may need to consume as much as twice as many calories per day compared to age-matched sedentary individuals. A similar rationale applies to children. Children playing in an after school soccer league may need to consume more calories than a child visiting the library for an after school reading program; although both activities provide distinct benefits, they require different amounts of energy. Principles of sports nutrition are similar for children and adults, but children and adolescents have specific nutritional requirements and differ from adults, particularly with respect to energy expenditure and fuel utilization. Like adults, young children need adequate energy to maintain active, healthy lifestyles. Specifically in children, sufficient energy is required for growth and body mass maintenance, while also important for fueling physical activity, specifically sporting activities, and activities of daily living (ADL). Chronic deficiency of adequate energy intake may result in delayed puberty, poor bone health, and increased risk of injury [8].

5.2.1 Differences between Adults and Children

So what characteristics make children different from adults in terms of energy requirements and usage? It has been determined that children have higher basal metabolic rates per kilogram of bodyweight when compared to adults, while differences between adults and children also occur in total body mechanical work and power production during locomotion. This includes differences in stride frequency, coordination of muscle activity, and their overall efficiency of energy utilization during movement tasks causing children to require more energy per kilogram of bodyweight to perform these tasks (Table 5.4).

Children are considered relatively "inefficient" energy users. The human body in general is an inefficient machine, losing 75% of energy produced as heat, while capturing 25% to produce and use ATP [61]. Higher relative energy use by children has been attributed to their novice motor control, resulting in extraneous movements. When considering a comparison between adults' and children's body mass in kilogram, the amount of energy per kilogram that it costs to walk or run at a given speed is considerably higher in children than adults, with younger children having an even higher relative cost to perform these tasks [6,21,42]. For example, a 6-year-old child would require 25%–30% more energy per kilogram of body mass than would a 26-year-old adult when they both perform a running task at the same speed [6]. You may be asking yourself, how and why does this occur? It appears that children seem to lack adequate coordination between their agonist and antagonist muscle groups. Particularly in the first 10 years of a child's life, the antagonist muscles of children do not seem to relax sufficiently when the agonists contract. This is commonly observed during walking and running in children.

While differences exist between adults and children in overall energy utilization and demand, the primary substrates providing energy are also different. Outside of long-term aerobic exercise, most of us think of carbohydrates, specifically glucose stored as glycogen, playing a major role in energy production. Children, however, possess unique macronutrient utilization characteristics, operating on fat to perform both low-intensity activities, such as a minor league baseball game, or high-intensity activities, such as basketball game, a sport requiring anaerobic capabilities [51].

Typically, carbohydrate (i.e., glycogen) storage capacity is lower in children than in adults [10], and enzymes involved in carbohydrate breakdown are less developed in young children. With a decreased overall capacity for storage and breakdown of carbohydrates, children appear to oxidize relatively more fat than carbohydrates, especially during exercise.

5.2.2 Fats: The Quarterback of Children's Metabolic Playing Field

It has been postulated that children use relatively more fat and less carbohydrate than do adolescents or adults. We could say carbohydrates act as the supporting teammates to fat, which acts as the quarterback, playing the primary role of supplying energy to active children participating in sports of all types. While currently we can only speculate as to why children utilize relatively more fat than adults when participating in physical activities, research analyzing metabolic enzyme activities

TABLE 5.4
Factors That Influence Energy Requirements of Children

Higher basal metabolic rate [7]
Locomotion, increased stride frequency [68]
Differences in total body mechanical work and power [68]
Increased co-contraction of opposing muscle groups, especially the leg muscles [25]

[27], respiration [46], and measuring concentrations of potential fat and carbohydrate sources in the blood [9] suggests that, during prolonged exercise specifically, children burn relatively more fat and less carbohydrate. Likewise, children performing short, intense activities also seem to rely more on aerobic energy metabolism during these tasks, operating with fat as the primary fuel source [30]. Typically short, intense activities rely on anaerobic energy metabolism, in which carbohydrates, such as glucose and glycogen, are the predominant energy sources in adults. Uniquely, with limited research being reported, the majority of evidence points toward children's metabolic systems favoring fat over carbohydrate, regardless of activity intensity.

Preferential fat oxidation in children may be designated by multiple factors, all of which may play an important role pertaining to increased fat utilization by children. Favored utilization of fat by children may be due to the greater concentration of plasma-free glycerol and FFAs found in their blood. Lactate, a by-product of carbohydrate metabolism and inhibitor of fatty acid mobilization and uptake, is consistently lower in children in all types of activity levels, submaximal, maximal, and supra-maximal exercise [30,44,46]. Young males, especially those in early stages of puberty, have been shown to burn more fat and produce less lactate at submaximal exercise intensities compared to late-pubertal and young adults. Differences in hormones also contribute to maturity-related differences in fuel metabolism. Sympathetic activity in children is decreased, affecting glycolytic metabolism, resulting in decreased carbohydrate use [22].

5.3 FAT SUPPLEMENTS AND HUMAN PERFORMANCE

People participate in sports and exercise for many different reasons. Whether the reasons are to become faster, stronger, or to improve overall fitness, many people desire rapid results and for this reason (among others) dietary supplements become a common alternative to ensure adequate levels of key nutrition are being delivered.

In the competitive world of youth and high school level sports, may athletes look for the edge that will help them cross the finish line faster, stay healthy, and train harder. This has led many young athletes to turn to dietary supplements. For example, investigators at one university found that, among a cohort of 270 high school athletes, 58% were using some form of dietary supplement [16]. A more developed discussion of research reporting on supplement use by youth athletes is discussed in Chapters 1 and 13 of this book.

While the majority of supplements target the ingestion of vitamins, minerals, protein, and amino acids, "fat" supplements have grown in popularity. These include medium-chain triglycerides (MCTs), long-chain triglycerides (LCTs), fish oil, and conjugated linoleic acids (CLAs). Although body stores of fat are very large, supplementing with fat has been examined, specifically supplementation prior to exercise or as a part of one's daily diet. As discussed throughout Chapters 1 and 3, the importance of muscle glycogen for shorter (20–60 min) bouts of strenuous to vigorous intensity activity as well as prolonged (>60 min) bouts of moderate intensity exercise is well known. For these reasons, supplementation with fat has increased in popularity to help reduce muscle glycogen breakdown by stimulating fat oxidation. Remember, per kilogram of body mass children expend more energy from fat than adults, therefore their consumption of fat supplements may not solely be based on maintenance of intramuscular glycogen stores, but instead to provide an additional supply of energy from fat. While research in this area is not extensive, especially in children, it is important to address the more popular fat supplements and how they work, as their consumption is becoming more common and eventually will start trickling down to teenage and adolescent children athletes. Table 5.5 lists popular claims made regarding fat supplements.

5.3.1 MEDIUM-CHAIN TRIGLYCERIDES

MCTs are a special type of fat in which the fatty acids that are joined to the glycerol are between 6 and 14 carbon molecules in length. Our diets typically consist of long-chain fatty acids that span

TABLE 5.5
Popular Claims Made Surrounding Fat Supplements

Fat Supplement	Common Ingestion Time	Claim
Medium-chain triglycerides (MCTs)	1 h prior to exercise	• Reduces muscle glycogen breakdown • Improves endurance capacity • Reduces body mass
Long-chain triglycerides (LCTs)	1–4 h prior to exercise	• Reduces muscle glycogen breakdown • Improves endurance capacity
Fish oil (EPA/DHA)	Daily/chronic (1–6 g/day)	• Increases RBC deformability • Increases VO_2 • Prevents or reduces muscle damage • Prevents or reduces inflammatory response • Reduces asthmatic symptoms • Improves metabolism
Conjugated linoleic acid (CLA)	Daily/chronic (1–9 g/day)	• Improves body composition

Source: Adapted from Jeukendrup AE and Aldred S. *Nutrition* 20: 678–688, 2004.

Note: Careful consideration of these claims is recommended as research provides little or no support for the claims listed below. The reader is encouraged to first seek ways within the diet to achieve required intakes of dietary fat before turning to supplementation.

16–22 carbons in length. Besides these obvious physical differences, key chemical differences exist in the breakdown and metabolism of MCTs as compared to LCTs, requiring less effort for the body to digest and use MCTs. Within the digestive tract, specifically the lumen of the intestines, MCTs require less bile and pancreatic juices for digestion compared to long-chain fatty acids. Moreover, MCTs can be taken up more easily into the mitochondria of cells and processed during oxidative metabolism into ATP.

MCTs, naturally found in coconut oils, are commonly prescribed to clinical patients who have complications associated with lipid digestion. Due to the physiological ease with which the body can digest MCTs, when compared to LCTs, researchers have explored the potential benefits of supplementing with MCTs on health and exercise performance (see Table 5.5). The United States Food and Drug Administration (FDA) have labeled MCTs as "generally recognized as safe (GRAS)." Amounts ranging from 30 to 100 g/day have been recommended. Research examining dosages and timing of consumption, such as before and after exercise, has been conducted. Ivy and colleagues reported that, although ranges of 30–100 g/day are suggested, several adverse symptoms have been associated with dosages higher than 50 g. These include nausea, vomiting, bloating, emesis, gastrointestinal discomfort, abdominal cramps, and diarrhea [34]. Alternatively, when 30 g of MCTs were given, only 10% of subjects reported side effects [24]. A tolerance seems to develop over time; however, current evidence suggests that children supplementing with MCTs should not use any dosages higher than 30 g/day [53].

The most beneficial outcome from MCT supplementation in an athletic setting appears to take place during prolonged exercise, allowing for increased fat availability. Research also indicates that adult athletes competing in sports requiring a specific body weight (i.e., benefit from being lean), such as wrestling, or athletes, such as endurance runners, may benefit from MCTs [15]. Compared to short, explosive sporting events, prolonged endurance events offer time to utilize a fat source. The most beneficial MCT supplementation appears to occur for athletes undergoing long cycling or running events. It should be acknowledged that the majority of these sporting events are being completed by adults, but yes, children are beginning to compete in events such as 100-mile ultramarathons. In 2013, both a 12- and 13-year-old boy from the Southwestern United States finished 100-mile ultramarathons. Therefore, MCTs consumed during an endurance event may prove beneficial to their overall performance, perhaps because of glycogen sparing potential. Research is needed to document whether this hypothesis may be true.

Supplementing with MCTs in order to reduce body mass has also been evaluated. Children competing in sports where they must propel their bodies over long distances or against gravity (jumps or hurdles for example) may have an advantage if they are lean [72]. Furthermore, the situation of athletes undergoing weight loss (see Chapters 11 and 12 for a more developed discussion) may be heightened in female athletes who already face social pressure to be thin, yet physiologically, females carry higher levels of essential body fat despite training at the level of males. The basis of MCTs and body mass reduction is centered around three major theories: (1) MCTs increase feelings of satiety, (2) MCTs have a high thermogenic effect, and (3) MCTs are more effectively and completely absorbed than long-chain fatty acids [15]. Research examining short-term (~1 week) MCT supplementation has revealed favorable results in both men and women [32,54]. MCT supplementation in two studies by St-Onge found reductions in body mass in men after 4 weeks [63,65]. Overall calorie consumption has also been reduced by supplementation with MCT. In a study of 12 adult males, energy intake was reduced in the groups consuming diets high in MCTs, as compared to monounsaturated LCTs and saturated LCTs [64].

Practical applications for MCT supplementation may benefit child athletes undergoing prolonged, endurance events or those looking for a healthy way to cut weight. Most commonly occurring in the sport of wrestling, weight cutting also occurs in the sports of gymnastics, ice skating, ballet, judo, jiu jitsu, and taekwondo. Consideration of diets high in MCTs could apply to a child who wrestles and needs to lose 10 lb in 1 week in order to wrestle in the 170 weight class. However, little research in children and adolescents has been published and more research needs to be conducted in this area to determine both safety and efficacy. Furthermore, parents, coaches, nutritionists, and dietitians should work closely to first educate themselves and their young athletes on how to safely modify the diet before relying too much upon dietary supplements for such adjustments.

5.3.2 LONG-CHAIN TRIGLYCERIDES

Remember, the majority of the fats consumed in the human diet are in the form of triglyceride molecules that contain long-chain fatty acids, containing 16 or more carbons. LCTs may either be saturated or unsaturated. The consumption of LCTs on exercise performance or energy production during exercise remains unclear [14,31,35,43,67]. LCTs that are ingested prior to exercise will reach the circulation in the form of chylomicrons. Chylomicrons do not play a vital role in energy production during exercise. In fact, research has found that fat oxidation during exercise was lower when LCTs were consumed prior to exercise when compared to that of a control group [20,59]. Hawley and colleagues also demonstrated a lack of evidence for improved performance while supplementing with LCTs. Plasma fatty acid concentrations were manipulated in subjects by intravenous infusion of LCTs. Subjects then exercised at 80% VO_2 Max followed by a time trial lasting approximately 30 min. Although fat availability was elevated in all study participants, there was little to no effect on performance. From these results, it seems fair to conclude that LCT ingestion before exercise will have little to no effect on exercise performance. Therefore, any claim that suggests pre-exercise supplemental LCT reduces muscle glycogen breakdown and improves endurance capacity (Table 5.5) should be taken with a grain of salt. Like MCTs, research on LCTs is scarce and future research must be conducted, especially before making specific suggestions to children (Box 5.1).

5.3.3 FISH OILS

Initial interests concerning the benefits of fish oil supplementation began when researchers found that Greenland Eskimos and other populations who consume diets rich in these fatty acids had

> **BOX 5.1 ARE HIGH-FAT DIETS CONSUMED OVER A LONG-TERM PERIOD EFFECTIVE IN ENHANCING PERFORMANCE?**
>
> Rather than supplementing short term with fats, there is a growing interest in whether the more abundant stores of fats in the body might be tapped for energy especially during endurance competitions [71]. The idea arose from two observations. First, human bodies store far more energy as fat than as carbohydrate (glycogen). Second, arctic explorers and Eskimos consume very little carbohydrate, and use fats as fuels for strenuous work lasting hours in the cold.
>
> Recent research in adults is exploring the idea of fat adaptation, which occurs when diets containing very low amounts of carbohydrates are consumed for 2 weeks to a month. Fat adaptation increases the enzymes needed for using fat as fuel for exercise. Emerging evidence suggests that dietary carbohydrate restriction and increased protein intake during training may support greater mitochondrial biogenesis allowing greater use of fat as fuel during exercise [45]. However, fat adaptation has also been shown to compromise carbohydrate use as fuel by adults during very intense exercise requiring very fast generation of ATP [29]. At present, there is no consensus on whether high-fat diets are effective in enhancing performance, particularly high-intensity performance. Research to date has not included investigations in children.

remarkably low incidence of common cardiovascular disease [23,75]. Multiple experimental and epidemiological studies [1,11,52] have since been conducted to examine the effects of fish oil supplementation for their cardioprotective ability, as well as their potential impact on sport performance and recovery. Fish oil supplementation in exercise and human performance has been a popular topic over the past few decades. Claims have been put forward that supplementation increases overall performance through different physiological mechanisms, such as red blood cell (RBC) deformability, improved VO_2, prevention or reductions in muscle damage and inflammation, improved immune function, reduced asthmatic symptoms, and improved metabolism. Each of these potential benefits will be briefly discussed as well as how fish oil supplementation may provide a benefit.

5.3.3.1 RBC Deformability and VO_2 Max

RBC deformability refers to the membrane properties of red blood cells (RBCs), which determine the degree of shape change under a given level of pressure. RBCs are able to change their shape or "deform" while passing through the microcirculation, the capillaries which are the smallest of blood vessels. Deformability of RBCs is beneficial to oxidative energy production, the process that is utilized to metabolize fats. During exercise, RBCs ability to deform decreases [26,69]. Decreases in RBC deformability are associated with slower transit time through capillaries [62,74]. In turn, this will reduce oxygen delivery and therefore, aerobic performance. A number of studies have shown that dietary fish oil increases the deformability of RBCs due to the incorporation of the highly PUFAs EPA and DHA into the RBC membrane [2,18]. In addition, fish oils have also been shown to facilitate the transport of RBCs through blood vessels, specifically the capillary beds [13]. As a result of both increased RBC deformability and faster transport time through capillaries, fish oil supplementation could lead to enhanced oxygen delivery to skeletal muscle and a subsequent improvement in exercise performance. In theory, this could enhance maximum oxygen utilization (VO_2 Max), ultimately resulting in improved exercise performance. Overall research indicates that fish oil supplementation in adults may increase RBC deformability during exercise, allowing for the potential rise in VO_2 Max. However, these effects appear rather small and may not be effective unless individuals are training consistently and for prolonged, endurance events [36]. It is important to note that no research on supplementation with fish oil in children involving exercise-related outcomes has been completed to date.

5.3.3.2 Muscle Damage, Inflammation, and Immune Function

Children undergoing multiple games in a weekend, such as three basketball games on a Saturday at an Amateur Athletic Union (AAU) tournament, and then another game on Sunday because their team makes it to the championship, may experience muscle fatigue, soreness, dehydration, muscle structural damage, inflammation, muscle swelling, and neutrophilia, which is a large number of white blood cells entering the circulation [5]. Inflammation is a physiological response to injury or tissue damage, such as muscle damage, that involves recruitment of the body's defense systems. The inflammatory response is characterized by an increased number of cytokines. Cytokines have the potential to trigger the release of acute phase proteins and inflammatory mediators (i.e., signaling molecules such as leukotrienes and prostaglandins) and to increase the number of circulating white blood cells. Moreover, oxidative stress increases after intense exercise. Increases in markers of oxidative stress are related to a reduction in immunity and increases risk for infection [12].

Omega-6 PUFA are precursors to inflammatory signaling molecules needed for fighting infections; however, when they are chronically produced they can have negative consequences. The long-chain omega-3 PUFA from fish oil, EPA, competitively inhibits the long-chain omega-6 PUFA AA from being used to generate inflammatory signals. In addition, the signaling molecules produced from EPA itself are less inflammatory. Therefore, consuming fish or fish oil results in partial replacement of AA by EPA in inflammatory cell membranes and may beneficially dampen inflammation following muscle damage occurring during exercise and prolonged physical activity (i.e., multiple games in a weekend) [37,60].

Similar to the anti-inflammatory benefits of EPA from fish oil in muscle that may be damaged during exercise, EPA also can protect lung airway linings. Consuming fish oil results in partial replacement of AA by EPA in inflammatory cell membranes lining the lung airways, and thus demonstrates a potential anti-inflammatory effect of n-3 PUFA [50].

5.3.3.3 Asthma and Exercise-Induced Asthma

The original studies examining diets high in fish oils also found that Greenland Eskimos reported a lower prevalence of asthma [23,75]. A reduction in the prevalence of asthma, along with the known potential anti-inflammatory effects of fish oil supplementation sparked interest in fish oil supplementation and asthma, specifically exercise-induced asthma (EIA). The results of fish oil supplementation on EIA and exercise-induced bronchitis are extremely important; however, due to the inconsistency of results concerning fish oil supplementation and asthma [47], more research is needed before conclusions can be drawn.

With regard to the clinical effectiveness of fish oil supplementation and asthma, research offers mixed reviews, specifically for EIA. However, the literature does point toward prophylactic and acute therapeutic effects of fish oil supplementation in inflammatory diseases such as asthma (i.e., EIA). It is possible that fish oil supplementation could provide an alternative treatment for EIA and that a combination of asthma treatment drugs and fish oils may confer greater anti-inflammatory benefits than either intervention alone [3,4,48–50], however further research is needed.

5.3.4 CONJUGATED LINOLEIC ACIDS

Conjugated linoleic acid (CLA) is a joint term used to describe linoleic acid containing conjugated double bonds. Conjugated double bonds are two double bonds separated by a single bond. This uncharacteristic arrangement can theoretically be in any position on the carbon backbone of the fat molecule, thus, multiple configurations of CLA can exist. The most common positions are between carbons 8 and 13. Predominant natural sources of CLAs in the human diet include meat, particularly grass-fed beef versus grain-fed beef and full fat dairy products such as cheese derived from ruminants, commonly sheep, goats, or cows [55].

CLA supplements for humans have been marketed primarily for resistance-training athletes in addition to individuals interested in weight loss and improving their body composition. Largely on the basis of animal research, CLA is promoted to improve lean body mass, minimize catabolism, and promote greater gains in strength and muscle mass during a training period. Human research on CLA is limited, with mixed results being reported over the years. Both animal and human studies have reported CLAs to decrease catabolism, increase bone density, reduce body weight, and enhance immunity.

Thom and colleagues found that both men and women who supplemented with 1.8 g/day of CLA for 12 weeks, while also exercising 90 min/day three times per week showed improved endurance performance and body composition [41]. Colakogula et al. [19] found the same improvements when examining 3.6 g/day of CLA and an exercise regimen of 30 min/day three times per week [19]. However, Lambert and colleagues [40] and Kreider and colleagues [17,38] concluded that CLAs did not possess any significant effects at the end of their individual supplementation periods. All studies were conducted on adults.

When considering children and CLAs, there is no standard dose for CLA and it would be best to consult a dietitian prior to supplementing. However, child athletes considering CLAs may consume many different animal products, such as milk, beef, and lamb, thus additional CLA through supplemental sources may not be necessary.

5.3.5 Fats and Testosterone

Testosterone is a steroid hormone with anabolic potential on a number of tissues, including muscle and can subsequently impact muscle growth and performance of athletes. Throughout puberty, a significant surge in the blood levels of testosterone occurs in children and can play a significant role in natural development of both boys and girls. Testosterone is responsible for male body features, such as facial hair and increased muscle size. Testosterone concentrations in females are much less, but important nonetheless for growth and maintenance of reproductive tissues. The effects of testosterone on athletic performance have been examined since the early 1980s [57]. Data suggest that testosterone may affect both anaerobic and aerobic performance, such as sprinting or cross-country running, respectively [28,66].

Particularly in males, ingested fat may have the potential to alter testosterone levels in the blood, a relationship due largely to the cholesterol content of various sources of dietary fat as and the cholesterol backbone found in all steroids [70]. Volek and colleagues demonstrated that consumption of MUFAs and saturated fatty acids were strong predictors of testosterone in males, but no significant relationship existed between PUFAs and testosterone. Research in resistance-trained males has also demonstrated that high-fat diets can lead to elevations in serum levels of testosterone [58]. Children who are undergoing or have undergone puberty may experience a decline in testosterone concentrations due to high volumes of training or ingestion of a diet low in dietary fat. For example, a wrestler consuming very few calories and not meeting the recommended intake for their given age may be at risk for low levels of testosterone. Consuming diets high in omega-3 fatty acids and CLAs has been proposed to cause an increase in testosterone, as well as promote an anabolic environment with rising levels of testosterone [41]. It is imperative that children and coaches understand the importance of natural testosterone production through a well-rounded diet. Anabolic steroids may mimic the effects of testosterone; however, research is consistent and conclusive that anabolic steroids containing testosterone accelerate pubertal changes, cause closure of growth plates, thus limiting full height growth, cause premature skeletal maturation, and affect the reproductive and immune systems, as well as many other important systems that are still developing in a young athlete's body [39].

5.4 FINDING THE RIGHT FATS AND OILS FOR THE CHILD ATHLETE

5.4.1 Fats Young Athletes Should Avoid and Ways to Avoid Them

Now that we understand how important fats are for child athletes, how do we properly fuel young athletes to maximize performance? Obtaining healthy sources of fat through dietary intake is simple and easy, but if you have ever driven down a business district full of fast food chains you may well remember the aroma of greasy burgers and French fries as it filled the air. Or perhaps you have stopped at a doughnut shop and enjoyed the sweet aroma as it fanned its way past you. As you prepare to satisfy your hunger with this appealing cuisine, you more than likely give no thought to how the food was prepared. Foods such as deep-fried chicken nuggets, deep-fried cheese balls, potato chips, French fries, and doughnuts are rich in trans fats. As we previously mentioned, trans fats are altered or damaged fats. Although they enhance flavor, texture, and shelf life, these artificially produced trans fats come with health risks and very well may lack some of the otherwise positive reasons for consuming other sources of fat. The key to fueling the child athlete is to not fuel them with deep-fried chicken rich in trans fats, but to fuel them with a well-balanced diet consisting of the right fats, at the right time. In order to do this, one first needs to be able to determine how much fat is in a given amount of food. Second, one needs to realize the difference between healthy and non-healthy fats, and finally select those food sources that only contain appropriate amounts of healthy fats.

5.4.2 Reading Food Labels for Fat

5.4.2.1 Find Out How Much Energy from Fat is in Food

Using food labels is a simple and easy method to calculate how much fat is in a given food. If you know how many grams of fat are in each serving of the food, clearly distinguishable on a food label, you can easily calculate fat calories using simple math. Each gram of fat has approximately 9 cal. If a serving of food contains 5 g of fat, that serving has 45 (9 cal/g × 5 g) cal from fat. An important point is to clearly understand the true size of a serving; many times a serving may be smaller than what you anticipate meaning that your actual fat and associated calorie consumption is higher than expected. You can also calculate the percentage of calories coming from fat. Simply divide the calories from fat by the total calories for the amount of food consumed. If your selected item (or portion of an item) has total calories 300 and 45 cal from fat, the percentage of calories from fat is determined by dividing 45 by 300 (i.e., 45 ÷ 300); this equals 0.15, or 15%.

5.4.2.2 How Much Fat Should the Child Athlete Consume?

Along with carbohydrate, fat is considered a protein-sparing energy nutrient. In other words, by consuming adequate calories from fat and carbohydrate, protein can be spared for its unique functions such as cell growth, turnover and repair and the production of enzymes, hormones, and antibodies. Young athletes should consume approximately 25%–35% of their daily calories from fat [33]. To estimate how many grams of fat this would be, multiply daily caloric intake by 0.25 or by 0.35 and divide the resulting number by 9 (there are 9 cal in a gram of fat). For example, if an athlete requires 2500 cal a day the fat intake should be 69–97 g of fat daily (2500 cal × 0.25 or 0.35 divided by 9).

5.4.2.3 The Facts about Zero Trans Fat

Being the health conscious shopper you are, you may reach for a product whose label boldly depicts zero trans fat! What you are really getting is a product that has less than 0.5 g of trans fats per serving. The FDA allows food companies to label their products with "0," as long as the products have less than 0.5 g of trans fat per serving. It is likely that instant soup packages, microwavable popcorn, frozen pizzas, and margarine or butters labeled with zero trans fats still contain trans fats, and this is important especially if you consume more than one serving. Nonetheless, fueling your child athlete with a zero trans fat cereal in the morning would be wise. Just remember, a "trans-fat free" cereal, plus a slice of cake after dinner and some microwavable popcorn prior to bed add up quickly (Box 5.2).

> **BOX 5.2 WHY IS THERE NO DAILY VALUE LISTED FOR TRANS FAT ON FOOD LABELS?**
>
> Researchers and scientists have not determined a safe level of consumption for trans fats so there is no daily value (DV) listed on food labels for trans fat. This means it is important to take extra caution when consuming trans fats, artificial trans fats in particular "to keep quantities consumed as low as possible." Notably, the FDA announced in June 2015 that all trans fats must be removed from foods within 3 years.

5.4.2.4 Trans Fats are Everywhere Though!

Unless you are eating a strict vegan diet (no animal products of any kind) you are going to consume some naturally occurring and artificial trans fats. And even if you are a strict vegan, foods such as peas and vegetables oils contain tiny amounts of natural trans fats too. When selecting foods for your child athlete, concern yourself with what are known as artificial trans fats, which are produced by partial hydrogenation of vegetable oils. Artificial trans fat is now found in almost 40% of the products available in grocery stores today. This means that out of 100,000 products found in the local grocery store, 40,000 of them contain some type of artificial trans fat!

Unfortunately, artificial trans fat is not recognized by your body as an "artificial" substance, so it is not discarded in the digestion process. Rather, your body absorbs trans fats and uses them in some chemical reactions. This means that the cell membranes, the lining of the arteries and veins, and the liver, brain, and kidneys are directed to utilize these artificial fatty acids, changing the functions and properties of your cells and of the enzymatic reactions that fuel our bodies. This is where the problem starts, and Table 5.6 highlights how trans fat affects the body.

5.4.2.5 Natural Trans Fats

Naturally occurring trans fat is created when bacteria in the stomach of ruminant animals, such as cows and sheep, transform some of the fats found in the plant materials they eat into a "trans" configuration. This means that products such as milk, cheese, and beef will have small amounts of naturally occurring trans fat. These natural fats are better for you, unlike artificial trans fats. In your blood stream some are transformed to CLA, which may have positive effects! However, they

TABLE 5.6
Purported Physiological Outcomes Related to Trans Fat Consumption

- Changes in hormone levels
- Increases LDL cholesterol levels
- Decreases HDL cholesterol levels
- Damages cell membranes
- Decreases nutrient absorption
- Reduces flexibility of capillaries and arteries
- Increases the level of insulin in the blood stream
- Contributes to weight gain
- Causes inflammation in cell walls and artery walls
- Increases the risk of all-cause mortality

Source: Adapted from Ivy JL. *Canadian Journal of Applied Physiology* (*Revue Canadienne de Physiologie Appliquee*) 26 (Suppl): S236–S245, 2001.

must be consumed in moderation because naturally occurring trans fats are found in dairy and meat products, which also are sources of saturated fats that also must be consumed in moderation.

5.4.2.6 Find and Avoid Those Artificial Trans Fats!

The most dangerous type of trans fats are those produced by hydrogenating vegetable oils and occur in manufactured foods, all of which must be labeled for sale. When examining a food label in the grocery store or at home, first look to see if the label states "0 g of trans fat." If it does, move to the ingredient list and look for the words "partially hydrogenated," "margarine," or "shortening." If these words are listed, the product does indeed contain some quantity of artificial trans fat. Food labels list their products in the ingredients list in order from highest amount to lowest amount. If the hydrogenated fat or margarine ingredients are listed near the start of the list, it is safe to assume the product contains close to 0.5 g of trans fat per serving. If these ingredients appear near the end of the list, there are probably close to 0–0.1 g of trans fat per serving. Some of the most common foods containing artificial trans fats are French fries and battered fried foods, packaged crackers and cookies, piecrusts made with shortening or stick margarines, cake or pancake mixes, canned frostings, and microwave popcorn. The rule of thumb is to keep consumption of all trans fats as low as possible while also limiting the amount of saturated fat. Table 5.7 lists amounts of trans and saturated fats in common foods (Box 5.3).

TABLE 5.7
Comparison of Trans Fats and Saturated Fats in Common Servings of Foods with Natural and Artificial Trans Fats

Food	Trans Fats (g)	Saturated Fats (g)	Total Trans and Saturated Fats (g)
Natural Trans Fats			
Butter (1 Tbsp[a])	0.5	7.3	7.8
Cheddar cheese (1 oz)	0.3	5.5	5.8
Ground beef (3 oz)	0.7	4.9	5.6
Pork rinds (3 oz)	0.0	8.1	8.1
Artificial Trans Fats			
Stick margarine (1 Tbsp)	2.1	2.1	4.2
Shortening (1 Tbsp)	1.7	3.2	4.9
Popcorn, microwave (1 bag)	8.5	6.3	14.8
Snack crackers (10)	2.2	2.0	4.2
Potato chips (8 oz bag)	0.5	12.5	13.0
French fries (medium serving)	0.2	4.2	4.4

[a] Tablespoon. U.S. Department of Agriculture, Agricultural Research Service. 2014. USDA National Nutrient Database for Standard Reference, Release 27. Nutrient Data Laboratory Home Page http://www.ars.usda.gov/ba/bhnrc/ndl.

BOX 5.3   SOME FOOD LABELS LIST "PARTIALLY HYDROGENATED" AND OTHERS LIST "HYDROGENATED," IS THERE A DIFFERENCE?

Food companies often use partially hydrogenated and hydrogenated interchangeably. It is best to avoid products that use either phrase. If the label states "fully hydrogenated" all of the unsaturated fat has been converted to saturated fat, so there is no trans fat, but remember it is also recommended to limit intake of saturated fat.

5.4.3 Snacks and Meal Recommendations for the Child Athlete

A common question that coaches, parents, or athletes may be wondering is whether or not young athletes should fuel with fat prior to a game? It is not uncommon for an athlete to become nervous or anxious prior to a match or game. The human digestive tract is sensitive to these emotions and may be slowed down when the athlete is emotionally charged with anticipation. To avoid intestinal and digestive tract discomfort, young athletes should fuel up with easily digestible meals. As a starting point, meals should be consumed 3 h prior to a game or match, with further adjustments in feeding time being due to individual variability that exists between the children. While research indicates that young children burn primarily fat during activity, it is not advised that children consume foods with substantial amounts of fat prior to participating in a game. Fats are more slowly digested than other nutrients. A child athlete participating with a high-fat meal in their stomach may develop significant gastrointestinal discomfort and end up fighting a losing battle. You may be asking yourself, well earlier it was discussed that young athletes burn or oxidize more fat than carbohydrate compared with adults during exercise at a given relative intensity, how is a young athlete going to perform at a high level if they do not fuel up with fat prior to their event? The answer lies in the human body's capability to store fat as discussed previously. During performance, these stores are mobilized to fuel the athlete. A well-rounded diet consumed on a consistent basis made up of fat, carbohydrates, and protein will ensure young athletes are fueled with the energy they need to perform at the highest level. Consequently, consuming meals or snacks comprising high amount of fat is not recommended. Athletes, coaches, and parents are recommended to closely read Chapters 15 and 16 as they are developed to help with decisions such as these.

Many ways exist to incorporate healthy fats into your diet. If baked goods are commonplace around your home, substitute oil (see Figure 5.1) for shortening or margarine when making muffins, bars, or cakes. Choosing vinaigrettes with healthy oils for salad dressings, rather than regular or low-fat salad dressings, is another easy way to incorporate healthy fats into your child's diet. Mix and match nuts, such as walnuts and pecans, in a casserole or salad to add a little extra crunch, or add olives or avocado to a turkey or deli sandwich. Additionally, two servings of fish from the list provided in Table 5.8 or adopting any of the approaches provided in Table 5.9 are effective strategies to maximize the intake of healthy fat into a young athlete's daily diet. Chapters 15 and 16 have been prepared with the intent of providing tips, guidelines, and recommendations to help coaches, parents, and healthcare providers to help athletes achieve all of the fueling recommendations provided throughout Chapters 3 through 5.

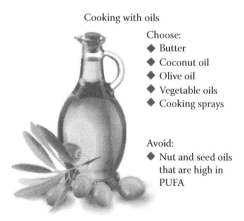

FIGURE 5.1 Cooking with oils, choose healthy fats! The fats listed under "Choose" withstand the temperatures used for cooking. Nut and seed oils that are high in PUFA are easily damaged by heat and should be used as salad dressings or added to hot vegetables just before serving.

TABLE 5.8
Grocery List for Foods Containing Healthy Fats, Especially Essential Fatty Acids of both the Omega-3 and Omega-6 Families

Healthy Fats Grocery List

Nuts	Seeds	Fish
Walnuts	Chia	Salmon
Almonds	Flax	Tuna
Cashews	Hemp	Trout
Pistachios	Sunflower	Herring
Hazelnuts	Pumpkin	Sardines
Peanut butter		

TABLE 5.9
Examples of Food Choices That Increase Intake of Healthy Fats

Breakfast	Lunch/Dinner	Snacks
• Add almonds to oatmeal	• Use oil and vinegar on salad	• Granola bar with nuts
• Peanut butter on toast	• Add nuts to a salad	• Peanut butter on crackers, pretzels
• Add ground flaxseed to cereal, yogurt, or muffins	• Cook with olive oil	• Nut medley
	• Fish (broiled, grilled, or steamed; not deep fat fried)	
	• Tuna sandwich	
	• Avocado in a salad or by itself	
	• Olives	
	• Soybeans	

5.4.4 Special Considerations

5.4.4.1 Fats for Vegetarian Athletes

Vegetarians do not eat meat, poultry, or fish while vegans consume only plant foods. If a child athlete consumes a vegan diet, it is still essential that the child consumes an adequate amount of fat each day to provide first for their normal growth and development needs as well as what is required of their athletic practice and participation. Vegan athletes should consider alternative sources of fat, including all nuts and seeds. These foods operate as easy-to-pack snacks for between games or matches during a busy sporting event day or for quick snacks while at home or on the road. Considering that vegans do not consume fish, vegan children should strive to maximize their consumption of good plant sources of omega-3 fatty acids by also consuming walnuts and ground flax seeds or flax oil, rich sources of alpha-linolenic acid. Soy products and canola oil also have small amounts of alpha-linolenic acid.

5.4.4.2 Fats for Female Athletes

Physically active postpubescent females may find that they have infrequent or diminished menstrual cycles. This is not uncommon for very active female teens and may serve as an indication to look closely at the athlete's diet. Sufficient body fat is needed for healthy estrogen levels, and very active teens tend to have lower body fat levels when compared to their nonathletic or nonactive peers, a formula for infrequent menstruation. Due to the link between menstruation and body fat, coaches, parents, and young female athletes need to make sure their body fat is kept at a healthy level. Diets with adequate amounts of healthy fats will help prevent cessation of a young female athlete's menstrual cycle, possibly preventing injury and detrimental health issues.

5.5 GUIDELINES FOR YOUNG ATHLETES FOR DAILY CONSUMPTION OF FATS

- Fats are not villains! Fats have many favorable functions. For example, fats provide a concentrated source of energy and serve as an energy reserve (fat stores). Fats serve a structural component of cell membranes and are key players in healthy brain and eye development while also serving as precursors to sex hormones, and help the absorption of fat-soluble vitamins.
- Children have higher basal metabolic rates per kilogram of body mass when compared to adults, and children require more fuel per kilogram of body mass for total body mechanical work and power production during locomotion. The preferred fuel for children during exercise and physical activity is oxidation of fat.
- Make sure children have enough fat as fuel to perform their daily activities while maintaining optimal growth.
- Children require an average of 25%–35% of their calories from fat; children may achieve this by eating larger quantities of low-fat or smaller quantities of moderate-fat foods, but not consuming nonfat foods.
- Young athletes should aim to consume less saturated and trans fats, and more unsaturated fats.

The best choices for young athletes to ensure intake of adequate EFA are healthy fats from fish, nuts, seeds, and plant oils.

REFERENCES

1. Adkins Y and Kelley DS. Mechanisms underlying the cardioprotective effects of omega-3 polyunsaturated fatty acids. *Journal of Nutrition and Biochemistry* 21: 781–792, 2010.
2. Andersson A, Nalsen C, Tengblad S, and Vessby B. Fatty acid composition of skeletal muscle reflects dietary fat composition in humans. *American Journal of Clinical Nutrition* 76: 1222–1229, 2002.
3. Arm JP, Horton CE, Mencia-Huerta JM, House F, Eiser NM, Clark TJ, Spur BW, and Lee TH. Effect of dietary supplementation with fish oil lipids on mild asthma. *Thorax* 43: 84–92, 1988.
4. Arm JP, Horton CE, Spur BW, Mencia-Huerta JM, and Lee TH. The effects of dietary supplementation with fish oil lipids on the airways response to inhaled allergen in bronchial asthma. *American Review of Respiratory Disease* 139: 1395–1400, 1989.
5. Armstrong RB, Warren GL, and Warren JA. Mechanisms of exercise-induced muscle fibre injury. *Sports Medicine* 12: 184–207, 1991.
6. Astrand P-O. *Experimental Studies of Physical Working Capacity in Relation to Sex and Age.* Copenhagen, Denmark: Munksgaard, 1952.
7. Bar-Or O, Rowland T. *Pediatric Exercise Medicine.* Champaign, IL: Human Kinetics, 2004.
8. Bass S, Inge K. Nutrition for special populations: Children and young athletes, in: *Clinical Sports Nutrition.* V Deakin, LM Burke, eds. Sydney, NSW: McGraw-Hill, 2006, pp. 589–632.
9. Berg A and Keul J. Biochemical changes during exercise in children, in: *Young Athletes/Biological, Psychological and Educational Perspectives.* RM Malina, ed. Champaign, IL: Human Kinetics, 1988, pp. 61–77.
10. Boisseau N and Delamarche P. Metabolic and hormonal responses to exercise in children and adolescents. *Sports Medicine* 30: 405–422, 2000.
11. Bonafini S, Antoniazzi F, Maffeis C, Minuz P, and Fava C. Beneficial effects of omega-3 PUFA in children on cardiovascular risk factors during childhood and adolescence. *Prostaglandins and Other Lipid Mediators* 120: 72–79, 2015.
12. Brenner IK, Shek PN, and Shephard RJ. Infection in athletes. *Sports Medicine* 17: 86–107, 1994.
13. Bruckner G, Webb P, Greenwell L, Chow C, and Richardson D. Fish oil increases peripheral capillary blood cell velocity in humans. *Atherosclerosis* 66: 237–245, 1987.

14. Burke LM and Read RS. Sports nutrition. Approaching the nineties. *Sports Medicine* 8: 80–100, 1989.
15. Calbet JA, Mooren FC, Burke LM, Stear SJ, and Castell LM. A-Z of nutritional supplements: Dietary supplements, sports nutrition foods and ergogenic aids for health and performance: Part 24. *British Journal of Sports Medicine* 45: 1005–1007, 2011.
16. Calfee R and Fadale P. Popular ergogenic drugs and supplements in young athletes. *Pediatrics* 117: e577–e589, 2006.
17. Campbell B and Kreider RB. Conjugated linoleic acids. *Current Sports Medicine Reports* 7: 237–241, 2008.
18. Cartwright IJ, Pockley AG, Galloway JH, Greaves M, and Preston FE. The effects of dietary omega-3 polyunsaturated fatty acids on erythrocyte membrane phospholipids, erythrocyte deformability and blood viscosity in healthy volunteers. *Atherosclerosis* 55: 267–281, 1985.
19. Colakoglu S, Colakoglu M, Taneli F, Cetinoz F, and Turkmen M. Cumulative effects of conjugated linoleic acid and exercise on endurance development, body composition, serum leptin and insulin levels. *Journal of Sports Medicine and Physical Fitness* 46: 570–577, 2006.
20. Costill DL, Coyle E, Dalsky G, Evans W, Fink W, and Hoopes D. Effects of elevated plasma FFA and insulin on muscle glycogen usage during exercise. *Journal of Applied Physiology: Respiratory, Environmental and Exercise Physiology* 43: 695–699, 1977.
21. Daniels J, Oldridge N, Nagle F, and White B. Differences and changes in VO_2 among young runners 10 to 18 years of age. *Medicine and Science in Sports* 10: 200–203, 1978.
22. Delamarche P, Monnier M, Gratas-Delamarche A, Koubi HE, Mayet MH, and Favier R. Glucose and free fatty acid utilization during prolonged exercise in prepubertal boys in relation to catecholamine responses. *European Journal of Applied Physiology and Occupational Physiology* 65: 66–72, 1992.
23. Dyerberg J, Bang HO, and Hjorne N. Fatty acid composition of the plasma lipids in Greenland Eskimos. *American Journal of Clinical Nutrition* 28: 958–966, 1975.
24. Eckel RH, Hanson AS, Chen AY, Berman JN, Yost TJ, and Brass EP. Dietary substitution of medium-chain triglycerides improves insulin-mediated glucose metabolism in NIDDM subjects. *Diabetes* 41: 641–647, 1992.
25. Frost G, Bar-Or O, Dowling J, and Dyson K. Explaining differences in the metabolic cost and efficiency of treadmill locomotion in children. *Journal of Sports Sciences* 20: 451–461, 2002.
26. Galea G and Davidson RJ. Hemorheology of marathon running. *International Journal of Sports Medicine* 6: 136–138, 1985.
27. Haralambie G. Skeletal muscle enzyme activities in female subjects of various ages. *Bulletin Europeen de Physiopathologie Respiratoire* 15: 259–268, 1979.
28. Hartgens F and Kuipers H. Effects of androgenic-anabolic steroids in athletes. *Sports Medicine* 34: 513–554, 2004.
29. Havemann L, West SJ, Goedecke JH, Macdonald IA, St Clair Gibson A, Noakes TD, and Lambert EV. Fat adaptation followed by carbohydrate loading compromises high-intensity sprint performance. *Journal of Applied Physiology* 100: 194–202, 2006.
30. Hebestreit H, Meyer F, Htay H, Heigenhauser GJ, and Bar-Or O. Plasma metabolites, volume and electrolytes following 30-s high-intensity exercise in boys and men. *European Journal of Applied Physiology and Occupational Physiology* 72: 563–569, 1996.
31. Herd SL, Kiens B, Boobis LH, and Hardman AE. Moderate exercise, postprandial lipemia, and skeletal muscle lipoprotein lipase activity. *Metabolism, Clinical and Experimental* 50: 756–762, 2001.
32. Hill JO, Peters JC, Yang D, Sharp T, Kaler M, Abumrad NN, and Greene HL. Thermogenesis in humans during overfeeding with medium-chain triglycerides. *Metabolism, Clinical and Experimental* 38: 641–648, 1989.
33. Institute of Medicine. Dietary Reference Intakes: The essential guide to nutrient requirements. Washington (DC): The National Academies Press; 2006.
34. Ivy J, Costill D, Fink W, and Maglischo E. Contribution of medium and long chain triglyceride intake to energy metabolism during prolonged exercise. *International Journal of Sports Medicine* 1: 15, 1980.
35. Ivy JL. Dietary strategies to promote glycogen synthesis after exercise. *Canadian Journal of Applied Physiology* (*Revue Canadienne de Physiologie Appliquee*) 26 (Suppl): S236–S245, 2001.
36. Jeukendrup A and Cronin L. Nutrition and elite young athletes. *Medicine and Sport Science* 56: 47–58, 2011.
37. Jeukendrup AE and Aldred S. Fat supplementation, health, and endurance performance. *Nutrition* 20: 678–688, 2004.

38. Kreider RB, Ferreira MP, Greenwood M, Wilson M, and Almada AL. Effects of conjugated linoleic acid supplementation during resistance training on body composition, bone density, strength, and selected hematological markers. *Journal of Strength and Conditioning Research/National Strength & Conditioning Association* 16: 325–334, 2002.
39. Lamb DR. Anabolic steroids in athletics: How well do they work and how dangerous are they? *American Journal of Sports Medicine* 12: 31–38, 1984.
40. Lambert EV, Goedecke JH, Bluett K, Heggie K, Claassen A, Rae DE et al. Conjugated linoleic acid versus high-oleic acid sunflower oil: Effects on energy metabolism, glucose tolerance, blood lipids, appetite and body composition in regularly exercising individuals. *British Journal of Nutrition* 97: 1001–1011, 2007.
41. Macaluso F, Barone R, Catanese P, Carini F, Rizzuto L, Farina F, and Di Felice V. Do fat supplements increase physical performance? *Nutrients* 5: 509–524, 2013.
42. MacDougall JD, Roche PD, Bar-Or O, and Moroz JR. Maximal aerobic capacity of Canadian school-children: Prediction based on age-related oxygen cost of running. *International Journal of Sports Medicine* 4: 194–198, 1983.
43. Magazanik A, Shapiro Y, Meytes D, and Meytes I. Enzyme blood levels and water balance during a marathon race. *Journal of Applied Physiology* 36: 214–217, 1974.
44. Mahon AD, Duncan GE, Howe CA, and Del Corral P. Blood lactate and perceived exertion relative to ventilatory threshold: Boys versus men. *Medicine & Science in Sports & Exercise* 29: 1332–1337, 1997.
45. Margolis LM and Pasiakos SM. Optimizing intramuscular adaptations to aerobic exercise: Effects of carbohydrate restriction and protein supplementation on mitochondrial biogenesis. *Advances in Nutrition* 4: 657–664, 2013.
46. Martinez LR and Haymes EM. Substrate utilization during treadmill running in prepubertal girls ar women. *Medicine & Science in Sports & Exercise* 24: 975–983, 1992.
47. Mickleborough TD. Omega-3 polyunsaturated fatty acids in physical performance optimization. *International Journal of Sport Nutrition and Exercise Metabolism* 23: 83–96, 2013.
48. Mickleborough TD, Lindley MR, Ionescu AA, and Fly AD. Protective effect of fish oil supplementation on exercise-induced bronchoconstriction in asthma. *Chest* 129: 39–49, 2006.
49. Mickleborough TD, Murray RL, Ionescu AA, and Lindley MR. Fish oil supplementation reduces severity of exercise-induced bronchoconstriction in elite athletes. *American Journal of Respiratory and Critical Care Medicine* 168: 1181–1189, 2003.
50. Mickleborough TD and Rundell KW. Dietary polyunsaturated fatty acids in asthma- and exercise-induced bronchoconstriction. *European Journal of Clinical Nutrition* 59: 1335–1346, 2005.
51. Montfort-Steiger V and Williams CA. Carbohydrate intake considerations for young athletes. *Journal of Sports Science & Medicine* 6: 343–352, 2007.
52. Mori TA. Omega-3 fatty acids and cardiovascular disease: Epidemiology and effects on cardiometabolic risk factors. *Food & Function* 5: 2004–2019, 2014.
53. Medium Chain Triglycerides (MCTs). Natural Medicines Comprehensive Database. Therapeutic Research Faculty, 8, 2013. http://naturaldatabase.therapeuticresearch.com/home.aspx?cs=&s=ND.
54. Papamandjaris AA, White MD, Raeini-Sarjaz M, and Jones PJ. Endogenous fat oxidation during medium chain versus long chain triglyceride feeding in healthy women. *International Journal of Obesity and Related Metabolic Disorders: Journal of the International Association for the Study of Obesity* 24: 1158–1166, 2000.
55. Ponnampalam EN, Mann NJ, and Sinclair AJ. Effect of feeding systems on omega-3 fatty acids, conjugated linoleic acid and trans fatty acids in Australian beef cuts: Potential impact on human health. *Asia Pacific Journal of Clinical Nutrition* 15: 21–29, 2006.
56. Prentice AM and Paul AA. Fat and energy needs of children in developing countries. *American Journal of Clinical Nutrition* 72: 1253S–1265S, 2000.
57. Ryan AJ. Anabolic steroids are fool's gold. *Federation Proceedings* 40: 2682–2688, 1981.
58. Sallinen J, Pakarinen A, Ahtiainen J, Kraemer WJ, Volek JS, and Hakkinen K. Relationship between diet and serum anabolic hormone responses to heavy-resistance exercise in men. *International Journal of Sports Medicine* 25: 627–633, 2004.
59. Satabin P, Portero P, Defer G, Bricout J, and Guezennec CY. Metabolic and hormonal responses to lipid and carbohydrate diets during exercise in man. *Medicine & Science in Sports & Exercise* 19: 218–223, 1987.
60. Sen CK, Atalay M, Agren J, Laaksonen DE, Roy S, and Hanninen O. Fish oil and vitamin E supplementation in oxidative stress at rest and after physical exercise. *Journal of Applied Physiology* 83: 189–195, 1997.

61. Sherwood L. *Fundamentals of Human Physiology.* Belmont, CA: Brooks/Cole, Cengage Learning, 2011.
62. Simchon S, Jan KM, and Chien S. Influence of reduced red cell deformability on regional blood flow. *American Journal of Physiology* 253: H898–H903, 1987.
63. St-Onge MP, Bourque C, Jones PJ, Ross R, and Parsons WE. Medium- versus long-chain triglycerides for 27 days increases fat oxidation and energy expenditure without resulting in changes in body composition in overweight women. *International Journal of Obesity and Related Metabolic Disorders: Journal of the International Association for the Study of Obesity* 27: 95–102, 2003.
64. St-Onge MP and Jones PJ. Physiological effects of medium-chain triglycerides: Potential agents in the prevention of obesity. *Journal of Nutrition* 132: 329–332, 2002.
65. St-Onge MP, Ross R, Parsons WD, and Jones PJ. Medium-chain triglycerides increase energy expenditure and decrease adiposity in overweight men. *Obesity Research* 11: 395–402, 2003.
66. Tamaki T, Uchiyama S, Uchiyama Y, Akatsuka A, Roy RR, and Edgerton VR. Anabolic steroids increase exercise tolerance. *American Journal of Physiology: Endocrinology and Metabolism* 280: E973–E981, 2001.
67. Tipton KD, Borsheim E, Wolf SE, Sanford AP, and Wolfe RR. Acute response of net muscle protein balance reflects 24-h balance after exercise and amino acid ingestion. *American Journal of Physiology: Endocrinology and Metabolism* 284: E76–E89, 2003.
68. Unnithan VB and Eston RG. Stride frequency and treadmill running economy in adults and children. *Pediatric Exercise Science* 2: 149–155, 1990.
69. van der Brug GE, Peters HP, Hardeman MR, Schep G, and Mosterd WL. Hemorheological response to prolonged exercise—No effects of different kinds of feedings. *International Journal of Sports Medicine* 16: 231–237, 1995.
70. Volek JS, Kraemer WJ, Bush JA, Incledon T, and Boetes M. Testosterone and cortisol in relationship to dietary nutrients and resistance exercise. *Journal of Applied Physiology* 82: 49–54, 1997.
71. Volek JS, Noakes T, and Phinney SD. Rethinking fat as a fuel for endurance exercise. *European Journal of Sport Science* 15: 13–20, 2015.
72. Wilmore J. Body weight and body composition, in: *Eating, Body Weight and Performance in Athletes.* J Rodin, KD Brownell, JH Wilmore, eds. Philadelphia: Lea & Febiger, 1992, pp. 77–93.
73. Wilmore JH and Costill DL. Physical energy: Fuel metabolism. *Nutrition Reviews* 59: S13–S16, 2001.
74. Yalcin O, Bor-Kucukatay M, Senturk UK, and Baskurt OK. Effects of swimming exercise on red blood cell rheology in trained and untrained rats. *Journal of Applied Physiology* 88: 2074–2080, 2000.
75. Yamori Y, Nara Y, Iritani N, Workman RJ, and Inagami T. Comparison of serum phospholipid fatty acids among fishing and farming Japanese populations and American inlanders. *Journal of Nutritional Science and Vitaminology* 31: 417–422, 1985.

6 Vitamin and Mineral Needs

Brad Schoenfeld and Alan Aragon

CONTENTS

Abstract 99
6.1 Vitamins 99
      6.1.1 Vitamin D 100
6.2 Minerals 102
      6.2.1 Iron 103
      6.2.2 Calcium 105
      6.2.3 Magnesium 106
      6.2.4 Zinc 107
6.3 Conclusion 108
References 109

ABSTRACT

Vitamins and minerals are important micronutrients required in the diet for sustaining health and performance in the child and adolescent athlete. Vitamins are organic compounds that are part of the broad spectrum of essential micronutrients that carry out a multitude of regulatory functions. Alternatively, minerals are inorganic compounds that carry out similar necessary physiological functions, often in synergism with vitamins. This chapter discusses the specific roles of vitamins and minerals as they pertain to the young athlete. In particular, vitamin D, iron, calcium, magnesium, and zinc, as these micronutrients have been especially well studied with respect to the target population. Evidence-based conclusions are drawn to provide guidance as to the requirements. Recommendations take into account the unique needs of the young athletic population throughout varying stages of physical development.

6.1 VITAMINS

Vitamins are organic compounds that are part of the broad spectrum of essential micronutrients with a multitude of regulatory functions. Unlike macronutrients, vitamins are not direct sources of energy. Rather, they catalyze numerous biochemical reactions that facilitate energy metabolism. As essential nutrients, they must be provided in adequate amounts through exogenous means (i.e., diet and/or environment), since the body cannot biosynthesize them in adequate amounts for survival. Vitamins have appropriately been referred to as "accessory growth factors" (Gropper et al. 2009).

There are two broad classifications of vitamins: water-soluble (vitamin C and the B complex) and fat-soluble vitamins (A, D, E, and K). In contrast to fat-soluble vitamins that are stored in the adipose tissue, the water-soluble vitamins with the exception of cobalamin (B12) have a higher physiological turnover rate. They are absorbed into the portal blood and do not stay in the system for long periods. The water-soluble vitamins contribute to the regulation of energy metabolism by modulating the synthesis and breakdown of the macronutrients and other bioactive compounds (National Research Council 1998). In contrast, the fat-soluble vitamins do not have a direct role in energy metabolism (Lukaski 2004). Their roles range from antioxidation (vitamin A and E) to bone formation (vitamin D and K).

Our understanding of the complexities of micronutrition is ever evolving, but incomplete. This is due to methodological challenges and ethical considerations preventing invasive and potentially harmful investigations that could answer lingering questions. As a result, a very limited body of information is available on the vitamin requirements of young athletes, and even less is available regarding the vitamin needs specific to each sport (Meyer et al. 2007). Despite these limitations, the march of scientific research has uncovered data worth serious consideration when forming practical applications. Although the full range of vitamins is crucial for sustaining life and health, vitamin D has received the most extensive study within the context of the child and adolescent athletic population. In addition to the material provided on vitamin D below, Tables 6.1 and 6.2 provide the recommended daily allowances for each vitamin across a wide array of ages, key functions of each vitamin, as well as optimal food sources.

6.1.1 Vitamin D

Vitamin D is a steroid hormone occurring in several forms, and is essential for regulating the metabolism of several minerals, most notably calcium for the purpose of maintaining skeletal growth and health. Other minerals with vitamin D-dependent functions include iron, magnesium, and zinc. Vitamin D also has numerous extraskeletal effects that it regulates by influencing an estimated 2000 genes (Wacker and Holick 2013). In addition to preventing rickets, osteoporosis,

TABLE 6.1
Recommended Daily Allowance (RDA), Functions, and Food Sources for Vitamins during Childhood and Adolescence

Vitamin	Childhood (Ages 4–8)[a]	Childhood (Ages 9–13) Males	Childhood (Ages 9–13) Females	Adolescence (Ages 14–18) Males	Adolescence (Ages 14–18) Females
Folate	200 mcg/day[b]	300 mcg/day[b]	300 mcg/day[b]	400 mcg[b]	400 mcg[b]
Niacin	8 mg/day[c]	12 mg/day[c]	12 mg/day[c]	16 mg[c]	14 mg[c]
Pantothenic acid	3 mg/day (AI)	4 mg/day (AI)	4 mg/day (AI)	5 mg (AI)	5 mg (AI)
Riboflavin	600 mcg/day	900 mcg/day	900 mcg/day	1.3 mg	1.0 mg
Thiamin	600 mcg/day	900 mcg/day	900 mcg/day	1.2 mg	1.0 mg
Vitamin A	400 mcg/day (1333 IU/day)[d]	600 mcg/day (2000 IU/day)[d]	600 mcg/day (2000 IU/day)[d]	900 mcg (3000 IU)[d]	700 mcg (2333 IU)[d]
Vitamin B_6	600 mcg/day	1 mg/day	1 mg/day	1.3 mg	1.2 mg
Vitamin B_{12}	1.2 mcg/day	1.8 mcg/day	1.8 mcg/day	2.4 mcg	2.4 mcg
Vitamin C	25 mg/day	45 mg/day	45 mg/day	75 mg	65 mg
Vitamin D	15 mcg/day (600 IU/day)	15 mcg/day (600 IU/day)	15 mcg/day (600 IU/day)	15 mcg (600 IU)	15 mcg (600 IU)
Vitamin E	7 mg/day (10.5 IU/day)[e]	11 mg/day (16.5 IU/day)[e]	11 mg/day (16.5 IU/day)[e]	15 mg (22.5 IU)[e]	15 mg (22.5 IU)[e]
Vitamin K	55 mcg/day (AI)	60 mcg/day (AI)	60 mcg/day (AI)	75 mcg (AI)	75 mcg (AI)

Source: Adapted from http://lpi.oregonstate.edu/mic/life-stages/children#vitamins, http://lpi.oregonstate.edu/mic/life-stages/adolescents, and http://www.nal.usda.gov/wicworks/Topics/FG/AppendixC_NutrientChart.pdf.

[a] Amount for both males and females; AI = adequate intake
[b] Dietary folate equivalents
[c] NE = niacin equivalent: 1-mg NE = 60-mg tryptophan = 1-mg niacin
[d] Retinol activity equivalents
[e] α-Tocopherol

TABLE 6.2
Key Functions and Food Sources for Vitamins during Childhood and Adolescence

Vitamin	Functions	Best Dietary Sources
Folate	Essential in the biosynthesis of nucleic acids; necessary for the normal maturation of red blood cells	Asparagus, Brussel sprouts, black-eyed peas, spinach, cantaloupe, and breakfast cereals
Niacin	Part of the enzyme system for oxidation, energy release, necessary for synthesis of glycogen, and for synthesis and breakdown of fatty acids	Liver, tuna, turkey, chicken, salmon, peanuts, milk, and wheat germ
Pantothenic acid	Functions in the synthesis and breakdown of many vital body compounds; essential in the intermediary metabolism of carbohydrate, fat, and protein	Avocado, broccoli, kale, eggs, legumes, lentils, milk, and mushrooms
Riboflavin	Essential for growth, plays an enzymatic role in tissue respiration, acts as a transporter of hydrogen ions, and synthesis of FMN and FAD	Milk and dairy products, liver, pork chop, collard greens, beef, broccoli, and eggs
Thiamin	Combines with phosphorus to form thiamin pyrophosphate (TPP) necessary for metabolism of protein, carbohydrate, and fat; essential for growth, normal appetite, digestion, and healthy nerves	Pork, sunflower seeds, bran flakes, beef, and ham
Vitamin A	Preserves integrity of epithelial cells; formation of rhodopsin for vision in dim light; and necessary for wound healing, growth, and normal immune function	Liver, crab, milk and dairy products, carrots, sweet potato, and pumpkin
Vitamin B_6	Aids in the synthesis and breakdown of amino acids and unsaturated fatty acids; essential for conversion of tryptophan into niacin; and essential for normal growth	Liver, salmon, split peas, banana, turnip greens, chicken, beef, pork, dried beans, and avocado
Vitamin B_{12}	Essential for biosynthesis of nucleic acids and nucleoproteins; red blood cell maturation; involved with folate metabolism; and central nervous system metabolism	Liver, trout, beef, clams, crab, lamb, tuna, and milk products
Vitamin C	Essential in the synthesis of collagen; iron absorption and transport; water-soluble antioxidant; and functions in folacin metabolism	Kiwi, green peppers, broccoli, oranges, cantaloupe, Brussel sprouts, and strawberries
Vitamin D	Necessary for the formation of a normal bone; promotes the absorption of calcium, and phosphorus in the intestines	Milk and dairy products, salmon, tuna, shrimp, beef, and chicken liver
Vitamin E	May function as an antioxidant in the tissues; may also have a role as a coenzyme; and neuromuscular function	Oils, nuts and seeds, sweet potato, wheat germ, and crab
Vitamin K	Catalyzes prothrombin synthesis, required in the synthesis of other blood-clotting factors and synthesis of intestinal bacteria	Green, leafy vegetables (kale, collards, spinach, turnip greens, Brussel sprouts, and broccoli)

Source: Adapted from http://lpi.oregonstate.edu/mic/life-stages/children#vitamins, http://lpi.oregonstate.edu/mic/life-stages/adolescents, and http://www.nal.usda.gov/wicworks/Topics/FG/AppendixC_NutrientChart.pdf.

and associated bone pathologies, a growing body of literature indicates the importance of adequate vitamin D status in the prevention of cardiovascular disease, diabetes, autoimmune diseases, and cancer (Holick 2004, Holick and Chen 2008, Wacker and Holick 2013). Furthermore, an emerging body of data suggests that vitamin D also plays a role in regulating skeletal muscle physiology, including the improvement of strength and recovery (Barker, Henriksen et al. 2013, Barker, Schneider et al. 2013).

Vitamin D is unique among the other vitamins since it can be synthesized cutaneously through exposure to the sun as well as derived from food sources. The exposure of human skin to sunlight converts 7-dehydroxycholesterol into previtamin D3 in the skin, which is then converted into the active D3 (cholecalciferol), commonly denoted in its simplified chemical formula of 25(OH)D. Thus, a significant source of vitamin D for most humans is exposure to sunlight. Vitamin D naturally occurs in significant amounts in only a few foods (i.e., oily fish such as herring, mackerel, and salmon). This natural lack of vitamin D in many foods common to the Western diet helps explain the fortification of foods common throughout the United States in milk products, various fruit beverages, and some cereal grain products (Holick and Chen 2008).

The normal range of serum 25 (OH)D is 30–74 ng/mL (Medline Plus 2012). To convert these units into nmol/L, multiply the values listed in ng/mL by 2.496. There is considerable debate over the proper clinical stratification of vitamin D status indicated by serum levels of 25(OH)D, but at least two sets of standards can be considered authoritative. The Institute of Medicine (IOM) (Ross, Manson et al. 2011) classifies severe deficiency as <5 ng/mL and deficiency as <15 ng/mL. Sufficiency begins at >20 ng/mL and risk of toxicity begins at >50 ng/mL. The Endocrine Society's thresholds are higher (Holick et al. 2011), classifying deficiency as <20 ng/mL, insufficiency as 21–29 ng/mL, sufficiency as >30 ng/mL, and toxicity as >150 ng/mL. These values vary according to geography, race, and culture (Hoch et al. 2008). The recommended dietary allowance (RDA) for vitamin D set by the IOM is 15 µg (600 IU) for a very broad age range (1–70 years) for both sexes (Ross, Taylor et al. 2011). It is debatable whether or not this target is sufficient. Vitamin D is potentially a case where significantly exceeding the RDA may be necessary to optimize several health endpoints. It has been suggested that supplementing the diet with 1000–2000 IU of D3 can provide protective benefits to the general population (Heaney 2008).

Vitamin D deficiency is regarded as a major public health problem throughout the world (Holick and Chen 2008). An estimated 30%–50% of children and adults in the general population are vitamin D deficient (Wacker and Holick 2013). A significantly larger segment of the population may be treading along at insufficient levels. Constantini and colleagues recently found that in a sample of 98 young athletes and dancers (age 14.7 ± 3.0 years), 73% had serum 25(OH)D levels that were insufficient (Constantini et al. 2010). Both basketball players and dancers had an insufficiency rate of 94%, which is reflective of the sports being played indoors. It is noteworthy that the overall high insufficiency rates were seen despite the study population living in a sunny country, suggesting that other factors need to be bolstered to prevent deficiency.

Vitamin D deficiency has been attributed to a number of possible etiological factors including insufficient sunlight exposure, decreased synthesis via darker pigmentation or physical/chemical agents blocking ultraviolet rays, malabsorption from various disease states including chronic liver disease, celiac disease, biliary obstruction, or increased degradation of cholecalciferol via drugs such as antibiotics, anticonvulsants, or glucocorticoids (Hoch et al. 2008). A potential cause of deficiency worth illuminating is decreased nutritional intake through restrictive or poorly constructed diets. Adolescent athletes sustaining hypocaloric conditions to reach a lower weight class or maintain a leaner physique are at a higher risk for insufficient dietary vitamin D. Successful oral vitamin D3 regimens for correcting deficiencies in individuals aged 1–18 years has been reported as a daily dose of 1000–5000 IU for 8–12 weeks, or a weekly dose of 50,000 IU for 8–12 weeks (Balasubramanian et al. 2013). It is important to underscore the necessity of proper counseling and dietary programming by a qualified health professional in matters where nutrient deficiency is suspected.

6.2 MINERALS

Minerals are required in the diet for normal body function and often have a synergist relationship with vitamins. Minerals are classified as either "major" or "trace" depending on the amount needed by the body to carry out normal function. Specifically, the major minerals (a.k.a. macrominerals) are required in amounts greater than 100 mg/day while requirements for the trace minerals are below this amount. Mineral status in athletes can play an important role in physical performance and general health and well-being. The four minerals that have been well studied with respect to the young athlete are iron, calcium, magnesium, and zinc. Therefore, these elements will be discussed

TABLE 6.3
RDA for Minerals during Childhood and Adolescence

Mineral	Childhood (Ages 4–8)[a]	Childhood (Ages 9–13)		Adolescence (Ages 14–18)	
		Males	Females	Males	Females
Biotin	12 mcg/day (AI)	20 mcg/day (AI)	20 mcg/day (AI)	25 mcg/day (AI)	25 mcg/day (AI)
Calcium	1000 mg/day	1300 mg/day	1300 mg/day	1300 mg	1300 mg
Chromium	15 mcg/day (AI)	25 mcg/day (AI)	21 mcg/day (AI)	35 mcg (AI)	24 mcg (AI)
Copper	440 mcg/day	700 mcg/day	700 mcg/day	890 mcg	890 mcg
Fluoride	1 mg/day (AI)	2 mg/day (AI)	2 mg/day (AI)	3 mg (AI)	3 mg (AI)
Iodine	90 mcg/day	120 mcg/day	120 mcg/day	150 mcg	150 mcg
Iron	10 mg/day	8 mg/day	8 mg/day	11 mg	15 mg
Magnesium	130 mg/day	240 mg/day	240 mg/day	410 mg	360 mg
Manganese	1.5 mg/day (AI)	1.9 mg/day (AI)	1.6 mg/day (AI)	2.2 mg (AI)	1.6 mg (AI)
Molybdenum	22 mcg/day	34 mcg/day	34 mcg/day	43 mcg	43 mcg
Phosphorus	500 mg/day	1250 mg/day	1250 mg/day	1250 mg	1250 mg
Potassium	3800 mg/day (AI)	4500 mg/day (AI)	4500 mg/day (AI)	4700 mg (AI)	4700 m (AI)
Selenium	30 mcg/day	40 mcg/day	40 mcg/day	55 mcg	55 mcg
Sodium	1200 mg/day (AI)	1500 mg/day (AI)	1500 mg/day (AI)	1500 mg (AI)	1500 mg (AI)
Zinc	5 mg/day	8 mg/day	8 mg/day	11 mg	9 mg

Source: Adapted from http://lpi.oregonstate.edu/mic/life-stages/children#vitamins, http://lpi.oregonstate.edu/mic/life-stages/adolescents, and http://www.nal.usda.gov/wicworks/Topics/FG/AppendixC_NutrientChart.pdf.

[a] Amount for both males and females; AI = adequate intake.

here in detail. In addition, Tables 6.3 and 6.4 provide the recommended daily allowances in children of varying ages, key functions, and food sources for all minerals.

6.2.1 IRON

Although technically classified as a "trace element," iron is arguably the most important micronutrient for athletic performance. Iron is responsible for numerous cellular processes including oxygen delivery to body tissues, adenosine triphosphate (ATP) production, and deoxyribonucleic acid (DNA) synthesis (Unnithan and Goulopoulou 2004). Approximately 70% of the body's iron is contained in hemoglobin and myoglobin, which facilitate oxygen delivery; the remaining amounts are stored as ferritin with a tiny amount found in mitochondrial heme compounds (Hoch et al. 2008). Iron status is predicated on a balance of consumption and absorption from what is lost during bodily processes. Given that humans do not possess a mechanism to alter iron excretion, its status in the body is regulated at the level of intestinal absorption (Hoch et al. 2008).

Absorption of iron from food depends on its chemical form. Heme iron, found mostly in animal-based products, is efficiently absorbed from the gastrointestinal tract (5%–35% of intake) (Lukaski 2004). In contrast, nonheme iron from plant-based foods is poorly absorbed, with only 2%–20% taken up from the gastrointestinal tract (Lukaski 2004). Thus, vegetarians who consume primarily iron in its nonheme form require almost double the intake of those consuming an animal-based diet (Hoch et al. 2008). This is particularly true in those who consume high amounts of soy, phytates, polyphenols, and tannins, which inhibit iron absorption (Hoch et al. 2008).

To meet daily needs, it is recommended that boys and girls who are 9–13 years of age consume 8 mg/day of iron (Institute of Medicine Food and Nutrition Board 2001). An increased need for iron during puberty exists to support increases in hemoglobin concentrations, lean body mass, and overall growth (Petrie et al. 2004). Requirements are even greater in pubescent girls due to the onset

TABLE 6.4
Key Functions and Food Sources for Minerals during Childhood and Adolescence

Mineral	Functions	Best Dietary Sources
Biotin	Essential component of enzymes; plays an important role in the metabolism of fatty acids and amino acids	Cereal, chocolate, egg yolk, legumes, milk, nuts, organ meats, pork, and yeast
Calcium	Builds and maintains bones and teeth; essential in clotting of blood; influences transmission of ions across cell membranes; and required in nerve transmission	Milk and dairy products, collard greens, tofu, spinach, and broccoli
Chromium	Required for normal glucose metabolism; insulin cofactor	Broccoli, grape juice, waffles, English muffin, bagels, and mashed potatoes
Copper	Facilitates the function of many enzymes and iron; may be an integral part of RNA and DNA molecules	Oyster, whole grains, beans, nuts, potatoes, and organ meats
Fluoride	Helps protect teeth against tooth decay; may minimize bone loss	Fluoridated water, seafood, tea, and gelatin
Iodine	Helps regulate thyroid hormones; important in the regulation of cellular oxidation and growth	Table salt, cod, sea bass, haddock, kelp, and dairy
Iron	Essential for the formation of hemoglobin and oxygen transport; increases resistance to infection	Liver, round steak, lean beef, baked beans, fortified cereals, prune juice, and spinach
Magnesium	Required for many coenzyme oxidation–phosphorylation reactions, nerve impulse transmissions, and muscle contraction	Peanuts, bran buds, lentils, split peas, wild rice, and bean sprouts
Manganese	Essential part of several enzyme systems involved in protein and energy metabolism	Pecans, brown rice, instant oatmeal, spinach, and pineapple
Molybdenum	Possibly helps reduce incidence of dental caries	Beans, lentils, peas, grain products, and nuts
Phosphorus	Builds and maintains bones and teeth; component of nucleic acids; phospholipids; functions as a coenzyme in energy metabolism; and buffers intracellular fluid	Milk and dairy products, pork, sunflower seeds, bran flakes, peanuts, beef, and tuna
Potassium	Helps regulate acid–base equilibrium and osmotic pressure of body fluids; influences muscle activity, especially cardiac muscle	Potato, avocado, bran buds, fish, banana, hamburger, and yogurt
Selenium	May be essential to tissue respiration; associated with fat metabolism and vitamin E; and acts as an antioxidant	Lobster, tuna, liver, shrimp, oysters, and eggs
Sodium	Helps regulate acid–base equilibrium and osmotic pressure of body fluids; plays a role in normal muscle irritability and contractility; and influences cell permeability	Salt, pickles, chicken broth, corned beef, ham, and canned fish
Zinc	Component of many enzyme systems and insulin	Liver, beef, fortified cereals, crab, lamb, and wheat germs

Source: Adapted from http://lpi.oregonstate.edu/mic/life-stages/children#vitamins, http://lpi.oregonstate.edu/mic/life-stages/adolescents, and http://www.nal.usda.gov/wicworks/Topics/FG/AppendixC_NutrientChart.pdf.

of menstruation. Recommended intake in girls aged 14–18 years is 15 mg/day while comparably aged boys require approximately 11 mg/day (Institute of Medicine Food and Nutrition Board 2001).

Iron needs in young athletes may be further increased due to losses associated with regular, intense exercise (Unnithan and Goulopoulou 2004). Mechanisms theorized to mediate these losses include increased sweat, fecal and urinary excretion, increased erythrocyte hemolysis and turnover, increased gastrointestinal blood losses, exercise-induced ischemia or organ movement, foot strike hemolysis, and thermohemolysis (Petrie et al. 2004, Suedekum and Dimeff 2005). Accordingly, research shows a high prevalence of nonanemic iron deficiency (defined as ferritin concentrations of <12 μg/L and transferrin saturation of <16%) in young athletes across a wide variety of sports including field hockey, cross-country skiing, crew, basketball, and softball (Lukaski 2004, Unnithan and Goulopoulou 2004). Spodaryk found that prepubertal boys aged 10–12 years engaged in intensive endurance-swimming exercise experienced a significant and progressive decline in serum ferritin levels over 8 months of training compared to age-matched, nonexercising controls despite comparable dietary intakes (Spodaryk 2002). Similar results were found in a group of adolescent male and female cross-country runners (Rowland et al. 1987). Over the course of a 11-week competitive season, serum ferritin levels fell in all nine female athletes and 14 of the 17 males studied. Overall incidence of iron deficiency by the end of the study was 17% in male athletes and 45% in the females.

While male athletes generally consume adequate iron through diet, intake in females tends to fall below recommended levels. Studies show that female runners have a low consumption of animal-based foods along with a high-fiber intake, thereby reducing iron bioavailability to approximately 10% (Lukaski 2004). Since losses from menstruation and sweat amount to about 0.9 and 0.5 mg/day, respectively, there is an increased risk for deficiency in this population (Lukaski 2004). There is evidence that even marginal iron status can impair optimal athletic performance due to an increased reliance on anaerobic glycolysis (Petrie et al. 2004). Research shows an increased incidence of gastrointestinal bleeding in cross-country runners who are deficient in iron (Unnithan and Goulopoulou 2004). In addition, iron deficiencies can impair an athlete's muscle metabolism and cognitive function (Meyer et al. 2007). When iron deficiency progresses to anemia, it can have a markedly detrimental effect on athletic performance (Unnithan and Goulopoulou 2004). Although the prevalence of anemia is not greater in athletes than the general population, female runners and cross-country skiers appear to be at increased risk (Lukaski 2004). It is common for moderately anemic athletes to feel completely normal during rest but show substantial declines in performance as a result of reduced oxygen-carrying capacity (Hoch et al. 2008). These impairments are most prevalent in endurance-based sports that heavily involve the aerobic energy system. Periodic screening of young athletes for iron deficiency, especially females, can help to address deficiencies before they reach anemic levels and thus prevent substantial reductions in performance (Hoch et al. 2008).

For those who have trouble consuming adequate iron from food sources, supplementation can be beneficial from an endurance performance standpoint even in cases of iron deficiency without anemia. Specifically, iron supplementation of 50–100 mg/day in iron-depleted women has been shown to significantly enhance performance in both ergometer cycling and dynamic knee extension exercise compared to nonsupplemented controls over the course of a 4–6-week training period (Hinton et al. 2000, Brownlie et al. 2002, Brutsaert et al. 2003). Supplementation should be approached conservatively as it increases the risk of iron toxicity. This is particularly true in males, in whom the risk of iron overload and associated liver failure is twice the risk of iron deficiency (Hoch et al. 2008).

6.2.2 Calcium

Calcium is an essential mineral responsible for a wide range of bodily functions that include carrying out muscle contraction and supporting bone health. Upward of 99% of the body's calcium stores are located in the skeleton, with the remaining amounts found in plasma and extravascular fluid (Greer, Krebs, and Nutrition American Academy of Pediatrics Committee on 2006). These stores are in a perpetual state of turnover, with net losses through the urine, feces, and sweat dictating the amount of dietary calcium needed to maintain optimal levels in the body (Hoch et al. 2008).

Calcium homeostasis is regulated by a variety of hormones including parathyroid hormone (PTH), calcitonin, and 1,25-dihydroxyvitamin D. Absorption of calcium is both a passive and an active process that takes place in the intestine (Greer, Krebs, and Nutrition American Academy of Pediatrics Committee on 2006). When calcium levels in the extracellular fluid are low, the parathyroid gland secretes PTH. PTH in turn serves to reestablish normal blood calcium levels by multiple mechanisms including increasing the conversion of vitamin D into its active form, increasing calcium absorption from the gut, and increasing bone resorption (Hoch et al. 2008).

Current recommendations for calcium intake in girls and boys aged 9–18 years are 1100 and 1300 mg/day, respectively (Abrams 2011), although it is believed that values change depending on the stage of adolescence (Hoch et al. 2008). These recommendations are dependent on sufficient vitamin D levels as bone resorption is increased when this hormone is deficient despite adequate calcium intake (Hoch et al. 2008). Ensuring adequate calcium intake is particularly important during adolescence, as approximately 40% of total bone mass is achieved during this period with peak accretion rates attained at 12.5 and 14 years of age in girls and boys, respectively (Greer, Krebs, and Nutrition American Academy of Pediatrics Committee on 2006). Studies show a correlation between peak bone mass achieved during adolescence and the risk for developing osteoporosis in adulthood, reinforcing the importance of consuming adequate calcium early in life (Hoch et al. 2008). Unfortunately, a majority of adolescents worldwide fail to consume recommended levels of the mineral (Mesias et al. 2011). In the United States, a mere 13.5% of teenage girls and 36.3% of teenage boys meet daily calcium requirements (Hoch et al. 2008). Deficiencies in young athletes are rampant and have been attributed to a decreased consumption of calcium-rich foods, especially dairy products (Hoch et al. 2008).

There is scant evidence that exercise increases calcium requirements. Although athletes may lose calcium via sweat, these losses do not appear to substantially affect dietary needs (Kunstel 2005). A prospective, cross-sectional study of Brazilian male adolescent tennis players found no correlation between bone mineral density (BMD) and calcium intake and exercise (Juzwiak et al. 2008). This was despite a mean daily calcium intake below recommended levels in all subjects.

However, some female athletes may benefit from increased consumption, particularly those involved in sports requiring low levels of body fat such as endurance running, figure skating, and gymnastics. These athletes often have an obsession with body weight, leading to low-energy intakes while simultaneously expending a substantial amount of calories during their respective sports. In combination, this can cause a disturbance in estrogen concentrations leading to a greater risk of osteopenia and stress fractures (Petrie et al. 2004). Thus, intakes of up to 1500 mg/day might be necessary in these athletes to help maintain bone health. In those who have trouble obtaining adequate calcium from food sources, supplementation can be beneficial in optimizing bone mineral accrual (Unnithan and Goulopoulou 2004). To maximize absorption, intake should be spread out over the day with doses kept to not more than 500 mg at a time (Hoch et al. 2008).

6.2.3 Magnesium

Magnesium is a major mineral that plays a role in a myriad of cellular actions across numerous physiological systems. Magnesium is intricately involved in over 300 enzymatic reactions that control a diverse array of metabolic processes including glycolysis, protein synthesis, ATP hydrolysis, and second-messenger functions (Lukaski 2004). Moreover, magnesium regulates many aspects of human performance including a variety of neuromuscular, cardiovascular, immune, and hormonal functions (Lukaski 2004). These diverse actions make magnesium intake an important consideration for the young athlete as a deficiency may serve to limit sports performance.

Approximately 60% of magnesium is found in the skeleton, with the balance contained primarily in soft tissues (Unnithan and Goulopoulou 2004). Less than 1% of total magnesium is contained in the blood, and these levels are tightly regulated, with the kidneys striving to maintain magnesium levels by modulating urinary excretion (Rude 2012). Given that the majority of magnesium is contained intracellularly, accurate assessment of magnesium status in the body is difficult (Rude 2012). It is recommended that children between the ages of 9 and 13 years obtain 240 mg/day through dietary means (Institute of Medicine Food and Nutrition Board 1997). Recommended dietary magnesium intake for girls and boys aged 14–18 years increases to 360 and 410 mg/day, respectively (Institute of Medicine Food and Nutrition Board 1997). With respect to the population as a whole, magnesium deficiencies in healthy children and adolescents are rare because the foods they eat are generally rich in these minerals (Unnithan and Goulopoulou 2004). Cross-sectional studies of athletic populations reveal that male participants generally consume adequate amounts of magnesium, but intake in females is only 60%–65% of current recommendations (Lukaski 2004). Irrespective of gender, athletes competing in aesthetic sports or those with weight classifications tend to consume well below the required amounts of magnesium, in some cases less than half of the recommended levels (Lukaski 2004).

Physical activity can acutely affect magnesium levels as magnesium is lost through sweat (Speich et al. 2001). Accordingly, activities of long duration can result in significant magnesium losses, particularly if the exercise is performed in hot climates. Marathon runners have been shown to display significant reductions in serum magnesium concentrations (Speich et al. 2001). Thus, athletes may need increased dietary magnesium intake due to greater urinary and surface losses (Finstad et al. 2001).

There is evidence that relatively mild alterations in magnesium status can have a substantial effect on athletic performance. A decreased serum magnesium concentration is associated with chronic muscle spasms, which is relieved in a matter of days with treatment of 500 mg/day of magnesium gluconate (Lukaski 2004). The efficacy of supplementation in an athletic population is equivocal. Several studies have shown improved performance following supplemental provision. In a double-blind study, Brilla and Haley (1992) supplemented a group of untrained males to bring the total magnesium intake up to 8 mg/kg/day while providing a placebo to another matched group. Both groups performed multiple sets of lower body resistance exercise 3 times a week for 7 weeks. Results showed that the supplemented group displayed a significantly greater increase in strength compared to controls. These findings suggest that a magnesium intake in excess of current recommendations may be beneficial in activities relying on anaerobic glycolysis. Several other studies have shown benefits of supplementation associated with endurance-oriented exercise (Brilla and Gunter 1995, Golf et al. 1998, Ripari et al. 1989). When taking the entire body of literature into account, however, the evidence does not seem to support the use of magnesium supplementation for enhancing strength-, anaerobic-lactacid-, or aerobic-related performance, as most studies fail to show significant effects (Newhouse and Finstad 2000). This may be specific to the population studied and their initial magnesium levels. Young athletes who are deficient and find it difficult to meet daily needs through food sources may indeed benefit from supplementation.

6.2.4 Zinc

Zinc is a trace mineral that is one of the most widely distributed elements in the body (Deuster et al. 1989). The functions of zinc are varied and involve numerous physiological systems such as immunity, reproduction, taste, wound healing, skeletal development, behavior, and gastrointestinal function (Lukaski 2004). Zinc is also responsible for a diverse array of bodily functions including nucleic acid and protein synthesis, cellular differentiation and replication, and glucose use and insulin secretion, and multiple aspects of hormone metabolism (Lukaski 2004). On the basis of these factors, it has been theorized that zinc plays a significant role in human performance.

In children, the RDA for zinc in children aged 9–13 years is 8 mg/day irrespective of gender (Institute of Medicine Food and Nutrition Board 2001). The recommendations rise during adolescence, with girls and boys aged 14–18 years requiring 9 and 11 mg/day, respectively (Institute of Medicine Food and Nutrition Board 2001). On average, zinc intake is below recommended levels in the general population for both children and adolescents (Munoz et al. 1997). Similarly, consumption of zinc in young athletes tends to be suboptimal, with low intakes more prevalent in female competitors compared to males (Lukaski 2004). Soric et al. (2008) found that 13% of prepubescent girls who competed in aesthetic sports had inadequate intakes of zinc. Moreover, female adolescent volleyball players were shown to consume only 7.4 mg/day—well below recommended levels for this age group (Beals 2002). However, there is evidence that when athletes consume at least 70% of the RDA for zinc, plasma concentrations fall within the range of normal values (Lukaski 2004).

Numerous studies show that physical activity can alter zinc status. Serum zinc concentrations generally increased in the immediate postexercise period, conceivably mediated by the movement of zinc from working skeletal muscle into plasma pursuant to proteolysis from the exercise bout (Lukaski 2000). On the other hand, exercise appears to suppress zinc levels chronically. Dressendorfer and Sockolov (1980) found that approximately 25% of competitive male runners displayed below-normal zinc levels, with values correlating to weekly training distance. Duester et al. (1989) compared zinc status in high trained versus untrained women before and after a 25-mg oral zinc load. Results showed that the highly trained subjects had significantly greater urinary zinc excretion than those who were not trained, which was attributed to the daily effects of exercise. These findings are consistent with those of Anderson et al. (1984), who reported that male runners had significantly greater zinc excretion on training days compared to nontraining days. Similar findings have been found in adolescent athletes. Karakukcu et al. (2013) carried out a multiphased study in teenage males that included an acute mineral status assessment following a 4-week boxing training program with and without zinc supplementation. Results showed that zinc levels were significantly decreased after 4 weeks of nonsupplemented boxing training.

In athletes, a zinc deficiency is associated with a number of disorders including anorexia, loss of body weight, latent fatigue, and an increased risk of osteoporosis (Micheletti et al. 2001). Zinc supplementation in this population has generally focused on its effects on immune and antioxidant function. A number of studies have shown that zinc supplementation can enhance immune-related factors in those who perform intense physical activity. Kara et al. (2011) found that zinc supplementation boosted the production of tumor necrosis factor-α, interleukin-2, and interpheron-γ levels in young wrestlers aged 15–17 years, suggesting a positive effect on immune function. de Oliveira Kde et al. (2009) showed a beneficial effect of 12 weeks of zinc supplementation on antioxidant status in a group of adolescent male football players. Given that altered immune function can impair recovery and thus negatively impact performance, these findings provide a theoretical basis for supplementation in young athletes. However, it is not clear whether supplementing with zinc actually translates into beneficial effects on human performance. In a double-blind, crossover design, women supplemented with 135 mg of zinc/day for 14 days displayed significantly greater increases in dynamic isokinetic strength and isometric endurance compared to placebo, suggesting that supplementation may be beneficial in improving activities relying heavily on fast-twitch muscle fiber involvement (Krotkiewski et al. 1982). Conversely, Peake et al. (2003) found no benefits from zinc supplementation during periods of moderately increased training volume in male runners. Overall, there is a paucity of research on the efficacy of zinc supplementation in an athletic population and its use in this regard remains speculative. Moreover, recent studies show that altering antioxidant status through supplementation can actually interfere with recovery from exercise, indicating a potential detrimental effect from supplemental zinc (Gomez-Cabrera et al. 2012). Importantly, a high zinc intake can have a negative effect on copper, magnesium, and iron status (de Oliveira Kde et al. 2009, Karakukcu et al. 2013). Supplementation with zinc should therefore be approached with caution.

6.3 CONCLUSION

The body of research underlying our knowledge of the essential micronutrient requirements of child and adolescent athletes is growing and evolving, but still vastly incomplete. Methodological, logistical, and ethical constraints will continue to challenge this area of study in terms of performing trials that can adequately address lingering questions. Young subjects are a diverse and dynamic population whose variables are inherently difficult to control. Nevertheless, the current data yield important practical implications for various therapeutic and preventive purposes, and they also provide considerations for future study.

An ongoing challenge is finding realistic, reliable ways to consume these essential nutrients via the diet, supplementation, or both. In the context of youth athletics, vitamin D has received perhaps the most extensive study. This is likely due to a combination of its very broad range of critical biological functions combined with its widespread deficiency across several populations. Vitamin D in substantial doses is also relatively uncommon in the food supply. This exacerbates the problem of inadequate intake, but it has also driven the study of supplementation as a simple, feasible intervention. However, despite the potential to increase force output of skeletal muscle via sensitizing calcium-binding sites on the sarcoplasmic reticulum (Dahlquist et al. 2015), it is unclear whether vitamin D supplementation can reliably impart ergogenic effects. It was recently seen that adolescent competitive swimmers with vitamin D insufficiency (serum 25 [OH]D <30 ng/mL) did not improve performance beyond placebo despite 12 weeks of D3 supplementation at 2000 IU/day (Dubnov-Raz et al. 2015). The research in this area is in its infancy, and further investigations of various sports and dose responses may provide more definitive conclusions.

Essential vitamins and minerals must be consumed from external sources since the body cannot biosynthesize them. Major challenges to meeting these needs are determining what the requirements are in the first place, and how these needs might be altered with varying modes and magnitudes of physical activity. It is clear that certain population subsets are at higher risk of deficiency than others. It is also clear that inadequate intakes can be free of outward manifestations, such as the case of iron deficiency as it progresses toward anemia. This highlights the importance of regularly monitoring the nutritional status of young athletes. It also highlights the importance of individualized patient/client care by a multidisciplinary team of health and medical professionals.

REFERENCES

Abrams, S. A. 2011. Calcium and vitamin D requirements for optimal bone mass during adolescence. *Curr Opin Clin Nutr Metab Care* 14 (6):605–9. doi: 10.1097/MCO.0b013e32834b2b01.

Anderson, R. A., M. M. Polansky, and N. A. Bryden. 1984. Acute effects on chromium, copper, zinc, and selected clinical variables in urine and serum of male runners. *Biol Trace Elem Res* 6 (4):327–36. doi: 10.1007/BF02989240.

Balasubramanian, S., K. Dhanalakshmi, and S. Amperayani. 2013. Vitamin D deficiency in childhood—A review of current guidelines on diagnosis and management. *Indian Pediatr* 50 (7):669–75.

Barker, T., V. T. Henriksen, T. B. Martins, H. R. Hill, C. R. Kjeldsberg, E. D. Schneider, B. M. Dixon, and L. K. Weaver. 2013. Higher serum 25-hydroxyvitamin D concentrations associate with a faster recovery of skeletal muscle strength after muscular injury. *Nutrients* 5 (4):1253–75. doi: 10.3390/nu5041253.

Barker, T., E. D. Schneider, B. M. Dixon, V. T. Henriksen, and L. K. Weaver. 2013. Supplemental vitamin D enhances the recovery in peak isometric force shortly after intense exercise. *Nutr Metab (Lond)* 10 (1):69. doi: 10.1186/1743-7075-10-69.

Beals, K. A. 2002. Eating behaviors, nutritional status, and menstrual function in elite female adolescent volleyball players. *J Am Diet Assoc* 102 (9):1293–6.

Brilla, L. R. and K. B. Gunter. 1995. Effect of magnesium supplementation on exercise time to exhaustion. *Med Exerc Nutr Health* 4:230–3.

Brilla, L. R. and T. F. Haley. 1992. Effect of magnesium supplementation on strength training in humans. *J Am Coll Nutr* 11 (3):326–9.

Brownlie, T., V. Utermohlen, P. S. Hinton, C. Giordano, and J. D. Haas. 2002. Marginal iron deficiency without anemia impairs aerobic adaptation among previously untrained women. *Am J Clin Nutr* 75 (4):734–42.

Brutsaert, T. D., S. Hernandez-Cordero, J. Rivera, T. Viola, G. Hughes, and J. D. Haas. 2003. Iron supplementation improves progressive fatigue resistance during dynamic knee extensor exercise in iron-depleted, nonanemic women. *Am J Clin Nutr* 77 (2):441–8.

Constantini, N. W., R. Arieli, G. Chodick, and G. Dubnov-Raz. 2010. High prevalence of vitamin D insufficiency in athletes and dancers. *Clin J Sport Med* 20 (5):368–71. doi: 10.1097/JSM.0b013e3181f207f2.

Dahlquist, D. T., B. P. Dieter, and M. S. Koehle. 2015. Plausible ergogenic effects of vitamin D on athletic performance and recovery. *J Int Soc Sports Nutr* 12:33. doi: 10.1186/s12970-015-0093-8.

de Oliveira Kde, J., C. M. Donangelo, A. V. de Oliveira Jr., C. L. da Silveira, and J. C. Koury. 2009. Effect of zinc supplementation on the antioxidant, copper, and iron status of physically active adolescents. *Cell Biochem Funct* 27 (3):162–6. doi: 10.1002/cbf.1550.

Deuster, P. A., B. A. Day, A. Singh, L. Douglass, and P. B. Moser-Veillon. 1989. Zinc status of highly trained women runners and untrained women. *Am J Clin Nutr* 49 (6):1295–301.

Dressendorfer, R. H., and R. Sockolov. 1980. Hypozincemia in runners. *Phys Sportsmed* 8:97–100.

Dubnov-Raz, G., N. Livne, R. Raz, A. H. Cohen, and N. W. Constantini. 2015. Vitamin D supplementation and physical performance in adolescent swimmers. *Int J Sport Nutr Exerc Metab* 25 (4):317–25. doi: 10.1123/ijsnem.2014-0180.

Finstad, E. W., I. J. Newhouse, H. C. Lukaski, J. E. McAuliffe, and C. R. Stewart. 2001. The effects of magnesium supplementation on exercise performance. *Med Sci Sports Exerc* 33 (3):493–8.

Golf, S. W., S. Bender, and J. Gruttner. 1998. On the significance of magnesium in extreme physical stress. *Cardiovasc Drugs Ther* 12 (Suppl 2):197–202.

Gomez-Cabrera, M. C., M. Ristow, and J. Vina. 2012. Antioxidant supplements in exercise: Worse than useless? *Am J Physiol Endocrinol Metab* 302 (4):E476–7; author reply E478–9. doi: 10.1152/ajpendo.00,567.2011.

Greer, F. R., N. F. Krebs, and Nutrition American Academy of Pediatrics Committee on. 2006. Optimizing bone health and calcium intakes of infants, children, and adolescents. *Pediatrics* 117 (2):578–85. doi: 10.1542/peds.2005-2822.

Gropper, S. S., J. L. Smith, and J. L. Groff. 2009. *Advanced Nutrition and Human Metabolism*. Belmont, CA: Wadsworth Cengage Learning.

Heaney, R. P. 2008. Vitamin D: Criteria for safety and efficacy. *Nutr Rev* 66 (10 Suppl 2):S178–81. doi: 10.1111/j.1753-4887.2008.00,102.x.

Hinton, P. S., C. Giordano, T. Brownlie, and J. D. Haas. 2000. Iron supplementation improves endurance after training in iron-depleted, nonanemic women. *J Appl Physiol (1985)* 88 (3):1103–11.

Hoch, A. Z., K. Goossen, and T. Kretschmer. 2008. Nutritional requirements of the child and teenage athlete. *Phys Med Rehabil Clin N Am* 19 (2):373–98, x. doi: 10.1016/j.pmr.2007.12.001.

Holick, M. F. 2004. Vitamin D: Importance in the prevention of cancers, type 1 diabetes, heart disease, and osteoporosis. *Am J Clin Nutr* 79 (3):362–71.

Holick, M. F., N. C. Binkley, H. A. Bischoff-Ferrari, C. M. Gordon, D. A. Hanley, R. P. Heaney, M. H. Murad, C. M. Weaver, and Society Endocrine. 2011. Evaluation, treatment, and prevention of vitamin D deficiency: An Endocrine Society clinical practice guideline. *J Clin Endocrinol Metab* 96 (7):1911–30. doi: 10.1210/jc.2011-0385.

Holick, M. F. and T. C. Chen. 2008. Vitamin D deficiency: A worldwide problem with health consequences. *Am J Clin Nutr* 87 (4):1080S–6S.

Institute of Medicine Food and Nutrition Board. 1997. *Dietary Reference Intakes: Calcium, Phosphorus, Magnesium, Vitamin D and Fluoride*. Washington, DC: National Academy Press.

Institute of Medicine Food and Nutrition Board. 2001. *Dietary Reference Intakes for Vitamin A, Vitamin K, Arsenic, Boron, Chromium, Copper, Iodine, Iron, Manganese, Molybdenum, Nickel, Silicon, Vanadium and Zinc*. Washington, DC: National Academy Press.

Juzwiak, C. R., O. M. Amancio, M. S. Vitalle, V. L. Szejnfeld, and M. M. Pinheiro. 2008. Effect of calcium intake, tennis playing, and body composition on bone–mineral density of Brazilian male adolescents. *Int J Sport Nutr Exerc Metab* 18 (5):524–38.

Kara, E., M. Ozal, M. Gunay, M. Kilic, A. K. Baltaci, and R. Mogulkoc. 2011. Effects of exercise and zinc supplementation on cytokine release in young wrestlers. *Biol Trace Elem Res* 143 (3):1435–40. doi: 10.1007/s12011-011-9005-1.

Karakukcu, C., Y. Polat, Y. A. Torun, and A. K. Pac. 2013. The effects of acute and regular exercise on calcium, phosphorus and trace elements in young amateur boxers. *Clin Lab* 59 (5–6):557–62.

Krotkiewski, M., M. Gudmundsson, P. Backstrom, and K. Mandroukas. 1982. Zinc and muscle strength and endurance. *Acta Physiol Scand* 116 (3):309–11. doi: 10.1111/j.1748-1716.1982.tb07146.x.

Kunstel, K. 2005. Calcium requirements for the athlete. *Curr Sports Med Rep* 4 (4):203–6.

Lukaski, H. C. 2000. Magnesium, zinc, and chromium nutriture and physical activity. *Am J Clin Nutr* 72 (2 Suppl):585S–93.

Lukaski, H. C. 2004. Vitamin and mineral status: Effects on physical performance. *Nutrition* 20 (7–8):632–44. doi: 10.1016/j.nut.2004.04.001.

Medline Plus. 2012. 25-Hydroxy vitamin D test. United States Library of Medicine. Accessed August 1, 2015. http://www.nlm.nih.gov/medlineplus/ency/article/003,569.htm.

Mesias, M., I. Seiquer, and M. P. Navarro. 2011. Calcium nutrition in adolescence. *Crit Rev Food Sci Nutr* 51 (3):195–209. doi: 10.1080/10408390903502872.

Meyer, F., H. O'Connor, and S. M. Shirreffs. 2007. Nutrition for the young athlete. *J Sports Sci* 25 (Suppl 1):S73–82. doi: 10.1080/02640410701607338.

Micheletti, A., R. Rossi, and S. Rufini. 2001. Zinc status in athletes: Relation to diet and exercise. *Sports Med* 31 (8):577–82.

Munoz, K. A., S. M. Krebs-Smith, R. Ballard-Barbash, and L. E. Cleveland. 1997. Food intakes of U.S. children and adolescents compared with recommendations. *Pediatrics* 100 (3 Pt 1):323–9.

National Research Council. 1998. *Dietary Reference Intakes for Thiamin, Riboflavin, Niacin, Vitamin B6, Folate, Vitamin B12, Pantothenic Acid, Biotin, and Choline*. Washington, DC: National Academy Press.

Newhouse, I. J. and E. W. Finstad. 2000. The effects of magnesium supplementation on exercise performance. *Clin J Sport Med* 10 (3):195–200.

Peake, J. M., D. F. Gerrard, and J. F. Griffin. 2003. Plasma zinc and immune markers in runners in response to a moderate increase in training volume. *Int J Sports Med* 24 (3):212–6. doi: 10.1055/s-2003-39,094.

Petrie, H. J., E. A. Stover, and C. A. Horswill. 2004. Nutritional concerns for the child and adolescent competitor. *Nutrition* 20 (7–8):620–31. doi: 10.1016/j.nut.2004.04.002.

Ripari, P., G. Pieralisi, M. A. Giamberardino, A. Resina, and L. Vecchiet. 1989. Effects of magnesium pidolate on cardiorespiratory submaximal effort parameters. *Magnes Res* 2:70–1.

Ross, A. C., J. E. Manson, S. A. Abrams, J. F. Aloia, P. M. Brannon, S. K. Clinton, R. A. Durazo-Arvizu et al. 2011. The 2011 report on dietary reference intakes for calcium and vitamin D from the Institute of Medicine: What clinicians need to know. *J Clin Endocrinol Metab* 96 (1):53–8. doi: 10.1210/jc.2010-2704.

Ross, A. C., C. L. Taylor, A. L. Yaktine, and H. B. Del Valle. 2011. *Dietary Reference Intakes for Calcium and Vitamin D*. Washington, DC: National Academy Press.

Rowland, T. W., S. A. Black, and J. F. Kelleher. 1987. Iron deficiency in adolescent endurance athletes. *J Adolesc Health Care* 8 (4):322–6.

Rude, R. K. 2012. Magnesium. In *Modern Nutrition in Health and Disease*, eds. A. C. Ross, B. Caballero, R. J. Cousins, K. L. Tucker, and T. R. Ziegler, 159–75. Baltimore, MD: Lippincott Williams & Wilkins.

Soric, M., M. Misigoj-Durakovic, and Z. Pedisic. 2008. Dietary intake and body composition of prepubescent female aesthetic athletes. *Int J Sport Nutr Exerc Metab* 18 (3):343–54.

Speich, M., A. Pineau, and F. Ballereau. 2001. Minerals, trace elements and related biological variables in athletes and during physical activity. *Clin Chim Acta* 312 (1–2):1–11.

Spodaryk, K. 2002. Iron metabolism in boys involved in intensive physical training. *Physiol Behav* 75 (1–2):201–6.

Suedekum, N. A. and R. J. Dimeff. 2005. Iron and the athlete. *Curr Sports Med Rep* 4 (4):199–202.

Unnithan, V. B., and S. Goulopoulou. 2004. Nutrition for the pediatric athlete. *Curr Sports Med Rep* 3 (4):206–11.

Wacker, M. and M. F. Holick. 2013. Vitamin D—Effects on skeletal and extraskeletal health and the need for supplementation. *Nutrients* 5 (1):111–48. doi: 10.3390/nu5010111.

7 The Importance of Proper Fluid and Hydration

Gabriela Tomedi Leites and Flavia Meyer

CONTENTS

Abstract 114
7.1 Introduction 114
7.2 Definitions and Classifications 115
    7.2.1 Hydration, Hypohydration, and Hyperhydration 115
    7.2.2 Exertional Heat Illness 115
7.3 Hypohydration and Performance 115
    7.3.1 Hypohydration and Aerobic Performance 115
    7.3.2 Hypohydration and High-Intensity Intermittent Efforts
          and Strength Performance 116
    7.3.3 Hypohydration and Cognitive Function 118
7.4 Factors Affecting Sweating Patterns 118
    7.4.1 Individual Factors 119
          7.4.1.1 Chronological Age and Biological Maturation, Sex, and Body
                 Composition 119
          7.4.1.2 Heat Acclimatization and Acclimation 119
    7.4.2 Exercise Pattern and Physical Training 120
    7.4.3 Environmental 120
          7.4.3.1 Clothing 120
7.5 Practical Considerations 121
    7.5.1 Estimation of Hydration Status and Sweating Responses 121
    7.5.2 Recommendations and Strategies for Fluid Replacement 122
          7.5.2.1 Before Exercise 122
          7.5.2.2 During Exercise 122
          7.5.2.3 After Exercise 123
7.6 Sports Drinks and Energy Drinks 123
7.7 Educational Intervention 123
7.8 Considerations of Hydration in Chronic Health Conditions 124
    7.8.1 Lung Conditions 124
          7.8.1.1 Asthma 124
          7.8.1.2 Cystic Fibrosis 125
    7.8.2 Metabolic Conditions 125
          7.8.2.1 Obesity 125
          7.8.2.2 Diabetes 126
7.9 Conclusions 126
References 126

ABSTRACT

Proper hydration for the exercising child and adolescent is important to guarantee optimal sport performance and avoid adverse health problems. While sweating is essential for body cooling, it increases the chances of dehydration during exercise. Hypohydration is associated with an increase in body core temperature and cardiovascular strain and a decrease in stroke volume during exercise. It may also affect metabolic responses, resulting in impaired aerobic and high-intensity endurance performance and premature fatigue. There is no single answer regarding the optimal drink volume and composition for adequate hydration as many factors interact to influence sweating rate, such as genetics, chronological age, biological maturation status, body composition, sex, heat acclimatization and acclimation, fitness levels, exercise intensity and modality, and environmental conditions. Practical considerations are necessary to guarantee proper fluid balance prior, during, and after exercise, and also implement educational intervention. Additionally, children and adolescents with well-controlled chronic diseases commonly participate in competitive athletic activities despite their fundamentally altered physiology. For clinical populations, extra caution is needed to monitor thermoregulatory and hydration responses and maintain proper hydration. Therefore, the purpose of this chapter is to review the importance of proper hydration and the physiological consequences of fluid imbalance in pediatric populations. This chapter will include definitions and classifications of hydration, hypohydration, hyperhydration, and exertional heat illnesses, followed by a discussion of the impact of hypohydration and performance in youth, factors affecting sweating patterns, practical considerations, and some recommendations and strategies for fluid replacement. Considerations for proper hydration for youth living with chronic diseases will also be discussed in the final section.

7.1 INTRODUCTION

Proper body fluid balance is required for young athletes to guarantee optimal sport performance and avoid adverse health problems (Bar-Or and Rowland 2004; Meyer et al. 2007, 2012). Children and adolescents—as is true with adults—may not ingest enough water, even when available, to compensate their losses during (Bar-Or et al. 1980, Rivera-Brown et al. 1999, Wilk and Bar-Or 1996) or after (Bergeron 2009) prolonged periods of exercise in the heat. Bergeron et al. (2009) showed that fit young athletes who fully rehydrate during rest from a prolonged strenuous exercise in the heat avoided the residual responses that would potentiate a greater thermal and cardiovascular strain in a subsequent exercise bout. Therefore, young athletes who properly rehydrate during and between training and competition events are more likely to guarantee their optimal performance.

Muscle contraction causes substantial production of heat, which should be transported by the vascular system to the skin in order to be dissipated (Rowell 1974; Fink et al. 1975). Sweat evaporation is the primary mechanism to dissipate heat during exercise, especially in warm conditions. While sweating is essential for body cooling through evaporation, it increases chances of dehydration (Casa et al. 2000). To match the volume of sweat losses and fluid intake, it is recommended to have an estimated sweat rate that can vary considerably among and within individuals and may depend on physical fitness, exercise, and thermal conditions (Casa et al. 2000; Maughan et al. 2007; Meyer et al. 2012).

In this chapter, we first clarify some definitions and classifications and then discuss the following aspects with a focus on youth:

- Hypohydration and performance
- Factors affecting sweating patterns
- Practical considerations
- Recommendations and strategies for fluid replacement
- Considerations of hydration in chronic health conditions

7.2 DEFINITIONS AND CLASSIFICATIONS

7.2.1 HYDRATION, HYPOHYDRATION, AND HYPERHYDRATION

Body hydration describes body water status, including euhydration, hypohydration, and hyperhydration (Armstrong 2006). Euhydration refers to the normal body water content. Under thermoneutral conditions, the body water content of a healthy active subject should change by about ±0.25%, and under heat conditions, body water deficit may increase by about 0.8%. Exercise-induced dehydration and hypohydration are often used synonymously, but dehydration is the active process of losing water and hypohydration refers to a state of body water deficit (Meyer et al. 2012). They are caused by a mismatch of overall water loss (sweating, urine, fecal, and breath) and intake (Mitchell et al. 1972; Bergeron et al. 2011). Involuntary dehydration is a term used to describe the behavior of insufficient fluid intake to replenish the losses, even when fluids are available to drink *ad libitum* (Greenleaf 1992; Bar-Or and Rowland 2004).

Hyperhydration is when body water content is above normal, and, as with hypohydration, is undesirable. Hyperhydration, although unusual in young athletes, is a concern when the excessive fluid ingestion involves low-sodium or sodium-free beverages and the resultant sweating from a prolonged event is excessive. Signs and symptoms of hyperhydration may start with light-headedness, nausea, vomiting, and headaches and, if severe, cramps, lethargy, mental confusion, and edema of the feet and hands.

7.2.2 EXERTIONAL HEAT ILLNESS

A Centers for Disease Control and Prevention (CDC 2011) report, based on data from the National Electronic Injury Surveillance System—All Injury Program reported that, between 2001 and 2009, heat illnesses caused by sports and recreation were more prevalent among males (72.5%) and among those aged 10–14 years (18.2%) and 15–19 years (35.6%). These conditions may be associated with body fluid imbalances, particularly under very hot or humid conditions and, therefore, are preventable.

Exertional heat illnesses usually refer to three categories: heat cramps, heat exhaustion, and heat stroke. Heat syncope and exertional hyponatremia may also be included. Although clinical manifestations may overlap, Table 7.1 summarizes the definition, signs, and symptoms of each of these exertional heat illnesses based on the study by Binkley et al. (2002).

7.3 HYPOHYDRATION AND PERFORMANCE

7.3.1 HYPOHYDRATION AND AEROBIC PERFORMANCE

Previous studies (Inbar et al. 2004; Rivera-Brown et al. 2006) pointed out that youth might present disadvantageous responses in comparison to those of adults while dehydrating during prolonged exercise in the heat. The direct association between hypohydration levels and core temperature as exercise continues is a reason to avoid body water deficits and risk of exertional heat injury (Bar-Or et al. 1980; Bar-Or 2001). A classic study (Bar-Or et al. 1980) showed that 1%–2% dehydration in children (10–12 years old) who exercised intermittently during 3.5 h in the heat increased rectal temperature by ~1°C. Such an increase in rectal temperature was twice as high as that observed in another study with adults (Bar-Or et al. 1976). It seems that under exercise and heat stress, dehydration at 1%–2% increases body temperature; at 3% decreases performance time; at 4%–6% cramps and heat exhaustion may occur, and above 6% increases the risk of heat stroke (Greenleaf 1992). However, it is unclear whether these thresholds can be extrapolated to young athletes. In laboratory settings, studies restrict dehydration levels at 2% in children and adolescents due to health constrains. However, a youth triathlon event in the tropical climate of Costa Rica demonstrated that a level up to 3% hypohydration can occur in children and adolescents (9–17 years old) without any apparent impairment in performance and health (Aragon-Vargas et al. 2013).

TABLE 7.1
Characteristics of Exertional Heat Illnesses by Categories

Illness	Characteristics
Heat cramps	Severe, spreading, and sustained painful muscle contractions (cramps) that result from prolonged exercise, usually at high ambient temperatures.
	Possible causes: dehydration, electrolyte imbalances, and neuromuscular fatigue. Signs and symptoms of dehydration include thirst and sweating.
Heat exhaustion	Inability to continue exercise. Presence of any combination of heavy sweating, dehydration, sodium loss, and energy depletion. Preventable by matching fluid intake with body fluid losses, including electrolytes (mainly sodium). Normal or elevated body core temperature.
	Signs and symptoms of dehydration, dizziness, light-headedness, syncope, headache, nausea, diarrhea, decreased urine output, persistent muscle cramps, pallor, profuse sweating, chills, cool and clammy skin, intestinal cramps, urge to defecate, weakness, and hyperventilation.
Exertional heat stroke	Elevated core temperature (>39°C) accompanied by signs of organ system failure due to hyperthermia.
	Central nervous system symptoms such as dizziness, irrational behavior, confusion, irritability, delirium, disorientation, seizures, loss of consciousness, and coma. Signs and symptoms of dehydration, weakness, hot and wet or dry skin, hypotension, hyperventilation, vomiting, and diarrhea.
Heat syncope	Condition caused by peripheral vasodilation, postural pooling of blood, diminished venous return and cardiac output, and cerebral ischemia. Usually involves exposure to a high ambient temperature, mainly if the person is not heat acclimatized and/or dehydrated. Main symptoms are fatigue, tunnel vision, pale or sweaty skin, decreased heart rate, dizziness, light-headedness, and fainting.
Exertional hyponatremia	When blood sodium concentration drops to levels below 130 mmol L^{-1}, which can occur due to one or a combination of (1) excessive sodium loss from heavy sweating, (2) excessive intake of drinks that have no or low sodium content, and (3) body water retention. It is uncommon, but when documented usually occurs in activities lasting more than 4 h. Signs and symptoms include body core temperature <40°C, nausea, vomiting, extremity (hands and feet) swelling, progressive headache, mental confusion and impairment, lethargy, altered consciousness, apathy, pulmonary edema, cerebral edema, seizures, and coma.

In adults, it is established that a level up to 3% hypohydration impairs aerobic exercise performance (Cheuvront et al. 2005, 2010; Sawka et al. 2007). Hypohydration can reduce muscle blood flow and modify skeletal muscle metabolism during prolonged exercise in the heat (Jentjens et al. 2002). On the other hand, a single bout of very intense exercise in a euhydrated person should not induce significant dehydration as it cannot be maintained for a long period (Cheuvront et al. 2010).

Hypohydration can increase body core temperature, leading to additional cardiovascular challenges during exercise. It may also affect metabolic responses, resulting in aerobic performance impairment and premature fatigue (Sawka 1992; Cheuvront et al. 2010). These detrimental responses were mostly observed in prolonged, and therefore, submaximal (~50%–70% VO_{2max}) exercise activities.

7.3.2 Hypohydration and High-Intensity Intermittent Efforts and Strength Performance

Most young athletes are involved in sport modalities characterized by high-intensity and intermittent exercise patterns such as cycling, basketball, soccer, football, gymnastics, and tennis. Young athletes may face difficulties in maintaining euhydration during practices and competitions in a variety of sport modalities such as basketball (Hoffman et al. 1995), triathlons (Aragon-Vargas et al. 2013), soccer (Decher et al. 2008), and judo (Artioli et al. 2010) during practices and competitions. Furthermore, hypohydration can potentially impair sport performance skills (Meyer et al. 2012).

A recent study (Wilk et al. 2013a) assessed the effect of 0%, 1%, and 2% hypohydration on high-intensity cycling performance in nine 10- to 12-year-old boys. Participants attended three sessions where 0%, 1%, and 2% dehydration were induced through cycling six 10-min bouts at 40%–45% VO_{2max} in the heat (35°C and 50% relative humidity) of a climatic clamber. After a 45-min recovery period, the boys were evaluated in a high-intensity (90% VO_{2max}) cycling performance test in the heat. The mean time to exhaustion was ~2 min earlier at 2% hypohydration (5.38 min) compared to boys who were euhydrated (7.35 min). However, performance time at 1% hypohydration (6.20 min) was not statistically different from that of 0% and 2% hypohydration sessions. The total mechanical work was 15.5% (42.3 kJ) and 23.3% (35.5 kJ) lower at 1% and 2% hypohydration in relation to the euhydrated session (49.3 kJ). This study indicates that even a mild dehydration may impair a high-intensity cycling performance in healthy, young boys in the heat.

Baker et al. (2007) evaluated the effect of 1%–4% dehydration versus euhydration with a carbohydrate solution on basketball performance in older adolescents and young adult players (17–28 years old). They completed six trials of 3 h walking on a treadmill in the heat (40°C and 20% relative humidity), and a progressive detriment in high-intensity and overall skill performance occurred as dehydration increased. The dehydration level at which performance decrement reached statistical significance was 2% for combined timed and shooting drills. At 3% dehydration, defensive slide time, sprinting defensive slide, and lay-up performance were impaired, and at 4%, repeated vertical jump and stationary shooting performance were impaired. In 15 boys, 12–15 years old (Dougherty et al. 2006), a 2% dehydration induced by exercise in the heat impaired performance and basketball skill drills, including various individual and combined shootings percentages, sprint, and lateral movement. On the other hand, Carvalho et al. (2011) showed that ~2.5% dehydration induced by exercise did not impair basketball drills (2-point, 3-point, and free-throw shooting, suicide sprints, and defensive zigzags) in adolescent athletes. No impairment occurred in anaerobic power, vertical jumping, and shooting performance at ~2% dehydration in 10 young basketball players (Hoffman et al. 1995). Another study (Cheuvront et al. 2010) examined vertical jump using a force platform in 15 active males (mean age 24 years) in three situations: euhydrated, hypohydrated (3.8%), and hypohydrated while wearing a weighted vest (lost water mass was replaced with a weighted vest). Jump height was similar between the euhydrated and hypohydrated status, but it was 4% lower while wearing a weighted vest compared to euhydrated. In sum, these studies indicate that detrimental effects may occur with varying levels of hypohydration on required skills for basketball performance. Hypohydration and performance in other youth sports are less documented. Decher et al. (2008) observed gradual dehydration according to urine specific gravity (USG) over 4 days of youth (age range 7–17 years) soccer and football games. On the 4th day, about 40% reached a moderate, and 30% a severe hypohydration according to their USG (1.025–1.029 and >1.030, respectively); but no apparent effect on performance was reported. In a regular 1–1.6-h training session in the heat (Perrone et al. 2011), dehydration levels of 21 soccer and 26 young futsal players was minimal (<1%) and probably of no biological significance to impair performance or health.

Combat sport modalities are a concern as athletes may intentionally dehydrate as they are classified according to their body mass to match opponents' physical characteristics. Studies have reported a high prevalence (60%–90%) of intentional rapid weight loss (2%–10% body mass) among high school, collegiate, and international style wrestling in an attempt to benefit by competing against lighter, smaller, and weaker opponents (Steen and Brownell 1990; Alderman et al. 2004; Franchini et al. 2012). The impact of weight loss on performance in young combat athletes is not clear. An investigation (Artioli et al. 2010), including 14 male judo athletes divided into weight loss (mean age 20 years) and control (mean age 22 years), showed that rapid weight loss (~5% body weight reduction in a self-selected regime) followed by a 4-h recovery (allowed to re-feed and rehydrate) had no effect on judo-related performance. In conclusion, the available data are inconsistent and insufficient to establish levels of dehydration that might impair high-intensity intermittent efforts and strength performance, specifically in child athletes.

7.3.3 Hypohydration and Cognitive Function

Sport performance may also depend on cognitive, technical, tactical, physical, and physiological factors (Stolen et al. 2005). Cognitive performance is required to make decisions during the match and allocate attention at different points of a dynamic scene (Faubert and Sidebottom 2012). During a game or sport situation, an athlete should integrate cognitive performance and complex moving patterns. Detriments in cognitive performance such as vigilance, perceived discrimination, long- (Cian et al. 2000) and short-term memory (Gopinathan et al. 1988; Cian et al. 2000), visual-motor tracking, and attention (Gopinathan et al. 1988) have been shown to occur from up to 2% dehydration in adults (Grandjean and Grandjean 2007). Not much information exists on the pediatric population. One study (Wilk et al. 2004) indicated that exercise-induced dehydration (~2%) did not affect cognitive functions of choice reaction time, choice movement time, selective attention goal-directed aiming, and short-term memory in 10- to 12-year-old nonathletic boys. However, one study (Bar-David et al. 2005) has shown that hypohydrated status compared to euhydrated status can impair cognitive function in the form of short-term memory, verbal analogy, and making groups.

7.4 FACTORS AFFECTING SWEATING PATTERNS

Sweating has a large ability to liberate heat (~580 kcal L^{-1}) and is controlled by the hypothalamus, specifically in the thermosensitive neurons, and is activated when skin and body core temperature increases (Shibasaki et al. 2006; Wilson 2013). Sweating patterns involve not only the amount and rate but also the characteristics of sweating threshold, sweat drop area, proportion of skin covered with sweat, and the density of heat-activated sweat glands. Sweating function is apparently fully developed by the third year of life, though children may present different sweating responses than adults due to their physical and physiological characteristics.

As shown in Table 7.2, many factors interact to influence sweating rate, such as individual influences (genetics, chronological age, biological maturation status, body composition, sex, heat acclimatization, and acclimation and fitness levels), exercise (intensity and modality), and environmental conditions (e.g., humidity, temperature, solar radiation, and clothing) (Maughan et al. 2007; Meyer et al. 2012).

TABLE 7.2
Individual, Exercise, and Environmental Factors That Affect Sweat Volume during Exercise

Factors	Sweat Volume	References
Individual		
Age/biological maturation	↑	Drinkwater et al. (1977), Araki et al. (1979), Bar-Or et al. (1980), Davies (1981), Inbar et al. (1981), Sato et al. (1987), Meyer et al. (1992), Falk et al. (1992a, 1992b), Armstrong and Maresh (1995)
Body composition (muscle mass)	↑	Bar-Or (1989)
Sex (male)	↑	Shapiro et al. (1980), Ichinose-Kuwahara et al. (2010)
Acclimatization and acclimation	↑	Wagner et al. (1972), Inbar et al. (1981), Falk et al. (1992b)
Endurance fitness levels/physical training	↑	Inbar et al. (1981), Buono and Sjoholm (1988)
Exercise		
Intensity	↑	Buono and Sjoholm (1988), Gagnon et al. (2013)
Aquatic ambient	↓	Henkin et al. (2010)
Environmental		
Clothing	↑	Bergeron et al. (2005)

Note: ↑ = increase, ↓ = decrease.

7.4.1 INDIVIDUAL FACTORS

7.4.1.1 Chronological Age and Biological Maturation, Sex, and Body Composition

The number of sweat glands is determined in childhood; thus, the density of glands at the skin surface decreases with growth (Falk 1998). The number of sweat glands (eccrine and apocrine) can vary, ranging from 1.6 to 4.0 million. Eccrine sweat glands are abundantly distributed throughout the body and are responsible for thermoregulatory sweating, which is present and functioning both in children and adults (Shibasaki et al. 2006). Apocrine glands are found mainly in the axilla and pubis, but may not be functional until puberty (Bar-Or and Rowland 2004).

Sweat volume presents great variability, as shown consistently both in youth (Meyer et al. 2012) and adults (Maughan et al. 2007). Children experience a lower absolute sweat rate as well as relative to the body surface area and the number of sweat glands (Meyer et al. 1994; Falk and Dotan 2008). On average, a child's sweat rate is about 40%–50% lower than that of an adult (Armstrong and Maresh 1995). During two 20-min cycling bouts in the heat, sweat rate was 3 mL m^{-2} min^{-1} for prepubescent boys and 6 mL m^{-2} min^{-1} for young male adults (Meyer et al. 1992). In a simulated duathlon, older boys (>15 years) had a higher sweat rate and greater relative rate (1.3 L h^{-1} and 1.95% body mass h^{-1}) than younger boys (<15 years) (0.64 L h^{-1} and 1.23% body mass h^{-1}), and both groups became dehydrated despite having water to ingest *ad libitum* (Luliano et al. 1998). Falk et al. (1992a) determined the associations among the sweat rate and heat-activated sweat glands and biological maturation during two 20-min bouts of exercise in the heat protocol. The prepubertal group presented the lowest sweat rate per surface area and the highest population density of heat-activated sweat glands (glands cm^{-2}) (4.95 and 128, respectively), followed by the mid-pubertal (5.79 and 97) and late-pubertal boys (6.70 and 74). In this study, physical growth and maturation were accompanied by a decreased density of heat-activated sweat glands. Other studies (Shibasaki et al. 1997; Inbar et al. 2004; Wilk et al. 2013b) also reported a higher density of heat-activated sweat glands in prepubertal boys compared to young and older men (Shibasaki et al. 1997; Inbar et al. 2004) and in prepubertal girls compared to pubertal girls (Wilk et al. 2013b). Therefore, it is possible that children, compared to adults, depend relatively more on cutaneous blood flow (convection), instead of the sweat evaporation, for body heat loss (Rowland 2005).

It is still unclear whether such maturational differences in sweating are present in females. One study showed no difference in sweat rates in prepubertal girls and young adult women (Drinkwater et al. 1977) when they ran on a treadmill under thermoneutral (28°C and 45% relative humidity), hot (35°C and 65% relative humidity), or very hot (48°C and 10% relative humidity) environmental conditions. Another study (Rivera-Brown et al. 2006) also showed no difference in sweating rate between prepubertal girls and women when they cycle in the heat. These studies indicate that the lower sweating rate of children compared to adults is more apparent in males than in females. Indeed, men usually have higher sweat rates that might lead to more fluid loss during exercise as compared with women (Sawka et al. 1983; Bar-Or 1989). In addition, men start sweating at a lower body core temperature threshold than women (Frye and Kamon 1981; Lopez et al. 1994; Eijsvogels et al. 2011). However, these differences could be related to other factors such as adiposity level or physical fitness rather than sex itself.

Heat production during exercise is associated with muscle mass, thereby affecting the magnitude of sweat production and dissipation, which are also dependent on body size (Bar-Or 1989; Falk 1998; Rowland 2005). A greater body surface area related to body mass (~40%) could be an advantage for an 8- to 9-year-old child compared to an adult (Bar-Or 1989; Falk 1998; Falk and Dotan 2008). In hot conditions, the child would absorb more heat from the environment and will depend on evaporative cooling as the main route for body heat elimination (Bar-Or and Rowland 2004; Maughan et al. 2007).

7.4.1.2 Heat Acclimatization and Acclimation

Heat acclimatization is a gradual process achieved by regular exposure to natural exercise-heat stress. Acclimation is a similar process, but when the exposure is induced under artificial conditions, usually in a climatic chamber (Bar-Or and Rowland 2004), this process induces various biological adaptations to help reduce the extra physiological strain from heat stress. Sweating adaptations include increases in sweat rate and heat-activated sweat glands, which improve heat loss and attenuate increases in body temperature, heart rate, and thermal discomfort. Despite the increase in sweat rate, heat acclimatization and acclimation also reduce the concentration of sodium in sweat, and apparently induce changes in the concentration of other electrolytes. A 10-day period of heat/exercise exposure in young adults (~20 years old) (Chinevere et al. 2008) showed a 6% increase in sweat rate was accompanied by a reduction in sweat sodium (~34%), calcium (~29%), copper (~50%), and magnesium (~43%), and a trend of lower sweat iron (~75%) and zinc (~23%) concentrations from the 1st to the 10th day. This study suggests that exercise-heat acclimation tends to conserve minerals by decreasing their concentration in sweat.

7.4.2 Exercise Pattern and Physical Training

Water loss through sweating is largely dependent on the exercise pattern such as intensity and duration, despite the ambient (land or aquatic) and thermal conditions. As aerobic fitness increases, thermoregulatory function and heat tolerance improve, which may be due to earlier onset and greater sweating (Drinkwater 1984; Jay et al. 2011; Gagnon et al. 2013). However, training duration may not be long enough to affect sweating responses until puberty. No differences in sweating responses were found between young, artistic gymnasts and nonathlete prepubescent girls cycling in the heat (Leites et al. 2013a). In early-pubertal boys (age 8–10 years), physiological adaptations due to heat acclimatization may be achieved either by exercise in heat (43°C) or by further training (~65% of VO_{2max}) even if the climate is neutral (24°C) (Inbar et al. 1981). Younger players may be training for a shorter period and present lower physical adaptations to the heat; therefore, they may be at a greater risk of heat illness (Bergeron et al. 2005).

Exercise intensity may affect sweat production during exercise. Recent studies (Jay et al. 2011; Gagnon et al. 2013) in adults suggest a given relative workload from that of the maximum determines sweat output during exercise-heat stress. In children, the use of relative or absolute (inducing similar metabolic heat production) exercise intensity to understand sweat responses has yet to be clarified (Haymes et al. 1975; Dougherty et al. 2010).

Sweating responses may be attenuated in aquatic sport modalities. Although aquatic training can generate substantial heat, the skin temperature should quickly reach thermal equilibrium with the surrounding water (Nadel et al. 1974). Therefore, exercising in the water helps dissipate body heat production through convection and conduction instead of evaporation, and a small loss of body weight due to sweating could make hydration during training unnecessary to maintain hydration status (Maughan et al. 2009). Swimmers likely do not need to sweat as much as athletes who train on land because they train in an aquatic environment. Henkin et al. (2010) compared 10 swimmers, 10 runners, and 10 nonathletes cycling in the heat (32°C and 40% relative humidity) for 30 min at similar intensity (10% below the second ventilatory threshold for each individual). The sweat volume of swimmers (~0.9 L) was similar to that of nonathletes (~0.6 L) and lower than that of runners (~1.5 L). Sodium and chloride concentrations of swimmers and nonathletes were higher than those of runners.

7.4.3 Environmental

7.4.3.1 Clothing

Wearing uniforms can increase metabolic heat production and decrease the effectiveness of heat loss mechanisms, especially evaporation (Bergeron et al. 2005). The protective equipment and clothing worn during sports such as football can create a microclimate above the skin surface, reducing heat dissipation. The helmet and pads cover ~50% of the skin surface area, and the remaining football uniform can cover more than 20% (Armstrong et al. 2010). One study

(Armstrong et al. 2010) evaluated high school and college football athletes not highly trained or heat acclimatized, using three different uniforms: control (socks, sneakers, and shorts), partial (uniform without a helmet and shoulder pads), and full uniform. They performed 10 min of repetitive box lifting, 10 min of rest, and up to 60 min of treadmill walking in the heat (~33°C and 48% RH). The resultant sweat rate with full uniform (2.05 L h^{-1}) was ~40% higher than that of the control (1.24 L h^{-1}) and 10% than that of the partial uniform (1.86 L h^{-1}). A practical implication based on this result is that, whenever possible, players should wear as little covering as possible and helmets should be taken off (e.g., during instruction). In addition, clothes with high wicking capacity may assist in evaporative heat loss.

7.5 PRACTICAL CONSIDERATIONS

7.5.1 Estimation of Hydration Status and Sweating Responses

Methods to identify body hydration status include changes (Δ) in body mass and laboratory markers. Measuring body mass is a practical way to verify acute changes in hydration status to calculate the % Δ of body weight; we use the following formula:

$$\frac{\text{Preexercise body weight} \times \text{Postexercise body weight}}{\text{Preexercise body weight}} \times 100$$

Up to 1% body mass change is still considered euhydration. During exercise, a decrease in body mass from 1% to 3% leads to mild hypohydration, from 3% to 5% moderate hypohydration, and >5% serious hypohydration. To verify sweat volume during exercise, it is necessary to measure nude body weight (or as little clothing as possible and dry body) before and after training, corrected by fluid consumed and a voided bladder. To calculate sweat rate, it is necessary to correct sweat volume per the total exercise time. Usually, a change in body mass is combined with laboratory markers such as urinary and blood indices. However, urine markers are not as sensitive to acute changes in hydration status as body mass and blood markers.

Among urinary indices, color, specific gravity, and osmolality are the most common markers used to determine hydration status. To verify urine color, a 1- to 8-level color chart (Armstrong et al. 1994) is used to classify individuals as well (1–2) hydrated, or with minimal (3–4), significant (5–6), and serious (>6) hypohydration. A refractometer is used to measure USG, which is the ratio of the densities between urine and water determined by the number of particles of a sample. No specific reference values have been identified for the pediatric population, so adult references are used for children and adolescents as well, whereby values <1.010 indicate euhydration, 1.010–1.020 mild hypohydration, 1.021–1.030 moderate hypohydration, and >1.030 significant hypohydration. The osmometer is considered a more accurate parameter as it indicates overall solute concentration by comparing the freezing point of the sample to the freezing point of water. Typical values for urine osmolality range from 500–800 mOsmol kg^{-1} (24 h) and 300–900 mOsmol kg^{-1} (random). According to the American College of Sports Medicine (ACSM) position stand (Sawka et al. 2007), a urine osmolality ≤700 mOsmol kg^{-1} is considered euhydration.

Blood markers are another way to evaluate hydration status. Plasma sodium concentration and osmolality tend to increase when the resulting dehydration is from exercise, as sweat is a hypotonic fluid compared to that of plasma. Studies show that plasma (Meyer et al. 1992; Armstrong et al. 1994), osmolality (Popowski et al. 2001), hemoglobin, and noradrenaline concentration (Hoffman et al. 1994) responded to the hydration changes when induced by exercise. In contrast, studies (Francesconi et al. 1987; Armstrong et al. 1994, 1998) showed that hematocrit, serum, testosterone, adrenaline, and cortisol concentrations seem not to be influenced by hypohydration during exercise in the heat.

7.5.2 Recommendations and Strategies for Fluid Replacement

Young athletes should adopt proper attitudes toward fluid ingestion to compensate for their body fluid losses from sweating. Educational and practical interventions can contribute to understanding specific needs and to individualize fluid intake recommendations (Kavouras 2002; McDermott et al. 2009; Kavouras et al. 2012).

To obtain sufficient replenishment during prolonged activities, fluids must be selected with the purpose of stimulating sufficient drinking, rather than quenching thirst (Bar-Or and Rowland 2004). Some fluid-related components can influence thirst perception and fluid consumption during exercise. Studies have shown that fluid flavor, color, and temperature could affect the beverage palatability of a drink and influence voluntary consumption. Plain water is an adequate beverage for fluid replenishment but it may instantaneously reduce thirst and may not stimulate further ingestion. When a grape flavor was added to water, it increased voluntary intake by 45% in boys during prolonged exercise in the heat (Meyer et al. 1994; Wilk and Bar-Or 1996). This volume ingestion, due to the effect of the drink flavoring on voluntary drink intake, maintained children who were euhydrated for a greater period during exercise.

Gastric emptying should be rapid to avoid gastrointestinal distress, as fluid stasis and gastric distension can occur. Exercise intensity, environmental conditions, and fluid volume, osmolality, and temperature can be important factors in gastric emptying and distension during exercise setting. Gastric emptying is thought to be negatively affected as exercise intensities reach over 70% VO_{2max}. Reduced blood flow during exercise to the intestine may impair the absorption of water, carbohydrates, and other nutrients. A study suggested the rate of gastric emptying was decreased in the heat compared with the cool trial (Jentjens et al. 2002). A high volume of fluids and hyperosmolar (carbohydrate-rich) solutions during exercise can delay gastric emptying (Clayton et al. 2013). In contrast, cold beverages could be an advantage compared with warm drinks, because they empty faster from the stomach and are more palatable (Costill and Saltin 1974; Burdon et al. 2012).

Guidelines suggest that appropriate fluids should be consumed before, during, and after training and competition to compensate for sweat loss and maintain the young athlete's euhydration status (Bergeron et al. 2011). Recommendations for young athletes should include monitoring prehydration status, hydration during exercise, and rehydration.

7.5.2.1 Before Exercise

Young athletes should begin exercise euhydrated. ACSM and the National Athletic Trainer's Association (NATA) recommend adding 400–600 mL of fluid 2–3 h before exercise. Body weight is dynamic, so additionally with the determination of the percentage difference between the current body weight and the hydrated baseline body weight, the measurement of USG is an easy and cheap method to determine hydration status before exercise.

7.5.2.2 During Exercise

As multiple factors can affect sweating responses, it is difficult to determine the optimal amount of fluids to drink. During exercise, it is preferable to drink small volumes (100–250 mL) periodically (every 20 min). This pattern helps to avoid abdominal cramps and the heaviness that usually accompanies a large amount of volume intake. In general, boys and girls should drink up to 1.0–1.5 L h^{-1} of exercise to reduce the sweating-induced body water loss, assuming their preexercise hydration status was adequate (Bergeron et al. 2011). A simple and effective practice is to replace body water losses, as almost 100% can be attributed to fluid losses.

Usually, water is enough to maintain proper hydration; however, during strenuous and prolonged exercise sessions, electrolyte-supplemented beverages that emphasize sodium can be more effective to maintain hydration or to rehydrate (Maughan et al. 1996; Bergeron et al. 2006). Adding flavor to water induced a 46% increase in voluntary drinking in nonacclimatized children exercising (50% of VO_2) 3 h intermittently in the heat (35°C and 45%–50% RH); additionally, adding 18 mmol L^{-1}

of NaCl, 2% glucose, and 4% sucrose induced a further 45% increase in voluntary drinking (Wilk and Bar-Or 1996). The flavored carbohydrate–electrolyte beverage helped to increase the amount of drinking during exercise in the heat in acclimatized adolescents (Rivera-Brown et al. 1999). The total amount was sufficient to replace sweat losses for nonacclimatized children as well as for acclimatized adolescents.

Recommendations suggest that the fluid-replacement beverages should be easily accessible in individual fluid containers and flavored to the athlete's preference. In addition, individual containers permit easier monitoring of fluid intake. Clear water bottles marked in 100-mL increments provide visual reminders to athletes to drink (Casa et al. 2000).

7.5.2.3 After Exercise

Athletes often do not consume enough fluids during exercise to balance fluid losses. Consuming up to 150% of weight lost during exercise may be necessary to cover body water losses through sweat and urine. Sodium is used to rehydrate reducing diuresis and maintain plasma osmolality (ACSM, ADA, and Dietitians of Canada 2000). Another recommendation states that a postexercise replenishment of 4 mL kg^{-1} is equally important in assuring a euhydrated state prior to subsequent bouts of exercise (Rowland 2011).

7.6 SPORTS DRINKS AND ENERGY DRINKS

Sports drinks and energy drinks are different products, so they should not be used interchangeably. Sports drinks are carbohydrate–electrolyte-flavored beverages, and sometimes have added protein, vitamins, and nutrients. For pediatric athletes, the purpose of sports drinks is the replacement of water and electrolytes lost in sweat during prolonged exercise, mainly in warm environments, and to improve performance. Despite the lower sweating sodium concentration and losses in children and adolescents compared with those of adults, the resulting sodium balance in response to exercise is expected to be negative, even when rehydration is achieved with a typical sports drink, because these beverages usually contain a lower sodium concentration (~20 mmol L^{-1}) than sweat (Meyer et al. 2012).

Energy drinks are beverages that contain substances such as caffeine, guarana, taurine, ginseng, L-carnitine, creatine, and/or glucorolactone, and are used as an ergogenic aid to enhance performance (Council on Sports Medicine and Fitness 2011). Energy drinks have more caffeine than is suggested for consumption in children and adolescents (2.5 mg kg^{-1} per day and 100 mg per day, respectively). Energy drink-related incidents include liver damage, kidney failure, respiratory disorders, agitation, confusion, seizures, psychotic conditions, rhabdomyolysis, tachycardia, cardiac dysrhythmias, hypertension, heart failure, and death (Seifert et al. 2011). The pediatric population needs to be aware of energy drinks, as there are potentially dangerous consequences of inappropriate use.

7.7 EDUCATIONAL INTERVENTION

Education intervention emphasizing fluid intake is important since in some individuals, thirst alone may be an insufficient compulsion to prevent dehydration during prolonged exercise in hot and humid conditions. Children generally consume fluid voluntarily during exercise to replace the high percentage of sweat water losses, even though voluntary dehydration remains after *ad libitum* intake. Adequate body fluid balance is achieved by a variety of specific responses coordinated by the central nervous system. These responses include the endocrine and neurophysiological responses from the autonomic nervous system and the perception and behavior effectors that lead to water and sodium intake (McKinley and Johnson 2004). Acute physiological and hormonal responses are regulated primarily by the kidneys in order to adjust for body water and sodium loss. In a classic study in animals, Gilman and Godman (1937) demonstrated that an intravenous infusion of hypertonic saline induced thirst due to intracellular dehydration. Other experiments (Kenney and Chiu

2001; Johnson 2007) showed that hypovolemia, or extracellular fluid depletion, also induces thirst. Thus, sweating from exercise can induce thirst and dehydration both from intra- and extracellular fluid compartments.

Educational intervention seems to be an effective tool to prevent body fluid imbalances in young athletes. Kavouras et al. (2012) showed that intervention that included the increase of water availability, lectures about hydration, and posting urine charts in bathrooms improved hydration in young volleyball and basketball athletes during a summer camp with outdoor exercise and warm environmental conditions. In addition, improving hydration status by *ad libitum* consumption of water enhanced aerobic performance in young children. Decher et al. (2008) reported that after an educational intervention during summer sports camps, including soccer and football, hydration knowledge improved, but no change in hydration behavior was observed. Cleary et al. (2012) investigated the effectiveness of education in modifying hydration behaviors in 36 female elite volleyball players (age ~15 years) in a one-time educational intervention and prescribed hydration intervention in a warm environment condition. A one-time education session alone was not successful in changing hydration behaviors. However, prescribing individualized hydration protocols improved hydration for adolescents exercising in a warm, humid environment, suggesting that coaches, camp staff, and athletes needed to develop and implement more effective hydration strategies.

An effective acclimatization process to prevent heat illness involves a satisfactory education intervention in young athletes. Prepubescent, compared to postpubescent, athletes may take longer to acclimate to the heat (Wagner et al. 1972; Falk et al. 1992b); thereby, the recommended acclimatization period is longer for younger children. Usually, the heat acclimatization/acclimation process is achieved by 1- to 3-h sessions, 3–7 times a week, for 1–2 weeks. It is retained for 7–10 days without further exposure, but afterwards the acclimated state is gradually lost (Bar-Or and Rowland 2004). Therefore, young athletes, especially football players, should start to acclimatize sufficiently in the early season to prevent exertional heat illnesses (Bergeron et al. 2005). The suggested duration to achieve acclimatization when physical activities happen in-field is ~14 days, and should involve progressive heat exposition and uniform use, such as in football, starting with helmets, followed by shoulder pads, then full pads, and finally the full uniform. Intervention programs may be successful to enhance hydration status and an effective acclimatization process, thereby avoiding dehydration and heat-related illnesses.

7.8 CONSIDERATIONS OF HYDRATION IN CHRONIC HEALTH CONDITIONS

Children and adolescents with well-controlled chronic diseases commonly participate in competitive athletic activities despite their fundamentally altered physiology. Evidence-based guidelines are specifically not available for exercising children and adolescents with chronic diseases. Owing to their altered physiology, extra caution is needed regarding their thermoregulatory and hydration responses.

7.8.1 Lung Conditions

7.8.1.1 Asthma

Physiological mechanisms of the regulation of lung fluid balance and water transport at pulmonary surfaces is related to hydration status. High fluid intake is strongly recommended in those with bronchopulmonary disorders (Kalhoff 2003) and usually can be prescribed as complementary therapy. Children and adolescents with asthma are often engaged in sports training and competitions despite their physiological challenges. Considerations regarding proper fluid and electrolyte balance are necessary for these young athletes, particularly during prolonged exercise. A study conducted by Oflu et al. (2010) showed that transepidermal water loss measurements (after an exercise protocol—resting) on the palmar surface were higher in children with asthma (22.8 g m^{-2} h^{-1})

compared with healthy children (15.2 g m^{-2} h^{-1}) (aged 8–18 years). In boys, all transepidermal water loss (palmar, volar, forehead, and back surfaces) were higher than their peers. An interesting finding was that asthmatic children using anti-inflammatories compared to those needing a bronchodilator presented lower water loss. Laitano et al. (2008) assessed sweat electrolyte concentration and losses in asthmatic children (average age 11 years) during exercise in the heat for 30 min, and no differences were observed in sweat [Na$^+$] (35 ± 12.9 and 43.4 ± 18 mmol L^{-1} asthmatic and control groups, respectively) and [Cl$^-$] (27.3 ± 10.4 and 38.5 ± 19.1 mmol L^{-1}).

7.8.1.2 Cystic Fibrosis

Overall, children with mild lung disease and appropriate growth were as active as control subjects (Orenstein and Higgins 2005). Mucus in children with cystic fibrosis is abnormally thick and sticky. This negatively impacts fluid balance and water transportation between bronchopulmonary compartments in the lung, where water is essential to homeostasis. In addition, sodium and chloride concentrations in sweat were 2–5 times as high as those found in other individuals. Cystic fibrosis individuals have been observed to drink less during exercise usually related to a decreased hyperosmotic trigger attenuating the thirst drive.

Excreting sweat that is nearly isotonic to plasma, cystic fibrosis individuals possibly are at a greater risk for heat-related illnesses, such as dehydration and hyponatremia, during prolonged exercise in the heat. Kaskavage and Sklansky (2012) reported exercise-induced hyponatremia and dehydration with rhabdomyolysis in a 14-year-old physically active boy with well-controlled cystic fibrosis. The boy was brought to the emergency room, complaining of severe muscle soreness in the calves, thighs, arms, and back, persisting for several hours after completing a football training session that lasted ~3 h on a warm summer morning (26–31°C). A minimal amount of water was ingested and he did not urinate ~8 h after voiding in the morning. His body mass was 4.4 kg (56.6 vs. 60 kg, 5.6%) lower than his last office visit 8 days prior. Serum sodium was 129 mmol L^{-1}, chloride 90 mmol L^{-1}, and creatine phosphokinase 1146 U L^{-1}. Aggressive hydration with intravenous 0.9% saline resulted in clinical improvement with no renal or muscular sequelae. High sodium concentration can be measured in the sweat from some apparently healthy individuals as well, with values approaching that of individuals with cystic fibrosis (Brown et al. 2011). A recent study (Lewis et al. 2013) showed no association between the presence of the single heterozygote cystic fibrosis gene that could lead to a defective chloride ion transport channel, and exercise-associated hyponatremia in endurance athletes, suggesting that salt replacement may not be necessary for these athletes.

7.8.2 Metabolic Conditions

7.8.2.1 Obesity

Studies have shown that during exercise in warm environment conditions obese children may present thermoregulatory disadvantages, both physiological (Haymes et al. 1975; Dougherty et al. 2009) and perceived (Dougherty et al. 2009, 2010; Sehl et al. 2012), compared with their lean peers. The obese have a smaller body surface area per unit of body mass than lean individuals, which could affect their ability to effectively exchange heat with the environment. Since fat has a specific heat that is approximately half of that of fat-free mass, the obese also can experience an insulative effect, where a given heat load will increase their body temperature more than that of a lean individual (Bar-Or et al. 1969). Otherwise, recent studies showed that even though obese children have greater difficulty acclimating (Dougherty et al. 2009) and higher body core temperature prior to exercise (Dougherty et al. 2009; Leites et al. 2013b), apparently, they are able to regulate their body core temperature and presented similar sweating responses to their lean pears. A study (Eijsvogels et al. 2011) evaluated lean and obese individuals who walked 30–50 km at a self-selected pace. Obese subjects tended to have a higher maximum core body temperature than lean controls and a significantly higher fluid intake and sweat rate, but lower urine output compared with lean subjects. Plasma-sodium concentration did not change in lean subjects after exercise, whereas plasma-sodium levels increased in overweight and obese subjects. Similarly, a higher sweat sodium concentration was observed in obese compared to lean girls during 30-min cycling in a hot environment (Meyer et al. 2013).

7.8.2.2 Diabetes

Individuals with diabetes can present greater rates of heat illness and heat stress compared to their nondiabetic peers during exposure to hot environments and physical activity that results in increased metabolic heat production (Yardley et al. 2013). Dehydration favors the development of hyperglycemia in individuals with diabetes mellitus, whereas fasting results in reduced glucose plasma concentrations (Burge et al. 2001). One study showed that, in children with diabetic ketoacidosis, serum osmolality level on emergency admission was the most important mortality predictor (Jayashree and Singhi 2004). In addition, poorly controlled type 1 diabetes may impair heat sensation, skin blood flow, and sweating responses and lead to a greater tendency toward dehydration compared to their healthy peers (Yardley et al. 2013).

7.9 CONCLUSIONS

Proper hydration is essential for young athletes to guarantee optimal physical and cognitive performance and avoid heat illnesses. Dehydration during exercise can lead to a higher increase in body core temperature, decreased cardiac output, and impaired sports performance. The only way to prevent becoming dehydrated is drinking the correct composition and amount of fluids before, during, and after exercise practice to compensate body water losses, mainly through sweating.

Many factors can affect sweating pattern, such as individual factors (age, biological maturation, sex acclimatization and acclimation, fitness levels) or factors related to exercise (intensity of training and aquatic ambience). In addition, during prolonged exercise in hot environments, additional attention to hydration status is needed. Periodical evaluation of hydration status during training and competitions, proper fluid availability, and educational programs regarding the importance of hydration are strongly recommended for young athletes.

REFERENCES

ACSM, ADA, and Dietitians of Canada. 2000. Joint Position Statement: Nutrition and athletic performance. American College of Sports Medicine, American Dietetic Association, and Dietitians of Canada. *Med Sci Sports Exerc* 32 (12):2130–45.

Alderman, B., D. M. Landers, J. Carlson, and J. R. Scott. 2004. Factors related to rapid weight loss practices among international-style wrestlers. *Med Sci Sports Exerc* 36 (2):249–52. doi: 10.1249/01.MSS.0000113668.03443.66.

Aragon-Vargas, L. F., B. Wilk, B. W. Timmons, and O. Bar-Or. 2013. Body weight changes in child and adolescent athletes during a triathlon competition. *Eur J Appl Physiol* 113 (1):233–9. doi: 10.1007/s00421-012-2431-8.

Araki, T., M. Inoue, and H. Fujiwara. 1979. Experiment studies on sweating for exercise prescription: Total body sweat rate in relation to work load in physically trained adult males. *J Hum Ergol (Tokyo)* 8 (2):91–9.

Armstrong, L. E., and C. M. Maresh. 1995. Exercise-heat tolerance of children and adolescents. *Pediatr Exerc Sci* 7:239–52.

Armstrong, L. E., C. M. Maresh, J. W. Castellani, M. F. Bergeron, R. W. Kenefick, K. E. LaGasse, and D. Riebe. 1994. Urinary indices of hydration status. *Int J Sport Nutr* 4 (3):265–79.

Armstrong, L. E., A. C. Pumerantz, K. A. Fiala, M. W. Roti, S. A. Kavouras, D. J. Casa, and C. M. Maresh. 2010. Human hydration indices: Acute and longitudinal reference values. *Int J Sport Nutr Exerc Metab* 20 (2):145–53.

Armstrong, L. E., J. A. Soto, F. T. Hacker, Jr., D. J. Casa, S. A. Kavouras, and C. M. Maresh. 1998. Urinary indices during dehydration, exercise, and rehydration. *Int J Sport Nutr* 8 (4):345–55.

Armstrong, N. 2006. *Paediatric Exercise Physiology*. Edinburgh: Churchill Livingstone.

Artioli, G. G., R. T. Iglesias, E. Franchini, B. Gualano, D. B. Kashiwagura, M. Y. Solis, F. B. Benatti, M. Fuchs, and A. H. Lancha Jr. 2010. Rapid weight loss followed by recovery time does not affect judo-related performance. *J Sports Sci* 28 (1):21–32. doi: 10.1080/02640410903428574.

Baker, L. B., K. A. Dougherty, M. Chow, and W. L. Kenney. 2007. Progressive dehydration causes a progressive decline in basketball skill performance. *Med Sci Sports Exerc* 39 (7):1114–23. doi: 10.1249/mss.0b013e3180574b02.

Bar-David, Y., J. Urkin, and E. Kozminsky. 2005. The effect of voluntary dehydration on cognitive functions of elementary school children. *Acta Paediatr* 94 (11):1667–73. doi: 10.1080/08035250500254670.

Bar-Or, O. 1989. Temperature regulation during exercise in children and adolescents. In *Perspectives in Exercise and Sports Medicine: Youth, Exercise, and Sports*, edited by C. V. Gisolfi and D. R. Lamb, 335–367. Indianapolis, IN: Benchmark Press.

Bar-Or, O. 2001. Nutritional considerations for the child athlete. *Can J Appl Physiol* 26 Suppl:S186–91.

Bar-Or, O., R. Dotan, O. Inbar, A. Rotshtein, and H. Zonder. 1980. Voluntary hypohydration in 10- to 12-year-old boys. *J Appl Physiol Respir Environ Exerc Physiol* 48 (1):104–8.

Bar-Or, O., D. Harris, V. Bergstein, and E. R. Buskirk. 1976. Progressive hypohydration in subjects who vary in adiposity. *Isr J Med Sci* 12 (8):800–3.

Bar-Or, O., H. M. Lundegren, and E. R. Buskirk. 1969. Heat tolerance of exercising obese and lean women. *J Appl Physiol* 26 (4):403–9.

Bar-Or, O., and T. W. Rowland. 2004. *Pediatric Exercise Medicine: From Physiologic Principles to Health Care Application*. Champaign, IL: Human Kinetics.

Bergeron, M. F. 2009. Youth sports in the heat: Recovery and scheduling considerations for tournament play. *Sports Med* 39 (7):513–22. doi: 10.2165/00007256-200939070-00001.

Bergeron, M. F., C. Devore, and S. G. Rice. 2011. Policy statement—Climatic heat stress and exercising children and adolescents. *Pediatrics* 128 (3):e741–7. doi: 10.1542/peds.2011-1664.

Bergeron, M. F., M. D. Laird, E. L. Marinik, J. S. Brenner, and J. L. Waller. 2009. Repeated-bout exercise in the heat in young athletes: Physiological strain and perceptual responses. *J Appl Physiol (1985)* 106 (2):476–85. doi: 10.1152/japplphysiol.00122.2008.

Bergeron, M. F., D. B. McKeag, D. J. Casa, P. M. Clarkson, R. W. Dick, E. R. Eichner, C. A. Horswill et al. 2005. Youth football: Heat stress and injury risk. *Med Sci Sports Exerc* 37 (8):1421–30.

Bergeron, M. F., J. L. Waller, and E. L. Marinik. 2006. Voluntary fluid intake and core temperature responses in adolescent tennis players: Sports beverage versus water. *Br J Sports Med* 40 (5):406–10. doi: 10.1136/bjsm.2005.023333.

Binkley, H. M., J. Beckett, D. J. Casa, D. M. Kleiner, and P. E. Plummer. 2002. National Athletic Trainers' Association Position Statement: Exertional heat illnesses. *J Athl Train* 37 (3):329–43.

Brown, M. B., N. A. McCarty, and M. Millard-Stafford. 2011. High-sweat Na^+ in cystic fibrosis and healthy individuals does not diminish thirst during exercise in the heat. *Am J Physiol Regul Integr Comp Physiol* 301 (4):R1177–85. doi: 10.1152/ajpregu.00551.2010.

Buono, M. J., and N. T. Sjoholm. 1988. Effect of physical training on peripheral sweat production. *J Appl Physiol (1985)* 65 (2):811–4.

Burdon, C. A., N. A. Johnson, P. G. Chapman, and H. T. O'Connor. 2012. Influence of beverage temperature on palatability and fluid ingestion during endurance exercise: A systematic review. *Int J Sport Nutr Exerc Metab* 22 (3):199–211.

Burge, M. R., N. Garcia, C. R. Qualls, and D. S. Schade. 2001. Differential effects of fasting and dehydration in the pathogenesis of diabetic ketoacidosis. *Metabolism* 50 (2):171–7. doi: 10.1053/meta.2001.20194.

Carvalho, P., B. Oliveira, R. Barros, P. Padrao, P. Moreira, and V. H. Teixeira. 2011. Impact of fluid restriction and ad libitum water intake or an 8% carbohydrate-electrolyte beverage on skill performance of elite adolescent basketball players. *Int J Sport Nutr Exerc Metab* 21 (3):214–21.

Casa, D. J., L. E. Armstrong, S. K. Hillman, S. J. Montain, R. V. Reiff, B. S. Rich, W. O. Roberts, and J. A. Stone. 2000. National athletic trainers' association position statement: Fluid replacement for athletes. *J Athl Train* 35 (2):212–24.

CDC. 2011. Nonfatal sports and recreation heat illness treated in hospital emergency departments—United States, 2001–2009. *MMWR Morb Mortal Wkly Rep* 60 (29):977–80.

Cheuvront, S. N., R. Carter, 3rd, J. W. Castellani, and M. N. Sawka. 2005. Hypohydration impairs endurance exercise performance in temperate but not cold air. *J Appl Physiol (1985)* 99 (5):1972–6. doi: 10.1152/japplphysiol.00329.2005.

Cheuvront, S. N., R. W. Kenefick, B. R. Ely, E. A. Harman, J. W. Castellani, P. N. Frykman, B. C. Nindl, and M. N. Sawka. 2010. Hypohydration reduces vertical ground reaction impulse but not jump height. *Eur J Appl Physiol* 109 (6):1163–70. doi: 10.1007/s00421-010-1458-y.

Chinevere, T. D., R. W. Kenefick, S. N. Cheuvront, H. C. Lukaski, and M. N. Sawka. 2008. Effect of heat acclimation on sweat minerals. *Med Sci Sports Exerc* 40 (5):886–91. doi: 10.1249/MSS.0b013e3181641c04.

Cian, C., P. A. Koulmann, P. A. Barraud, C. Raphel, C. Jimenez, and B. Melin. 2000. Influence of variations of body hydration on cognitive performance. *Int J Psychophysiol* 14 (1):29–36.

Clayton, D. J., G. H. Evans, and L. J. James. 2013. Effect of drink carbohydrate content on post-exercise gastric emptying, rehydration and the calculation of net fluid balance. *Int J Sport Nutr Exerc Metab* 24 (1):79–89. doi: 10.1123/ijsnem.2013-0024.

Cleary, M. A., R. K. Hetzler, D. Wasson, J. J. Wages, C. Stickley, and I. F. Kimura. 2012. Hydration behaviors before and after an educational and prescribed hydration intervention in adolescent athletes. *J Athl Train* 47 (3):273–81. doi: 10.4085/1062-6050-47.3.05.

Costill, D. L., and B. Saltin. 1974. Factors limiting gastric emptying during rest and exercise. *J Appl Physiol* 37 (5):679–83.

Council on Sports Medicine and Fitness. 2011. Sports drinks and energy drinks for children and adolescents: Are they appropriate? *Pediatrics* 127 (6):1182–9. doi: 10.1542/peds.2011-0965.

Davies, C. T. 1981. Thermal responses to exercise in children. *Ergonomics* 24 (1):55–61. doi: 10.1080/00140138108924830.

Decher, N. R., D. J. Casa, S. W. Yeargin, M. S. Ganio, M. L. Levreault, C. L. Dann, C. T. James, M. A. McCaffrey, C. B. Oconnor, and S. W. Brown. 2008. Hydration status, knowledge, and behavior in youths at summer sports camps. *Int J Sports Physiol Perform* 3 (3):262–78.

Dougherty, K. A., L. B. Baker, M. Chow, and W. L. Kenney. 2006. Two percent dehydration impairs and six percent carbohydrate drink improves boys basketball skills. *Med Sci Sports Exerc* 38 (9):1650–8. doi: 10.1249/01.mss.0000227640.60736.8e.

Dougherty, K. A., M. Chow, and W. L. Kenney. 2009. Responses of lean and obese boys to repeated summer exercise in the heat bouts. *Med Sci Sports Exerc* 41 (2):279–89. doi: 10.1249/MSS.0b013e318185d341.

Dougherty, K. A., M. Chow, and W. L. Kenney. 2010. Critical environmental limits for exercising heat-acclimated lean and obese boys. *Eur J Appl Physiol* 108 (4):779–89. doi: 10.1007/s00421-009-1290-4.

Drinkwater, B. L. 1984. Women and exercise: Physiological aspects. *Exerc Sport Sci Rev* 12:21–51.

Drinkwater, B. L., I. C. Kupprat, J. E. Denton, J. L. Crist, and S. M. Horvath. 1977. Response of prepubertal girls and college women to work in the heat. *J Appl Physiol Respir Environ Exerc Physiol* 43 (6):1046–53.

Eijsvogels, T. M., M. T. Veltmeijer, T. H. Schreuder, F. Poelkens, D. H. Thijssen, and M. T. Hopman. 2011. The impact of obesity on physiological responses during prolonged exercise. *Int J Obes (Lond)* 35 (11):1404–12. doi: 10.1038/ijo.2010.277.

Falk, B. 1998. Effects of thermal stress during rest and exercise in the paediatric population. *Sports Med* 25 (4):221–40.

Falk, B., O. Bar-Or, R. Calvert, and J. D. MacDougall. 1992a. Sweat gland response to exercise in the heat among pre-, mid-, and late-pubertal boys. *Med Sci Sports Exerc* 24 (3):313–9.

Falk, B., O. Bar-Or, and J. D. MacDougall. 1992b. Thermoregulatory responses of pre-, mid-, and late-pubertal boys to exercise in dry heat. *Med Sci Sports Exerc* 24 (6):688–94.

Falk, B., and R. Dotan. 2008. Children's thermoregulation during exercise in the heat: A revisit. *Appl Physiol Nutr Metab* 33 (2):420–7. doi: 10.1139/H07-185.

Faubert, J., and L. Sidebottom. 2012. Perceptual-cognitive training of athletes. *Clin Sport Psychol* 6:85–102.

Fink, W. J., D. L. Costill, and P. J. Van Handel. 1975. Leg muscle metabolism during exercise in the heat and cold. *Eur J Appl Physiol Occup Physiol* 34 (3):183–90.

Francesconi, R. P., R. W. Hubbard, P. C. Szlyk, D. Schnakenberg, D. Carlson, N. Leva, I. Sils et al. 1987. Urinary and hematologic indexes of hypohydration. *J Appl Physiol (1985)* 62 (3):1271–6.

Franchini, E., C. J. Brito, and G. G. Artioli. 2012. Weight loss in combat sports: Physiological, psychological and performance effects. *J Int Soc Sports Nutr* 9 (1):52. doi: 10.1186/1550-2783-9-52.

Frye, A. J., and E. Kamon. 1981. Responses to dry heat of men and women with similar aerobic capacities. *J Appl Physiol Respir Environ Exerc Physiol* 50 (1):65–70.

Gagnon, D., O. Jay, and G. P. Kenny. 2013. The evaporative requirement for heat balance determines whole-body sweat rate during exercise under conditions permitting full evaporation. *J Physiol* 591 (Pt 11):2925–35. doi: 10.1113/jphysiol.2012.248823.

Gilman, A., and L. Goodman. 1937. The secretory response of the posterior pituitary to the need for water conservation. *J Physiol* 90 (2):113–24.

Gopinathan, P. M., G. Pichan, and V. M. Sharma. 1988. Role of dehydration in heat stress-induced variations in mental performance. *Arch Environ Health* 43 (1):15–7. doi: 10.1080/00039896.1988.9934367.

Grandjean, A. C., and N. R. Grandjean. 2007. Dehydration and cognitive performance. *J Am Coll Nutr* 26 (5 Suppl):549S–54S.

Greenleaf, J. E. 1992. Problem: Thirst, drinking behavior, and involuntary dehydration. *Med Sci Sports Exerc* 24 (6):645–56.

Haymes, E. M., R. J. McCormick, and E. R. Buskirk. 1975. Heat tolerance of exercising lean and obese prepubertal boys. *J Appl Physiol* 39 (3):457–61.

Henkin, S. D., P. L. Sehl, and F. Meyer. 2010. Sweat rate and electrolyte concentration in swimmers, runners, and nonathletes. *Int J Sports Physiol Perform* 5 (3):359–66.

Hoffman, J. R., C. M. Maresh, L. E. Armstrong, C. L. Gabaree, M. F. Bergeron, R. W. Kenefick, J. W. Castellani, L. E. Ahlquist, and A. Ward. 1994. Effects of hydration state on plasma testosterone, cortisol and catecholamine concentrations before and during mild exercise at elevated temperature. *Eur J Appl Physiol Occup Physiol* 69 (4):294–300.

Hoffman, J. R., H. Stavsky, and B. Falk. 1995. The effect of water restriction on anaerobic power and vertical jumping height in basketball players. *Int J Sports Med* 16 (4):214–8. doi: 10.1055/s-2007-972994.

Ichinose-Kuwahara, T., Y. Inoue, Y. Iseki, S. Hara, Y. Ogura, and N. Kondo. 2010. Sex differences in the effects of physical training on sweat gland responses during a graded exercise. *Exp Physiol* 95 (10):1026–32. doi: 10.1113/expphysiol.2010.053710.

Inbar, O., O. Bar-Or, R. Dotan, and B. Gutin. 1981. Conditioning versus exercise in heat as methods for acclimatizing 8- to 10-yr-old boys to dry heat. *J Appl Physiol Respir Environ Exerc Physiol* 50 (2):406–11.

Inbar, O., N. Morris, Y. Epstein, and G. Gass. 2004. Comparison of thermoregulatory responses to exercise in dry heat among prepubertal boys, young adults and older males. *Exp Physiol* 89 (6):691–700. doi: 10.1113/expphysiol.2004.027979.

Jay, O., A. R. Bain, T. M. Deren, M. Sacheli, and M. N. Cramer. 2011. Large differences in peak oxygen uptake do not independently alter changes in core temperature and sweating during exercise. *Am J Physiol Regul Integr Comp Physiol* 301 (3):R832–41. doi: 10.1152/ajpregu.00257.2011.

Jayashree, M., and S. Singhi. 2004. Diabetic ketoacidosis: Predictors of outcome in a pediatric intensive care unit of a developing country. *Pediatr Crit Care Med* 5 (5):427–33.

Jentjens, R. L., A. J. Wagenmakers, and A. E. Jeukendrup. 2002. Heat stress increases muscle glycogen use but reduces the oxidation of ingested carbohydrates during exercise. *J Appl Physiol (1985)* 92 (4):1562–72. doi: 10.1152/japplphysiol.00482.2001.

Johnson, A. K. 2007. The sensory psychobiology of thirst and salt appetite. *Med Sci Sports Exerc* 39 (8):1388–400. doi: 10.1249/mss.0b013e3180686de8.

Kalhoff, H. 2003. Mild dehydration: A risk factor of broncho-pulmonary disorders? *Eur J Clin Nutr* 57 Suppl 2:S81–7. doi: 10.1038/sj.ejcn.1601906.

Kaskavage, J., and D. Sklansky. 2012. Hyponatremia-associated rhabdomyolysis following exercise in an adolescent with cystic fibrosis. *Pediatrics* 130 (1):e220–3. doi: 10.1542/peds.2011-1200.

Kavouras, S. A. 2002. Assessing hydration status. *Curr Opin Clin Nutr Metab Care* 5 (5):519–24.

Kavouras, S. A., G. Arnaoutis, M. Makrillos, C. Garagouni, E. Nikolaou, O. Chira, E. Ellinikaki, and L. S. Sidossis. 2012. Educational intervention on water intake improves hydration status and enhances exercise performance in athletic youth. *Scand J Med Sci Sports* 22 (5):684–9. doi: 10.1111/j.1600-0838.2011.01296.x.

Kenney, W. L., and P. Chiu. 2001. Influence of age on thirst and fluid intake. *Med Sci Sports Exerc* 33 (9):1524–32.

Laitano, O., J. Martins, R. Mattiello, C. Perrone, G. B. Fischer, and F. Meyer. 2008. Sweat electrolyte loss in asthmatic children during exercise in the heat. *Pediatr Exerc Sci* 20 (2):121–8.

Leites, G. T., P. L. Sehl, G. S. Cunha, A. Detoni Filho, and F. Meyer. 2013a. Thermoregulatory responses of artistic gymnast young athletes and non-athlete girls during exercise in the heat. In: *Children and Exercise XXVIII*, edited by M.J. Cupido-dos-Santos Coelho-e-Silva, A. Figueiredo, A.J. Ferreira, J.P., and Armstrong, N., 97–101. London and New York: Routledge.

Leites, G. T., P. L. Sehl, G. D. Cunha, A. Detoni Filho, and F. Meyer. 2013b. Responses of obese and lean girls exercising under heat and thermoneutral conditions. *J Pediatr* 162 (5):1054–60. doi: 10.1016/j.jpeds.2012.10.047.

Lewis, D. P., M. D. Hoffman, K. J. Stuempfle, B. E. Owen, I. R. Rogers, J. G. Verbalis, and T. Hew-Butler. 2013. The need for salt: Does a relationship exist between cystic fibrosis and exercise-associated hyponatremia? *J Strength Cond Res.* doi: 10.1519/JSC.0b013e3182a35dbd.

Lopez, M., D. I. Sessler, K. Walter, T. Emerick, and M. Ozaki. 1994. Rate and gender dependence of the sweating, vasoconstriction, and shivering thresholds in humans. *Anesthesiology* 80 (4):780–8.

Luliano, S., G. Naughton, G. Collier, and J. Carlson. 1998. Examination of the self-selected fluid intake practices by junior athletes during a simulated duathlon event. *Int J Sport Nutr* 8 (1):10–23.

Maughan, R. J., L. A. Dargavel, R. Hares, and S. M. Shirreffs. 2009. Water and salt balance of well-trained swimmers in training. *Int J Sport Nutr Exerc Metab* 19 (6):598–606.

Maughan, R. J., J. B. Leiper, and S. M. Shirreffs. 1996. Restoration of fluid balance after exercise-induced dehydration: Effects of food and fluid intake. *Eur J Appl Physiol Occup Physiol* 73 (3–4):317–25.

Maughan, R. J., S. M. Shirreffs, and J. B. Leiper. 2007. Errors in the estimation of hydration status from changes in body mass. *J Sports Sci* 25 (7):797–804. doi: 10.1080/02640410600875143.

McDermott, B. P., D. J. Casa, S. W. Yeargin, M. S. Ganio, R. M. Lopez, and E. A. Mooradian. 2009. Hydration status, sweat rates, and rehydration education of youth football campers. *J Sport Rehabil* 18 (4):535–52.

McKinley, M. J., and A. K. Johnson. 2004. The physiological regulation of thirst and fluid intake. *News Physiol Sci* 19:1–6.

Meyer, F., O. Bar-Or, D. MacDougall, and G. J. Heigenhauser. 1992. Sweat electrolyte loss during exercise in the heat: Effects of gender and maturation. *Med Sci Sports Exerc* 24 (7):776–81.

Meyer, F., O. Bar-Or, A. Salsberg, and D. Passe. 1994. Hypohydration during exercise in children: Effect on thirst, drink preferences, and rehydration. *Int J Sport Nutr* 4 (1):22–35.

Meyer, F., G. T. Leites, P. L. Sehl, A. Detoni Filho, and G. S. Cunha. 2013. Fatness alone does not affect children's sweating responses during exercise in the heat. In *Book of Abstracts Pediatric Work Physiology Meeting*, Faculty of Sports Sciences and Physical Education University of Coimbra, Coimbra, 114.

Meyer, F., H. O'Connor, and S. M. Shirreffs. 2007. Nutrition for the young athlete. *J Sports Sci* 25 (Suppl 1):S73–82. doi: 10.1080/02640410701607338.

Meyer, F., K. A. Volterman, B. Timmons, and B. Wilk. 2012. Fluid balance and dehydration in the young athlete: Assessment considerations and effects on health and performance. *Am J Lifestyle Med* 6 (6):489–501.

Mitchell, J. W., E. R. Nadel, and J. A. Stolwijk. 1972. Respiratory weight losses during exercise. *J Appl Physiol* 32 (4):474–6.

Nadel, E. R., I. Holmer, U. Bergh, P. O. Astrand, and J. A. Stolwijk. 1974. Energy exchanges of swimming man. *J Appl Physiol* 36 (4):465–71.

Oflu, A., O. U. Soyer, A. Tuncer, C. Sackesen, and O. Kalayci. 2010. Eccrine sweat response in children with asthma. *Allergy* 65 (5):645–8. doi: 10.1111/j.1398-9995.2009.02226.x.

Orenstein, D. M., and L. W. Higgins. 2005. Update on the role of exercise in cystic fibrosis. *Curr Opin Pulm Med* 11 (6):519–23.

Perrone, C. A., P. L. Sehl, J. B. Martins, and F. Meyer. 2011. Hydration status and sweating responses of boys playing soccer and futsal. *Med Sport* 15 (3):188–93.

Popowski, L. A., R. A. Oppliger, G. Patrick Lambert, R. F. Johnson, A. Kim Johnson, and C. V. Gisolf. 2001. Blood and urinary measures of hydration status during progressive acute dehydration. *Med Sci Sports Exerc* 33 (5):747–53.

Rivera-Brown, A. M., R. Gutierrez, J. C. Gutierrez, W. R. Frontera, and O. Bar-Or. 1999. Drink composition, voluntary drinking, and fluid balance in exercising, trained, heat-acclimatized boys. *J Appl Physiol (1985)* 86 (1):78–84.

Rivera-Brown, A. M., T. W. Rowland, F. A. Ramirez-Marrero, G. Santacana, and A. Vann. 2006. Exercise tolerance in a hot and humid climate in heat-acclimatized girls and women. *Int J Sports Med* 27 (12):943–50. doi: 10.1055/s-2006-923863.

Rowell, L. B. 1974. Human cardiovascular adjustments to exercise and thermal stress. *Physiol Rev* 54 (1):75–159.

Rowland, T. 2011. Fluid replacement requirements for child athletes. *Sports Med* 41 (4):279–88. doi: 10.2165/11584320-000000000-00000.

Rowland, T. W. 2005. *Children's Exercise Physiology*. Champaign, IL: Human Kinetics.

Sato, K., R. Leidal, and F. Sato. 1987. Morphology and development of an apoeccrine sweat gland in human axillae. *Am J Physiol* 252 (1 Pt 2):R166–80.

Sawka, M. N. 1992. Physiological consequences of hypohydration: Exercise performance and thermoregulation. *Med Sci Sports Exerc* 24 (6):657–70.

Sawka, M. N., L. M. Burke, E. R. Eichner, R. J. Maughan, S. J. Montain, and N. S. Stachenfeld. 2007. American College of Sports Medicine position stand. Exercise and fluid replacement. *Med Sci Sports Exerc* 39 (2):377–90. doi: 10.1249/mss.0b013e31802ca597.

Sawka, M. N., M. M. Toner, R. P. Francesconi, and K. B. Pandolf. 1983. Hypohydration and exercise: Effects of heat acclimation, gender, and environment. *J Appl Physiol Respir Environ Exerc Physiol* 55 (4):1147–53.

Sehl, P. L., G. T. Leites, J. B. Martins, and F. Meyer. 2012. Responses of obese and non-obese boys cycling in the heat. *Int J Sports Med* 33 (6):497–501. doi: 10.1055/s-0031-1301314.

Seifert, S. M., J. L. Schaechter, E. R. Hershorin, and S. E. Lipshultz. 2011. Health effects of energy drinks on children, adolescents, and young adults. *Pediatrics* 127 (3):511–28. doi: 10.1542/peds.2009-3592.

Shapiro, Y., K. B. Pandolf, and R. F. Goldman. 1980. Sex differences in acclimation to a hot-dry environment. *Ergonomics* 23 (7):635–42. doi: 10.1080/00140138008924778.

Shibasaki, M., Y. Inoue, N. Kondo, and A. Iwata. 1997. Thermoregulatory responses of prepubertal boys and young men during moderate exercise. *Eur J Appl Physiol Occup Physiol* 75 (3):212–8.

Shibasaki, M., T. E. Wilson, and C. G. Crandall. 2006. Neural control and mechanisms of eccrine sweating during heat stress and exercise. *J Appl Physiol (1985)* 100 (5):1692–701. doi: 10.1152/japplphysiol.01124.2005.

Steen, S. N., and K. D. Brownell. 1990. Patterns of weight loss and regain in wrestlers: Has the tradition changed?. *Med Sci Sports Exerc* 22 (6):762–8.

Stolen, T., K. Chamari, C. Castagna, and U. Wisloff. 2005. Physiology of soccer: An update. *Sports Med* 35 (6):501–36.

Wagner, J. A., S. Robinson, S. P. Tzankoff, and R. P. Marino. 1972. Heat tolerance and acclimatization to work in the heat in relation to age. *J Appl Physiol* 33 (5):616–22.

Wilk, B., and O. Bar-Or. 1996. Effect of drink flavor and NaCl on voluntary drinking and hydration in boys exercising in the heat. *J Appl Physiol (1985)* 80 (4):1112–7.

Wilk, B., F. Meyer, O. Bar-Or, and B. W. Timmons. 2013a. Mild to moderate hypohydration reduces boys' high-intensity cycling performance in the heat. *Eur J Appl Physiol* doi: 10.1007/s00421-013-2803-8.

Wilk, B., D. Pascale, O. Bar-Or, L. Tremblay, S. Dominic, and D. Elliott. 2004. Cognitive and perceptual-motor responses to exercise induced dehydration in boys. In *Book of Abstracts 9th Annual Congress, European College of Sport Science*, edited by E., Coudert Van Praagh, J. Fellmann, N.; Duche, P., 145. Clermont-Ferrand, France.

Wilk, B., N. Pender, K. Volterman, O. Bar-Or, and B. W. Timmons. 2013b. Influence of pubertal stage on local sweating patterns of girls exercising in the heat. *Pediatr Exerc Sci* 25 (2):212–20.

Wilson, T. E. 2013. Sweating the details: What really drives eccrine output during exercise-heat stress. *J Physiol* 591 (Pt 11):2777–0. doi: 10.1113/jphysiol.2013.255430.

Yardley, J. E., J. M. Stapleton, R. J. Sigal, and G. P. Kenny. 2013. Do heat events pose a greater health risk for individuals with type 2 diabetes? *Diabetes Technol Ther* 15 (6):520–9. doi: 10.1089/dia.2012.0324.

Section II

Special Considerations in Child and Adolescent Athletes

8 Effects of Caffeine, Nicotine, Alcohol, and Marijuana on Exercise Performance

Dominik H. Pesta, Siddhartha S. Angadi, Martin Burtscher, and Christian K. Roberts

CONTENTS

Abstract 135
8.1 Introduction 136
8.2 Caffeine 136
    8.2.1 History 136
    8.2.2 Overview 136
    8.2.3 Effects on Performance 137
    8.2.4 Legal Status 138
    8.2.5 Summary 138
8.3 Nicotine 138
    8.3.1 History 138
    8.3.2 Overview 139
    8.3.3 Effect on Performance 139
    8.3.4 Legal Status 141
    8.3.5 Summary 141
8.4 Ethanol (Alcohol) 142
    8.4.1 History 142
    8.4.2 Overview 142
    8.4.3 Effects on Health and Performance 142
    8.4.4 Legal Status 144
    8.4.5 Summary 144
8.5 Marijuana 145
    8.5.1 History 145
    8.5.2 Overview 145
    8.5.3 Effects on Performance 145
    8.5.4 Legal Status 146
    8.5.5 Summary 146
8.6 Drug Interactions 146
8.7 Conclusion and Perspectives 147
References 147

ABSTRACT

Caffeine, nicotine, ethanol (alcohol), and tetrahydrocannabinol (marijuana) are among the most prevalent and culturally accepted drugs in Western society. For example, in Europe and North America up to 90% of the adult population drinks coffee daily and, although less prevalent, the other drugs are also used extensively. Smoked tobacco, excessive alcohol consumption, and marijuana (cannabis) smoking are addictive and exhibit adverse health effects. These drugs are not only common in the general population, but have also made their way into elite sports because of their purported performance-altering potential. Only one of the drugs (i.e., caffeine) has enough scientific evidence indicating an ergogenic effect. There is some preliminary evidence for nicotine as an ergogenic aid, but further study is required; cannabis and alcohol can exhibit ergogenic potential under specific circumstances but are in general believed to be ergolytic for sports performance. These drugs are currently (THC, ethanol) or have been (caffeine) on the prohibited list of the World Anti-Doping Agency or are being monitored (caffeine, nicotine) due to their potential ergogenic or ergolytic effects. Throughout this chapter, the terms "alcohol" and "marijuana" will be used to refer to ethanol and tetrahydrocannabinol, respectively. The aim of this chapter is to evaluate the effects of caffeine, nicotine, alcohol, and marijuana by (1) examining evidence supporting the ergogenic or ergolytic effects; (2) providing an overview of the mechanism(s) of action and physiological effects; and (3) where appropriate, reviewing their impact as performance-altering aids used in recreational and elite sports.

8.1 INTRODUCTION

Caffeine, nicotine, alcohol, and marijuana are widely consumed substances in today's society (Crocq 2003, Robinson and Pritchard 1992). Drugs such as smoked tobacco, excessive alcohol, or marijuana pose a serious problem for public health and the healthcare system (Sturm 2002). Further, these substances are also related, as they are or have been on the prohibited list of the World Anti-Doping Agency (WADA) or are monitored due to their potential performance-altering effect and misuse in sport (WADA 2016). It is therefore important to discuss their potential to alter performance, as these substances are not only of significant importance for the general public but also for competitive athletes. Much like other topics in this research, the overwhelming majority of literature has been conducted on adults and not in the targeted age group of child and adolescent athletes. Nonetheless, the purpose of this chapter is to provide an overview of the evidence supporting the ergogenic or ergolytic effects of the most prevalent drugs in Western society.

8.2 CAFFEINE

8.2.1 History

Today, caffeine is considered the world's most popular drug (Pendergrast 2010). The history of coffee goes at least as far back as the thirteenth century. Today it is grown in many countries around the world, the most important being Asia, Africa, Central and South America, and the islands of the Caribbean, while Brazil continues to be one of the world's major suppliers of coffee. The two most important varieties of the genus *Coffea* are *Coffea arabica* and *Coffea canephora* var. robusta, conveniently referred to as Arabica and Robusta, respectively (Pendergrast 2010). Arabica coffee accounts for the majority of coffee produced and consumed (70%). The raw coffee is called green coffee and contains about 8%–12% water. By roasting the bean it loses its water and also changes the chemical composition. After roasting, the coffee beans are packed and ready to be ground for brewing coffee as we know it.

8.2.2 Overview

Apart from water, tea and coffee are among the most popular beverages consumed worldwide. The main pharmacologically active substance in both beverages is the purine alkaloid of the xanthine class, 1,3,7,-trimethylxanthine or caffeine. According to European and North American statistics, ~90% of the adult population consider themselves as daily coffee users, with an average daily caffeine consumption of about 200 mg or 2.4 mg/kg per day (about 2 cups of coffee) (Chou 1992). It is therefore considered the world's most widely consumed pharmacologically active substance. Caffeine is both water and fat soluble and is quickly distributed in the body after absorption mainly by the small intestine and the stomach, with peaking plasma levels after 15–120 min and a half-life of about 5–6 h with individual variation (Statland and Demas 1980).

As for many pharmacological substances, there is generally more than one potential mechanism explaining the ergogenic effects. This is also true for caffeine which might affect both the central nervous system (CNS) and skeletal muscle (Goldstein et al. 2010). Although questionable, a potential downside is that caffeine has diuretic properties, which can exert ergolytic effects during prolonged endurance events (Osswald and Schnermann 2011). Caffeine intake at very high doses (>500–600 mg or 4–7 cups/day) can cause restlessness, tremor, and tachycardia (Nawrot et al. 2003).

8.2.3 Effects on Performance

Caffeine reduces fatigue and increases concentration and alertness, and athletes regularly use it as an ergogenic aid (Paluska 2003). Caffeine-induced increases in performance have been observed in aerobic as well as anaerobic sports. For reviews, see Tarnopolsky (1994), Davis and Green (2009), and Goldstein et al. (2010). Trained athletes seem to benefit from a moderate dose of 5 mg/kg (Woolf et al. 2008); however, even lower doses of caffeine (1–2 mg/kg) may improve performance (Cox et al. 2002). Some groups found significantly improved time trial performance (Mc Naughton et al. 2008) or maximal cycling power (Del Coso et al. 2008), most likely related to a greater reliance on fat metabolism and decreased neuromuscular fatigue, respectively. The effect of caffeine on fat oxidation, however, may only be significant during lower exercise intensities and may be blocked at higher intensities (Gonzalez and Stevenson 2012). Spriet et al. (1992) found that ingestion of a high dose of caffeine before exercise reduced muscle glycogenolysis in the initial 15 min of exercise by increasing free fatty acid (FFA) levels, which inhibit glycolysis and spare glycogen for later use. Caffeine's effect on inhibition of glycogen phosphorylase has also been shown in vitro (Rush and Spriet 2001) as well as its effect on increasing hormone-sensitive lipase (HSL) activity (Donsmark et al. 2003). The effect of caffeine on adipose triglyceride lipase (Zimmermann et al. 2004) has not been studied and warrants investigation.

Augmented postexercise recovery by increased rates of muscle glycogen resynthesis has been observed (Pedersen et al. 2008, Taylor et al. 2011). Pedersen et al. (2008) found higher rates of muscle glycogen accumulation after the co-ingestion of caffeine with carbohydrates during recovery in highly trained subjects. Finally, not only does caffeine impact endurance, it has also been reported to benefit cognitive function and fine motor skills (Foskett et al. 2009).

While the performance-enhancing effects of caffeine in moderate-to-highly trained endurance athletes are quite clear and well documented, its effects on anaerobic, high-intensity tasks are less well investigated. Whereas caffeine supplementation did not yield significant performance increases in a Wingate test in untrained subjects (Collomp et al. 1991, Lorino et al. 2006), Mora-Rodriguez et al. (2012) report that caffeine ingestion of 3 mg/kg could counter reductions in maximum dynamic strength and muscle power output in the morning (2.5%–7.0%), thereby increasing muscle performance to the levels found in the afternoon. A possible explanation for the diverging effect of caffeine on anaerobic performance is that caffeine seems to benefit trained athletes who show specific physiological adaptations whereas performance gains in untrained subjects might be lost or masked by a high variability in performance.

Additionally, another reason for the widespread use of caffeine within the exercise community might be its small, but significant analgesic effect (Derry et al. 2012), possibly mediated by augmenting plasma endorphin concentrations (Grossman and Sutton 1985). It is also established that caffeine reduces the rate of perceived exertion during exercise (Doherty and Smith 2005), suggesting that athletes are able to sustain higher intensities but do not perceive this effort to be different from placebo conditions. Some studies used caffeine-naïve study participants whereas others used caffeine-habituated subjects. There seems to be a higher increase in plasma adrenaline in caffeine-naïve individuals compared to caffeine-habituated subjects after caffeine ingestion (Van Soeren et al. 1993). However, no differences between habitual caffeine intake and 1500 m running performance (Wiles et al. 1992) or force of contraction (Tarnopolsky and Cupido 2000) could be observed. For both caffeine-naïve as well as caffeine-habituated subjects, moderate-to-high doses of caffeine are ergogenic during prolonged moderate intense exercise (Mottram 1996). Although there is clearly the need to study caffeine habituation further, the differences between users and nonusers do not seem to be major.

In specific reference to adolescent athletes and caffeine use, Abian-Vicen and colleagues had 16 young (14.9 ± 0.8 years) basketball players complete a free throw and three-point shooting test in addition to a single and repeated vertical jump and an intermittent run test after consuming either a placebo solution or a solution containing 3 mg/kg of caffeine (Abian-Vicen et al. 2014). No impact of caffeine was seen on both free throw and three-point shooting as well as the distance covered during the intermittent running test (Yo-yo IR1). Caffeine ingestion did impact jump height during a countermovement jump and mean jump height during 15 s of repetitive jumping. Further, urinary excretion of caffeine after a single 3 mg/kg dose was well below thresholds employed for punitive action stemming from caffeine use.

8.2.4 Legal Status

From 1962 to 2003, caffeine found its way on and off the list of banned substances by WADA. One of the reasons caffeine was removed from the prohibited list was that many experts believe it to be ubiquitous in beverages and food and that having a threshold might lead to athletes being sanctioned for social or dietary consumption of caffeine (Mottram and Chester 2014). Furthermore, caffeine is metabolized at very different rates in individuals (Fenster et al. 1998) and hence urinary concentrations can vary considerably and do not always correlate to the dose ingested. In addition, caffeine is added to a wide range of popular food products (Temple 2009) such as coffee, tea, energy drinks and bars, and chocolate.

8.2.5 Summary

In summary, caffeine, even at physiological doses (3–6 mg/kg) has proven to be ergogenic and as such—in most exercise situations, especially in endurance-type events—is clearly work-enhancing (Goldstein et al. 2010). It most likely has a peripheral effect targeting skeletal muscle metabolism as well as a central effect targeting the brain to enhance performance, especially during endurance events (see Table 8.1). Also for anaerobic tasks, the effect of caffeine on the CNS might be most relevant. Further, postexercise caffeine intake seems to benefit recovery by increasing rates of glycogen resynthesis.

8.3 NICOTINE

8.3.1 History

Nicotine is the most important alkaloid of the tobacco plant *Nicotiana* (Solanaceae), which was named in honor of Jean Nicot, a French ambassador to Portugal at around 1560. More than 60 species of Nicotiana are known and most of them are native to the Americas (Charlton 2004, Goodspeed 1954). Whereas *Nicotiana tabacum*, primarily used for commercial tobacco production, likely comes from South America, *Nicotiana rustica* is of North American origin (Charlton 2004). Out of the more than 4000 chemicals generated when burning tobacco leaves, nicotine is by far the most extensively investigated compound isolated in 1828 by Posselt and Reimann (1828). The investigation of isolated effects of nicotine revealed that nicotine stimulates the nervous system by small doses and acts as a depressant at larger ones but most importantly, it causes smokers to

TABLE 8.1
Summary Table of the Effects of Caffeine on Performance

Legal (WADA) Status: Since 2004 Being Monitored (Stimulants—In Competition Only), Banned from 1962 to 1972 and again from 1984 to 2003 at Urinary Caffeine Concentrations >12 µg/mL

Acute Effect	Effect on Performance	Caffeine Dose	References
Greater reliance on fat metabolism; increased FFA, lower respiratory exchange ratio (RER)	Increased time-trial performance	6 mg/kg body mass	McNaughton et al. (2008)
Counteract central fatigue, directed effect on the CNS	3% PMAX increase, increase in voluntary activation, maintenance of maximum voluntary contraction	6 mg/kg body mass	Del Coso et al. (2008)
No clear mechanism, effect on CNS (greater motor unit recruitment and altered neurotransmitter function) or direct effect on skeletal muscle	Enhanced time-trial performance	6 mg/kg caffeine 1 h pre-exercise and ~1.5 mg/kg after 2 h of exercise	Cox et al. (2002)
No mechanism proposed	No significant effects observed on performance	1.5 or 3 mg/kg body mass of caffeine 1 h before cycling	Desbrow et al. (2009)
Direct effect on skeletal muscle, interaction with ryanodine receptor, potentiated calcium release from the SR	Increase in contraction force at low-frequency stimulation (20 Hz)	6 mg/kg 100 min before stimulation	Tarnopolsky et al. (2000)
Blunted pain response	Significantly higher reps during leg press set 3 with caffeine, same rate of perceived exertion	6 mg/kg 1 h prior to 10-RM bench and leg press	Green et al. (2007)
Glycogen-sparing effect and increased utilization of intramuscular TGs and plasma FFAs with caffeine	Increased cycling time trial performance with caffeine	9 mg/kg body mass 1 h before exercise	Spriet et al. (1992)

become addicted (Charlton 2004). Although most of the hazards on our health are caused by other chemicals in smoke than nicotine, for example, by carcinogenic polycyclic aromatic hydrocarbons and *N*-nitroso compounds (Brandt 1990), one must not forget that the addictive effect of nicotine is seriously hampering attempts to quit smoking. A complex political and cultural conflict about risk and responsibility of nicotine use continues up to date.

8.3.2 Overview

Nicotine or 3-(1-methyl-2-pyrrolidinyl) pyridine is a naturally occurring alkaloid and one of the most widely used psychostimulants in the world (Boutrel and Koob 2004). Cigarettes are the most common source of nicotine. Smoked tobacco contains additional harmful constituents and chemicals, which have detrimental effects on the respiratory system (Amann 2012). Due to worldwide smoking restrictions, the tobacco industry has developed a number of smokeless alternatives, often containing much higher nicotine concentrations than regular cigarettes. These represent an alternative for some athletes as they do not pose a risk of adversely affecting the respiratory system.

8.3.3 Effect on Performance

While it is clear that smoking can lead to the development of respiratory, cardiovascular, and skin diseases, as well as a number of tobacco-related cancers (Taioli 2008), there are other forms of application such as the use of alternative smokeless tobacco (snus), which is gaining popularity among athletes (Martinsen and Sundgot-Borgen 2014), as it bypasses the respiratory system. Snus and cigarette consumers show similar peak blood nicotine levels after use with a tendency for higher cotinine (the predominant metabolite of nicotine) levels in the former (Holm et al. 1992).

Nicotine activates the sympathoadrenal system, which leads to increased heart rate, contractility, vasoconstriction, and a rise in blood pressure and circulating catecholamines during light exercise (Walker et al. 1999). Nicotine also increases muscle blood flow (Weber et al. 1989) and lipolysis due to enhanced circulating levels of norepinephrine and epinephrine as well as direct action on nicotinic cholinergic receptors in adipose tissue (Andersson and Arner 2001).

The effects exerted by nicotine may be beneficial in a wide variety of sports and it is suggested that nicotine is abused by athletes (Martinsen and Sundgot-Borgen 2014). According to Marclay et al. (2011), cumulative exposure to nicotine metabolites were found in 26%–56% of urine samples that were subjected to screening for tobacco alkaloids. After correcting for exposure to second-hand smoke, 15% of the athletes were considered active nicotine consumers. Among athletes, this is high considering the World Health Organization's 25% worldwide estimate of smoking prevalence. It can be hypothesized that the metabolites stem mostly from smokeless tobacco due to the adverse effects of conventional cigarettes for athletes, which most severely effects athletes engaging in endurance-type sports (Alaranta et al. 2006).

Further, a large number of human and animal studies have found nicotine-induced improvements in several aspects of cognitive function, including learning and memory (Levin et al. 2006), reaction time (Marzilli et al. 2006), and fine motor abilities (see Table 8.2). Studies addressing the question of a direct performance-enhancing effect of nicotine are rare but will be summarized here; none have employed child or adolescents athletes as study participants. Sports most affected include ice hockey, skiing, biathlon, bobsleigh, skating, football, basketball, volleyball, rugby, American football, wrestling, and gymnastics. These sports seem to gain performance benefits from the stimulating effect of nicotine as evident from the use of other prohibited stimulants according to the Anti-Doping Database (ADDB 2012). Mundel and Jones (2006) found a 17% improvement in time-to-exhaustion after nicotine patch application compared to a placebo without affecting cardiovascular and respiratory parameters or substrate metabolism. In this sense, nicotine seems to exert similar effects as caffeine by delaying the development of central fatigue, as impaired central drive is an important factor contributing to fatigue during exercise. To date, no improvements in anaerobic performance (Wingate Test) have been reported (see Table 8.2).

Additionally, although nicotine may have ergogenic potential, it is also highly addictive, reportedly as addictive as heroin and cocaine (Stolerman and Jarvis 1995). Therefore, detrimental effects on motor performance can be altered after a short abstinence duration. Burtscher et al. (1994) noted that motor performance declines in heavy smokers after a short period of abstinence appears, this decline being similar to the motor symptoms of Parkinsonism. The abstinence symptoms are ameliorated by cigarette smoking. It is important to consider the concerning addictive potential with following deterioration of motor performance upon abstinence. Interestingly, however, it was noted that moderate and vigorous exercise led to significant reductions in the desire to smoke among abstaining smokers, possibly via reductions in cortisol (Scerbo et al. 2010). A recent meta-analysis showed that exercise has the potential to acutely reduce cigarette cravings and could therefore be a promising strategy to attenuate withdrawal symptoms in smokers (Haasova et al. 2013). It is also important to mention that the vasoconstriction mediated by nicotine could limit exercise performance in a hot environment. As skin blood flow increases during exercise to transfer heat, impaired nicotine-induced skin blood flow may be ergolytic.

A recent meta-analysis conducted by Heishman and colleagues clearly suggests significant effects of nicotine on fine motor abilities, including attention and memory (Heishman et al. 2010). Participants of the studies included in the meta-analysis were mainly nonsmokers, therefore avoiding confounding of nicotine withdrawal. Finally, nicotine's effect on increased pain tolerance might

TABLE 8.2
Summary of the Effects of Nicotine on Performance

Legal (WADA) Status: In Order to Detect Potential Patterns of Abuse, Nicotine Has Been Placed on WADA's Monitoring Program Since 2012

Acute Effect	Effect on Performance	Nicotine Dose	References
Likely delayed development of (central) fatigue by nicotine receptor activation and/or dopaminergic pathways; no evidence of altered substrate metabolism or cardiorespiratory effects	17% improvement in time to exhaustion	7 mg nicotine patch per 24 h	Mundel et al. (2006)
No mechanism proposed	No effect on anaerobic performance (Wingate test)	Nicotine gum	Meier (2006)
Unclear	Improvement in the degree in a real-life motor task, that is, handwriting (more pronounced in smokers than nonsmokers)	Nicotine gum (2 and 4 mg)	Tucha et al. (2004)
No mechanism proposed	No effect on cognitive functioning	Nicotine gum (2 and 4 mg)	Heishman et al. (1993)
No mechanism proposed	No effect on speed and accuracy of motor activity among nonsmokers (but improvements in smokers)	Nicotine gum (2 and 4 mg)	Hindmarch et al. (1990)
Likely by the action of nicotine on cholinergic pathways	Positive effects on fine motor abilities like finger tapping	Intranasal (2 mg)	West et al. (1986)

be of advantage in a wide variety of sports (Jamner et al. 1998). Further research will hopefully fill the gap to evaluate nicotine's effects on exercise performance.

8.3.4 LEGAL STATUS

In response to scattered reports of nicotine use, in 2012 has included nicotine, categorized as a stimulant and "in-competition only," in its monitoring program (WADA 2012). For this purpose, the World Anti-Doping Code (Article 4.5, page 36) states: "WADA, in consultation with signatories and governments, shall establish a monitoring program regarding substances which are not on the Prohibited List, but which WADA wishes to monitor in order to detect patterns of misuse in sport." Thus, nicotine use is not illegal, but is being monitored for misuse and other potential concerns.

8.3.5 SUMMARY

In summary, nicotine seems to have ergogenic potential. Athletes appear to benefit from activation of the sympathoadrenal system with increased catecholamine release and subsequent increases in muscle blood flow and lipolysis. There is evidence for the abuse of nicotine by athletes. Although the sale of snus is illegal within the European Union (Gray 2005), anecdotal observations by coaches and research from Scandinavia show a high prevalence of snus use among athletes (Mattila et al. 2012, Martinsen and Sundgot-Borgen 2014). It might therefore be reasonable to assume that smoking cigarettes will not be an issue for athletes. Instead, as there are several nicotine alternatives, many of the negative effects of cigarettes can be circumvented. In this respect, it is prudent to advise and make parents, coaches, and healthcare providers aware as to increase their awareness and heighten their vigilance to ensure the health and safety of young athletes regarding nicotine in the form of cigarettes and other alternative forms.

8.4 ETHANOL (ALCOHOL)

8.4.1 History

Alcohol was known as the "elixir of life" in ancient times. Sport and alcohol have enjoyed a close and almost symbiotic relationship in the United Kingdom since at least the sixteenth century (Collins and Vamplew 2002). Back then, the ale house was the main arena for staging sporting events. The property on which these ale houses were situated provided the spaces in which diverse sports such as boxing, wrestling, tennis, and cricket were played (Collins and Vamplew 2002). Even in America by 1882, an upstart baseball organization called the "Beer and Whiskey League" or the "Beer Ball League," arose to challenge the National league which at the time disallowed alcohol sales in ballparks (Nemec 2004). The new league was founded by the brewers and distillers in St. Louis, Milwaukee, Cincinnati, Baltimore, Louisville, and Pittsburgh. By the nineteenth century the selling and enjoying of beer and liquor became a symbol of baseball in and of itself (Riess 1991). In fact, the classic trophy awarded to winners is the "cup," which is designed to facilitate the consumption of alcohol by the winners (Collins and Vamplew 2002). These days nary a day goes by without a sporting event that enjoys alcohol sponsorship or advertising. It is within this rich historical context that the modern athlete exists. To this day, alcohol consumption is reported by a vast majority of college and elite athletes.

8.4.2 Overview

Alcohol (ethanol; here referred to as alcohol or EtOH) is and has been one the most commonly consumed and abused drugs for a substantial period in human history. Alcohol is a dependence-producing drug, which affects a host of organ systems and one that increases the risk of morbidity and mortality from different diseases when abused (El-Sayed et al. 2005). Indeed, some authors have suggested that alcohol is harmful, similar to drugs such as heroin or cocaine and, that excessive alcohol consumption is a serious worldwide health risk (Nutt et al. 2010). Although the detrimental effects of alcohol on human physiology are well known, even elite athletes consume alcohol. When looking at the effects of alcohol on overall health, it is, however, important to distinguish between chronic, moderate alcohol consumption versus alcohol abuse.

The link between alcohol consumption and mortality is subject to a J-shaped curve (i.e., improved longevity with moderate consumption with increasing intake resulting in greater mortality risk) (Poikolainen 1995). Indeed, dietary guidelines from the American Heart Association recommend moderation of alcohol intake, as it has been associated with a lower risk of cardiovascular events (Lichtenstein et al. 2006).

Alcohol use is fairly widespread among the athletic population with 88% of intercollegiate American athletes reporting the use of alcohol (O'Brien and Lyons 2000). It is also noteworthy that many athletes consume alcohol prior to sporting events (Gutgesell and Canterbury 1999). However, it is important to note that scientific evidence suggests that the consumption of alcohol has some detrimental effects on exercise performance (El-Sayed et al. 2005, O'Brien and Lyons 2000). It is fairly obvious that it is unlikely for competitive athletes to be alcohol abusers and most performance studies have focused on the acute ergolytic effects of EtOH consumption. The chronic studies merely reinforce the point that EtOH is profoundly ergolytic in the long-term setting. They also serve to reinforce that chronic EtOH use can be toxic to cardiac and skeletal muscle.

8.4.3 Effects on Health and Performance

Chronic alcohol abuse has significant detrimental effects on the human cardiac muscle (Richardson et al. 1996) and one of the putative mechanisms via which alcohol may induce cardiac dysfunction is through the induction of increased oxidative stress. Acute alcohol use can also have effects on cardiovascular determinants of exercise performance. Lang et al. (1985) examined the effects of acute alcohol administration on left ventricular contractility using echocardiography and found that alcohol had a significant depressant effect on the myocardium. Alcohol has significant effects on skeletal muscle substrate utilization during exercise. Specifically, it has been demonstrated that alcohol consumption decreases glucose and amino acid utilization, which can have adverse effects on energy supply to exercising muscle (Spolarics et al. 1994, Trounce et al. 1990, Vila et al. 2001). Ethanol consumption induces hypoglycemia and decreases glucose appearance in plasma by decreasing hepatic gluconeogenesis (Vella and Cameron-Smith 2010). Ethanol administration has been shown to worsen skeletal muscle determinants of exercise performance such as muscle capillary density and muscle fiber cross-sectional area (Vila et al. 2001). Finally, it was shown in vitro that alcohol can inhibit sarcolemmal calcium channel actions, thereby potentially impairing excitation–contraction coupling and diminishing muscular performance (Cofan et al. 2000).

In addition to a number of physical impacts, acute alcohol consumption is associated with the deterioration of psychomotor skills. A significant difference exists in injury rates between drinkers and nondrinkers in athletic populations. Further, athletes who consume alcohol at least once a week have almost a twofold higher risk of injury compared to nondrinkers and this elevated injury rate holds true for the majority of sports examined (O'Brien and Lyons 2000). Alcohol may also interfere with the body's ability to recover from injury. Barnes et al. (2010) examined the effects of 1 g/kg body weight alcohol consumption on recovery from eccentric exercise-induced muscle injury. The authors measured peak and average peak isokinetic and isometric torque produced by the quadriceps. Alcohol consumption was associated with significantly greater decreases in torque production (40%–44%) 36 h into recovery. The authors concluded that the consumption of a moderate amount of alcohol after damaging exercise magnified the loss of muscle force production potential.

Alcohol has direct and demonstrable effects on athletic performance which may be due to its cardiovascular effects. McNaughton and Preece (1986) demonstrated significant ergolytic effects in short- and middle-distance runners. The adverse effects were most prominent in events that were more dependent upon aerobic capacity (i.e., 800 and 1500 m). However, there were no adverse effects observed in the 100 m run. Similarly, Kendrick et al. (1993) demonstrated a significant impairment in 60-min treadmill time-trial performance in trained athletes following alcohol ingestion. Heart rate and VO_2 were significantly elevated in subjects after alcohol ingestion and only one out of four subjects could complete the run. This may be due, in part, to the significant hypoglycemia that the subjects experienced at the 60 min time point.

Acute alcohol consumption may also result in small but significant reductions in sustained power output. Lecoultre and Schutz (2009) demonstrated that acute ethanol ingestion resulted in an ~4% reduction in average cycling power output during a 60 min time-trial. Consumption of alcohol 24 h prior to exercise has also been shown to reduce aerobic performance by 11% (O'Brien and Lyons 2000). Some studies have failed to show reductions in exercise performance following alcohol consumption (Bond et al. 1983, Houmard et al. 1987). However, this may be due to limitations in their experimental design as well as type of exercise used. For instance, the lack of ergolytic effects on exercise performance during bicycle ergometer testing may be due to the fact that using a stationary bicycle ergometer does not place significant motor coordination demands as compared to running.

Alcohol can also impair recovery following exercise. It has been shown that alcohol can impair glycogen resynthesis after prolonged cycling (Burke et al. 2003). More importantly, alcohol seems to interfere with protein synthesis, most likely by suppressing the mTOR pathway, which is critical to facilitate repair and hypertrophy following strength training (Lang et al. 2009); similarly, acute ethanol ingestion has been shown to hinder testosterone metabolism and physiology (Vingren et al. 2005, 2013).

Although alcohol seems to have an overall ergolytic effect on exercise performance, a well-known athlete reportedly consumed alcohol before a downhill skiing competition (Winterfeldt 2007). This is potentially a dangerous precedent especially since alcohol has significant effects on executive functions such as judgment and decision making, while also having significant adverse effects on motor control and coordination. This has to be considered in sports requiring a high level of boldness (downhill skiing, downhill mountain biking) and may have implications for pre-participation testing. In addition, the effects of an alcohol-induced hangover are poorly quantified and as such are relatively unknown and subject to further investigation in humans.

8.4.4 Legal Status

Alcohol is prohibited by WADA in competition only (there is competition testing; alcohol is allowed in training and only banned in competition). Detection is conducted by analysis of breath and/or blood. The doping violation threshold (hematological values) is 0.10 g/L through detection in breath or blood. By 2016, alcohol is banned in the following sports: air sports, automobile sports, archery, and powerboating. Additionally, alcohol consumption in society is widespread, but is also illegal in certain quantities while operating many motor-driven vehicles. While this chapter is intended to focus upon the impact of alcohol on exercise performance, particularly in child or adolescent populations, research is lacking in these groups for a number of social and ethical reasons. To this point, the social implications and safety concerns of alcohol consumption for adolescent individuals is and will continue to be an area of concern for parents, coaches, healthcare providers, and school personnel, but is notably beyond the scope of this book and chapter.

8.4.5 Summary

Alcohol is the most commonly consumed drug in athletic communities. The American College of Sports Medicine (ACSM) concludes in its position stand that alcohol consumption adversely affects psychomotor skills and exercise performance while resulting in minimal reductions in maximal oxygen consumption (see also Table 8.3). The ACSM also recommends that if an athlete must consume alcohol, they should refrain from alcohol consumption for at least 48 h prior to competition

TABLE 8.3
Summary of the Effects of Alcohol (EtOH) on Performance

Legal (WADA) Status: Alcohol is Prohibited by WADA in Competition Only. The Doping Violation Threshold is 0.1 g/L. As of 2016, Alcohol is Banned in the Following Sports: Air Sports (FAI), Automobile (FIA), Archery (WA), and Powerboating (UIM)

Acute Effect	Chronic Effect	Effect on Performance	EtOH Dose	References
Reduced left ventricular contractility	Increased left ventricular dimensions and worsened left ventricular dysfunction	Negative effects on cardiac output	1.15 g/kg body weight	Delgado et al. (1975)
No mechanism proposed, authors speculate that decreased performance due to reduced myocardial contractility and reduced lung ventilation		Increased 800–1500 m run times	0.05–0.1 mg/mL blood alcohol concentration	McNaughton et al. (1986)
Hypoglycemia at 60-min time point		Reduced 60-min, treadmill time-trial performance	25 mL in 150 mL grapefruit juice	Kendrick et al. (1993)
No mechanism proposed		Reductions in sustained power output during cycling times trials	0.5 mL/kg FFM	Lecoulre et al. (2009)

while also understanding that alcohol consumption after competition or practice will hinder their ability to recovery and subsequent performance in the next 48–72 h. Chronic alcohol abuse is associated with significant impairments in cardiac and skeletal muscle as well as also slows postexercise recovery by inhibiting protein synthesis. Thus, alcohol is a uniformly ergolytic agent that has significant detrimental effects on exercise performance and use of the same during competitive activity should be minimized for athlete safety and to maximize athletic performance.

8.5 MARIJUANA

8.5.1 History

Cannabis (*Cannabis sativa*) is likely one of the most studied plants in human history. Although its origins remain unclear, it is indigenous to Central and South Asia, and recorded use dates as far back as ~3000 BC. Its genus was classified in 1753 by Carolus Linnaeus, the father of modern taxonomy (Booth 2003). Over the past 5000 years its use has ranged from part of spiritual and religious rites, to medicinal and recreational. In more recent times, the drug became illicit, and illegal in most countries as a result of its containing psychoactive cannabinoids. Although the medical consequences of cannabis use are well known, as of August 2013, 24 states including the District of Columbia have legalized marijuana for medical purposes, with five having legalized marijuana for nonmedical use and others considering the same (Gordon et al. 2013).

8.5.2 Overview

Cannabis is known for its widespread use worldwide. In total, more than 400 different compounds, distributed by 18 chemical groups—including its most active substance, tetrahydrocannabinol (Δ^9-THC)—have been detected in different species of cannabis plants. Consumption of THC-containing cannabis products, such as marijuana (herbal cannabis) and hashish (resinous cannabis) are commonly consumed in the form of cigarettes or even in small pipes. In addition, dronabinol, a THC synthetic product, has been approved in many countries to treat medical conditions such as HIV and cancer. The widespread popularity of use of substances derived from cannabis, such as marijuana, among young athletes has led to its high detection frequency. In 2012, 7.6 million individuals 12 years of age or older used marijuana on 20 or more days in the past month (HHS 2013).

8.5.3 Effects on Performance

The ergogenic effects of marijuana are questionable, as its performance-enhancing effects, if any, have yet to be established. Along these lines, very few studies have tested the effects of marijuana on performance. One of the first studies to evaluate the effects of marijuana smoking on exercise performance was performed by Steadward and Singh (1975), who tested the effects of marijuana smoking compared to placebo on several indices of exercise performance. Resting heart rate, systolic, and diastolic blood pressure were significantly elevated at rest after marijuana consumption compared to both control and placebo. Although there was no significant decrease in grip strength, physical work capacity at a heart rate of 170 decreased by 25% compared to placebo. Renaud and Cormier (1986) tested subjects 10 min after smoking a marijuana cigarette (containing 1.7% of Δ^9-THC) of 7 mg/kg of body weight, and noted a slight, but significant decrease in cycle ergometry time to exhaustion. Avakian et al. (1979) demonstrated that double-blind administration of marijuana as 7.5 mg of Δ^9-THC or placebo did not affect blood pressure, ventilation, or oxygen uptake during submaximal exercise (15 min at 50% of VO_{2max}); however, it did increase heart rate and rate–pressure product at rest and during both exercise and recovery. Tashkin et al. (1978) hypothesized that the decrease in exercise performance may be due to its chronotropic effect leading to achievement of maximum heart rate at reduced workloads. Furthermore, detrimental effects on other aspects of performance have also been demonstrated. When subjects were acutely given THC orally (215 µg/kg), significant deficits in general performance, standing steadiness, reaction time, and psychomotor performance were observed over a 5-h period post-ingestion (Bird et al. 1980). Interestingly, in a case report (Lach and Schachter 1979), it was documented that in a patient with asthma, a condition characterized by bronchoconstriction, smoking marijuana prior to exercise testing led to bronchodilation and no defect in pulmonary function (Tashkin et al. 1975, Vachon et al. 1973). Thus, if there is any positive effect of marijuana, it likely only indirectly improves performance.

It is conceivable that cannabis may reduce an athlete's feelings of pre-competition stress and anxiety as a result of the euphoric effect it may produce. Also, because cannabis diminishes alertness and has relaxing and sedative properties, use may be driven by the effects of relaxation, well-being, and improved sleep quality. For example, it has been reported that relaxing, pleasure, and improved sleeping were the main motives to use cannabis (Lorente et al. 2005), with the rationale that adequate sleep and being relaxed before competition may lead to optimal performance. However, due to the trade-off of decreased exercise performance, possibly secondary to increases in heart rate and blood pressure, which may alter perceived exertion, marijuana may be considered an ergolytic agent.

8.5.4 Legal Status

The International Olympic Committee (IOC) included cannabis in the banned substance list beginning in 1989. The WADA has prohibited its use for all sports competition since 2004. (Thevis et al. 2009). As of 2016, cannabinoids are substances prohibited in-competition only. Moreover, the National Collegiate Athletic Association (NCAA) also bans marijuana use as does many high school sporting associations. Finally, even though a growing movement to legalize marijuana exists, it still is considered illegal in 27 states in the United States.

8.5.5 Summary

Overall, it appears that cannabis does not have ergogenic potential in sports activities and thus, its inclusion on the banned list is likely a function of its illicitness. As cannabis smoking impairs exercise and psychomotor performance (such as its sedative effect, slower reaction times, and other psychomotor effects), its ability to serve as an ergogenic aid has been questioned, and is generally considered to be an ergolytic drug (see Table 8.4). This is likely due to the increase in heart rate and blood pressure, the decline of cardiac output, and the reduction in psychomotor activity that have been demonstrated in prior studies.

8.6 DRUG INTERACTIONS

Alcohol acts as a depressant and caffeine as a stimulant of the CNS. If the two substances are consumed together, the psychostimulatory effect of caffeine seems to antagonize the depressive effect of alcohol via incomplete antagonism. Indeed, ingestion of a combination of alcohol and caffeine showed no significant difference from placebo when simple reaction time was measured and the amplitude of the evoked potentials were assessed (Azcona et al. 1995). However, the subject's feeling of intoxication persisted. The interaction of caffeine with cannabis seems to be more complex. When caffeine and cannabis were given to rats, memory deficits induced by THC were not attenuated but actually exacerbated (Panlilio et al. 2012). In the presence of nicotine, caffeine exhibits a shorter half-life and faster metabolism (Brown et al. 1988). Ethanol, on the other hand, has been shown to slow caffeine metabolism and increases its half-life (George et al. 1986). Co-ingestion of caffeine and nicotine exhibit additive effects on cardiovascular parameters such as blood pressure during baseline conditions, but less than additive effects during conditions of physical and mental

TABLE 8.4
Summary of the Effect of THC on Performance

Legal (WADA) Status: The International Olympic Committee Included Cannabis in the Banned Substance List Beginning in 1989 and Since 2004 the World Anti-Doping Agency has Prohibited Its Use for All Sports Competition [166]

Acute Effect	Effect on Performance	THC Dose	References
Resting heart rate and both systolic/diastolic blood pressure were significantly elevated at rest	Physical work capacity at a heart rate of 170 decreased by 25% compared to placebo	18.2 mg of Δ^9-THC	Steadward and Singh (1975)
Induced tachycardia at rest	VE, VO_2, and VCO_2 were increased above control at ≥50% max effort; small, but significant reduction in maximal exercise duration; tachycardia up to 80% of maximum effort and during recovery	7 mg/kg marijuana (containing 1.7% Δ^9-THC)	Renaud and Cormier (1986)
Increased heart rate and the rate–pressure product at rest	No effect on blood pressure, ventilation or oxygen uptake during submaximal exercise (15 min at 50% of VO_{2max}); increased heart rate and the rate–pressure product during recovery	Smoking 7.5 mg of Δ^9-THC	Avakian et al. (1979)

stress and sympathoadrenal stimulation (Smits et al. 1993). While more research is needed to fully understand the potential interactions that exist between these drugs, it is safe to recommend caution and concern when these drugs are consumed and particularly if co-ingestion occurs.

8.7 CONCLUSION AND PERSPECTIVES

The physiological effects of the abovementioned substances are well established in adults. However, the ergogenic effect of some of the discussed drugs may be questioned and one has to consider the cohort tested for every specific substance. For these reasons and other social reasons, use of these drugs by adolescents and other young adults pose problems as they relate to health and performance. Only caffeine has enough strength of evidence to be considered an ergogenic aid. Marijuana and alcohol are ergolytic for sports performance, and nicotine needs confirmation with further research. It is well known that there is intersubject variability in response to every drug (Evans and Johnson 2001), thus one drug may have very different effects in different young adult individuals.

REFERENCES

Abian-Vicen, J., C. Puente, J. J. Salinero, C. Gonzalez-Millan, F. Areces, G. Munoz, J. Munoz-Guerra, and J. Del Coso. 2014. A caffeinated energy drink improves jump performance in adolescent basketball players. *Amino Acids* 46 (5):1333–41. doi: 10.1007/s00726-014-1702-6.

ADDB. 2012. Trond Husø. Anti-Doping Database. http://www.dopinglist.com/

Alaranta, A., H. Alaranta, K. Patja, P. Palmu, R. Prattala, T. Martelin, and I. Helenius. 2006. Snuff use and smoking in Finnish Olympic athletes. *International Journal of Sports Medicine* 27 (7):581–6.

Amann, M. 2012. Pulmonary system limitations to endurance exercise performance in humans. *Experimental Physiology* 97 (3):311–8. doi: 10.1113/expphysiol.2011.058800.

Andersson, K. and P. Arner. 2001. Systemic nicotine stimulates human adipose tissue lipolysis through local cholinergic and catecholaminergic receptors. *International Journal of Obesity and Related Metabolic Disorders* 25 (8):1225–32. doi: 10.1038/sj.ijo.0801654.

Avakian, E. V., S. M. Horvath, E. D. Michael, and S. Jacobs. 1979. Effect of marijuana on cardiorespiratory responses to submaximal exercise. *Clinical Pharmacology and Therapeutics* 26 (6):777–81.

Azcona, O., M. J. Barbanoj, J. Torrent, and F. Jane. 1995. Evaluation of the central effects of alcohol and caffeine interaction. *British Journal of Clinical Pharmacology* 40 (4):393–400.

Barnes, M. J., T. Mundel, and S. R. Stannard. 2010. Post-exercise alcohol ingestion exacerbates eccentric-exercise induced losses in performance. *European Journal of Applied Physiology* 108 (5):1009–14. doi: 10.1007/s00421-009-1311-3.

Bird, K. D., T. Boleyn, G. B. Chesher, D. M. Jackson, G. A. Starmer, and R. K. Teo. 1980. Intercannabinoid and cannabinoid-ethanol interactions on human performance. *Psychopharmacology* 71 (2):181–8.

Bond, V., B. D. Franks, and E. T. Howley. 1983. Effects of small and moderate doses of alcohol on submaximal cardiorespiratory function, perceived exertion and endurance performance in abstainers and moderate drinkers. *Journal of Sports Medicine and Physical Fitness* 23 (2):221–8.

Booth, M. 2003. *Cannabis: A History*. London, UK: Transworld Publishers Limited.

Boutrel, B. and G. F. Koob. 2004. What keeps us awake: The neuropharmacology of stimulants and wakefulness-promoting medications. *Sleep* 27 (6):1181–94.

Brandt, A. M. 1990. The cigarette, risk, and American culture. *Daedalus* 119 (4):155–76.

Brown, C. R., P. Jacob, 3rd, M. Wilson, and N. L. Benowitz. 1988. Changes in rate and pattern of caffeine metabolism after cigarette abstinence. *Clinical Pharmacology and Therapeutics* 43 (5):488–91.

Burke, L. M., G. R. Collier, E. M. Broad, P. G. Davis, D. T. Martin, A. J. Sanigorski, and M. Hargreaves. 2003. Effect of alcohol intake on muscle glycogen storage after prolonged exercise. *Journal of Applied Physiology* 95 (3):983–90.

Burtscher, M., R. Likar, C. Pechlaner, F. Kunz, and M. Philadelphy. 1994. Motor symptoms similar to parkinsonism in heavy smokers. *International Journal of Sports Medicine* 15 (4):207–12.

Charlton, A. 2004. Medicinal uses of tobacco in history. *Journal of the Royal Society of Medicine* 97 (6):292–6.

Chou, T. 1992. Wake up and smell the coffee. Caffeine, coffee, and the medical consequences. *Western Journal of Medicine* 157 (5):544–53.

Cofan, M., J. M. Nicolas, J. Fernandez-Sola, J. Robert, E. Tobias, E. Sacanella, R. Estruch, and A. Urbano-Marquez. 2000. Acute ethanol treatment decreases intracellular calcium-ion transients in mouse single skeletal muscle fibres in vitro. *Alcohol and Alcoholism* 35 (2):134–8.

Collins, T. and W. Vamplew. 2002. *Mud, Sweat and Beers: A Cultural History of Sport and Alcohol*. Oxford, England: Berg.

Collomp, K., S. Ahmaidi, M. Audran, J. L. Chanal, and C. Prefaut. 1991. Effects of caffeine ingestion on performance and anaerobic metabolism during the Wingate Test. *International Journal of Sports Medicine* 12 (5):439–43.

Cox, G. R., B. Desbrow, P. G. Montgomery, M. E. Anderson, C. R. Bruce, T. A. Macrides et al. 2002. Effect of different protocols of caffeine intake on metabolism and endurance performance. *Journal of Applied Physiology* 93 (3):990–9.

Crocq, M. A. 2003. Alcohol, nicotine, caffeine, and mental disorders. *Dialogues in Clinical Neuroscience* 5 (2):175–85.

Davis, J. K. and J. M. Green. 2009. Caffeine and anaerobic performance: Ergogenic value and mechanisms of action. *Sports Medicine* 39 (10):813–32. doi: 10.2165/11317770-000000000-00000.

Del Coso, J., E. Estevez, and R. Mora-Rodriguez. 2008. Caffeine effects on short-term performance during prolonged exercise in the heat. *Medicine & Science in Sports & Exercise* 40 (4):744–51. doi: 10.1249/MSS.0b013e3181621336.

Delgado, C. E., Gortuin, N. J., Ross, R. S. 1975. Acute effects of low doses of alcohol on left ventricular function by echocardiography. *Circulation* 51:535–40.

Derry, C. J., S. Derry, and R. A. Moore. 2012. Caffeine as an analgesic adjuvant for acute pain in adults. *Cochrane Database of Systematic Reviews* 3:CD009281. doi: 10.1002/14651858.CD009281.pub2.

Desbrow, B., Barrett, C. M., Minahan, C. L., Grant, G. D., and Leveritt, M. D. 2009. Caffeine, cycling performance, and exogenous CHO oxidation: A dose–response study. *Medicine & Science in Sports & Exercise* 41:1744–51.

Doherty, M. and P. M. Smith. 2005. Effects of caffeine ingestion on rating of perceived exertion during and after exercise: A meta-analysis. *Scandinavian Journal of Medicine and Science in Sports* 15 (2):69–78. doi: 10.1111/j.1600-0838.2005.00445.x.

Donsmark, M., J. Langfort, C. Holm, T. Ploug, and H. Galbo. 2003. Contractions activate hormone-sensitive lipase in rat muscle by protein kinase C and mitogen-activated protein kinase. *Journal of Physiology* 550 (Pt 3):845–54. doi: 10.1113/jphysiol.2003.042333.

El-Sayed, M. S., N. Ali, and Z. El-Sayed Ali. 2005. Interaction between alcohol and exercise: Physiological and haematological implications. *Sports Medicine* 35 (3):257–69.

Evans, W. E. and J. A. Johnson. 2001. Pharmacogenomics: The inherited basis for interindividual differences in drug response. *Annual Review of Genomics and Human Genetics* 2:9–39.

Fenster, L., C. Quale, R. A. Hiatt, M. Wilson, G. C. Windham, and N. L. Benowitz. 1998. Rate of caffeine metabolism and risk of spontaneous abortion. *American Journal of Epidemiology* 147 (5):503–10.

Foskett, A., A. Ali, and N. Gant. 2009. Caffeine enhances cognitive function and skill performance during simulated soccer activity. *International Journal of Sport Nutrition and Exercise Metabolism* 19 (4):410–23.

George, J., T. Murphy, R. Roberts, W. G. Cooksley, J. W. Halliday, and L. W. Powell. 1986. Influence of alcohol and caffeine consumption on caffeine elimination. *Clinical and Experimental Pharmacology and Physiology* 13 (10):731–6.

Goldstein, E. R., T. Ziegenfuss, D. Kalman, R. Kreider, B. Campbell, C. Wilborn et al. 2010. International Society of Sports Nutrition Position Stand: Caffeine and performance. *Journal of the International Society of Sports Nutrition* 7 (1):5. doi: 10.1186/1550-2783-7-5.

Gonzalez, J. T. and E. J. Stevenson. 2012. New perspectives on nutritional interventions to augment lipid utilisation during exercise. *British Journal of Nutrition* 107 (3):339–49.

Goodspeed, T. H. 1954. *The Genus Nicotiana; Origins, Relationships, and Evolution of Its Species in the Light of Their Distribution, Morphology, and Cytogenetics.* Waltham, MA: Chronica Botanica Co.

Gordon, A. J., J. W. Conley, and J. M. Gordon. 2013. Medical consequences of marijuana use: A review of current literature. *Current Psychiatry Reports* 15 (12):419.

Gray, N. 2005. Mixed feelings on snus. *Lancet* 366 (9490):966–7. doi: 10.1016/S0140-6736(05)67352-7.

Green, J. M., Wickwire, P. J., McLester, J. R., Gendle, S., Hudson, G., Pritchett, R. C., and Laurent, C. M. 2007. Effects of caffeine on repetitions to failure and ratings of perceived exertion during resistance training. *International Journal of Sports Physiology and Performance* 2:250–9.

Grossman, A. and J. R. Sutton. 1985. Endorphins: What are they? How are they measured? What is their role in exercise? *Medicine & Science in Sports & Exercise* 17 (1):74–81.

Gutgesell, M. and R. Canterbury. 1999. Alcohol usage in sport and exercise. *Addiction Biology* 4 (4):373–83. doi: 10.1080/13556219971353.

Haasova, M., F. C. Warren, M. Ussher, K. Janse Van Rensburg, G. Faulkner, M. Cropley, J. Byron-Daniel, E. S. Everson-Hock, H. Oh, and A. H. Taylor. 2013. The acute effects of physical activity on cigarette cravings: Systematic review and meta-analysis with individual participant data. *Addiction* 108 (1):26–37. doi: 10.1111/j.1360-0443.2012.04034.x.

Heishman, S. J., Snyder, F. R., and Henningfield, J.E. 1993. Performance, subjective, and physiological effects of nicotine in non-smokers. *Drug and Alcohol Dependence* 34:11–18.

Heishman, S. J., B. A. Kleykamp, and E. G. Singleton. 2010. Meta-analysis of the acute effects of nicotine and smoking on human performance. *Psychopharmacology (Berl)* 210 (4):453–69. doi: 10.1007/s00213-010-1848-1.

HHS. 2013. Substance Abuse and Mental Health Services Administration. Results from the 2012 National Survey on Drug Use and Health: Summary of National Findings. Edited by Substance Abuse and Mental Health Services Administration, NSDUH Series. Rockville, MD: HHS Publication No. (SMA) 13.

Hindmarch, I., Kerr, J. S., and Sherwood, N. 1990. Effects of nicotine gum on psychomotor performance in smokers and non-smokers. *Psychopharmacology (Berl)* 100:535–41.

Holm, H., M. J. Jarvis, M. A. Russell, and C. Feyerabend. 1992. Nicotine intake and dependence in Swedish snuff takers. *Psychopharmacology* 108 (4):507–11.

Houmard, J. A., M. E. Langenfeld, R. L. Wiley, and J. Siefert. 1987. Effects of the acute ingestion of small amounts of alcohol upon 5-mile run times. *Journal of Sports Medicine and Physical Fitness* 27 (2):253.

Jamner, L. D., S. S. Girdler, D. Shapiro, and M. E. Jarvik. 1998. Pain inhibition, nicotine, and gender. *Experimental and Clinical Psychopharmacology* 6 (1):96–106.

Kendrick, Z. V., M. B. Affrime, and D. T. Lowenthal. 1993. Effect of ethanol on metabolic responses to treadmill running in well-trained men. *Journal of Clinical Pharmacology* 33 (2):136–9.

Lach, E. and E. N. Schachter. 1979. Marijuana and exercise testing. *New England Journal of Medicine* 301 (8):438.

Lang, C. H., A. M. Pruznak, G. J. Nystrom, and T. C. Vary. 2009. Alcohol-induced decrease in muscle protein synthesis associated with increased binding of mTOR and raptor: Comparable effects in young and mature rats. *Nutrition & Metabolism (London)* 6:4.

Lang, R. M., K. M. Borow, A. Neumann, and T. Feldman. 1985. Adverse cardiac effects of acute alcohol ingestion in young adults. *Annals of Internal Medicine* 102 (6):742–7.

Lecoultre, V. and Y. Schutz. 2009. Effect of a small dose of alcohol on the endurance performance of trained cyclists. *Alcohol and Alcoholism* 44 (3):278–83. doi: 10.1093/alcalc/agn108.

Levin, E. D., F. J. McClernon, and A. H. Rezvani. 2006. Nicotinic effects on cognitive function: Behavioral characterization, pharmacological specification, and anatomic localization. *Psychopharmacology* 184 (3–4):523–39. doi: 10.1007/s00213-005-0164-7.

Lichtenstein, A. H., L. J. Appel, M. Brands, M. Carnethon, S. Daniels, H. A. Franch et al. 2006. Diet and lifestyle recommendations revision 2006: A scientific statement from the American Heart Association Nutrition Committee. *Circulation* 114 (1):82–96. doi: 10.1161/CIRCULATIONAHA.106.176158.

Lorente, F. O., P. Peretti-Watel, and L. Grelot. 2005. Cannabis use to enhance sportive and non-sportive performances among French sport students. *Addictive Behaviors* 30 (7):1382–91. doi: 10.1016/j.addbeh.2005.01.019.

Lorino, A. J., L. K. Lloyd, S. H. Crixell, and J. L. Walker. 2006. The effects of caffeine on athletic agility. *Journal of Strength and Conditioning Research* 20 (4):851–4.

Marclay, F., E. Grata, L. Perrenoud, and M. Saugy. 2011. A one-year monitoring of nicotine use in sport: Frontier between potential performance enhancement and addiction issues. *Forensic Science International* 213 (1–3):73–84.

Martinsen M., Sundgot-Borgen J. 2014. Adolescent elite athletes' cigarette smoking, use of snus, and alcohol. *Scandinavian Journal of Medicine and Science in Sports* 24 (2):439–46.

Marzilli, T. S., K. F. Willhoit, and M. Guadagnoli. 2006. Effects of information processing load in abstinent and nonabstinent smokers' psychomotor task performance. *Nicotine & Tobacco Research* 8 (3):425–33. doi: 10.1080/14622200600672757.

Mattila, V. M., S. Raisamo, H. Pihlajamaki, M. Mantysaari, and A. Rimpela. 2012. Sports activity and the use of cigarettes and snus among young males in Finland in 1999–2010. *BMC Public Health* 12:230. doi: 10.1186/1471-2458-12-230.

McNaughton, L. and D. Preece. 1986. Alcohol and its effects on sprint and middle distance running. *British Journal of Sports Medicine* 20 (2):56–9.

McNaughton, L. R., R. J. Lovell, J. C. Siegler, A. W. Midgley, M. Sandstrom, and D. J. Bentley. 2008. The effects of caffeine ingestion on time trial cycling performance. *Journal of Sports Medicine and Physical Fitness* 48 (3):320–5.

Meier, J. 2006. Effect of nicotine and muscle performance using a Wingate anaerobic tests of collegiate football players. Wisconsin: The University of Wisconsin Whitewater.

Mora-Rodriguez, R., J. Garcia Pallares, A. Lopez-Samanes, J. F. Ortega, and V. E. Fernandez-Elias. 2012. Caffeine ingestion reverses the circadian rhythm effects on neuromuscular performance in highly resistance-trained men. *PLoS One* 7 (4):e33807.

Mottram, D. R. 1996. *Drugs in Sport*, 2nd ed. London, New York: E & FN Spon, an imprint of Chapman & Hall.

Mottram, D. R. and N. Chester (Eds). 2014. *Drugs in Sport*, 6th ed. Oxon, UK: Routledge.

Mundel, T. and D. A. Jones. 2006. Effect of transdermal nicotine administration on exercise endurance in men. *Experimental Physiology* 91 (4):705–13. doi: 10.1113/expphysiol.2006.033373.

Nawrot, P., S. Jordan, J. Eastwood, J. Rotstein, A. Hugenholtz, and M. Feeley. 2003. Effects of caffeine on human health. *Food Additives & Contaminants* 20 (1):1–30. doi: 10.1080/0265203021000007840.

Nemec, D. 2004. *The Beer and Whisky League: The Illustrated History of the American Association—Baseball's Renegade Major League*. Guilford, Connecticut: Globe Pequot.

Nutt, D. J., L. A. King, and L. D. Phillips. 2010. Drug harms in the UK: A multicriteria decision analysis. *Lancet* 376 (9752):1558–65.

O'Brien, C. P. and F. Lyons. 2000. Alcohol and the athlete. *Sports Medicine* 29 (5):295–300.

Osswald, H., and J. Schnermann. 2011. Methylxanthines and the kidney. *Handbook of Experimental Pharmacology* (200):391–412.

Paluska, S. A. 2003. Caffeine and exercise. *Current Sports Medicine Reports* 2 (4):213–9.

Panlilio, L. V., S. Ferre, S. Yasar, E. B. Thorndike, C. W. Schindler, and S. R. Goldberg. 2012. Combined effects of THC and caffeine on working memory in rats. *British Journal of Pharmacology* 165 (8):2529–38. doi: 10.1111/j.1476-5381.2011.01554.x.

Pedersen, D. J., S. J. Lessard, V. G. Coffey, E. G. Churchley, A. M. Wootton, T. Ng, M. J. Watt, and J. A. Hawley. 2008. High rates of muscle glycogen resynthesis after exhaustive exercise when carbohydrate is coingested with caffeine. *Journal of Applied Physiology* 105 (1):7–13. doi: 10.1152/japplphysiol.01121.2007.

Pendergrast, M. 2010. *Uncommon Grounds: The History of Coffee and How It Transformed Our World*. Rev. ed. New York: Basic Books.

Poikolainen, K. 1995. Alcohol and mortality: A review. *Journal of Clinical Epidemiology* 48 (4):455–65.

Posselt, W, and L. Reimann. 1828. Chemische Untersuchungen des Tabaks und Darstellung des eigentlichen wirksamen Prinzips dieser Pflanze. *Geigers Magazin der Pharmazie* 24:138–61.

Renaud, A. M. and Y. Cormier. 1986. Acute effects of marijuana smoking on maximal exercise performance. *Medicine & Science in Sports & Exercise* 18 (6):685–9.

Richardson, P., W. McKenna, M. Bristow, B. Maisch, B. Mautner, J. O'Connell et al. 1996. Report of the 1995 World Health Organization/International Society and Federation of Cardiology Task Force on the definition and classification of cardiomyopathies. *Circulation* 93 (5):841–2.

Riess, S. A. 1991. *City Games: The Evolution of American Urban Society and the Rise of Sports*. Illinois, USA: University of Illinois Press.

Robinson, J. H. and W. S. Pritchard. 1992. The role of nicotine in tobacco use. *Psychopharmacology* 108 (4):397–407.

Rush, J. W. and L. L. Spriet. 2001. Skeletal muscle glycogen phosphorylase a kinetics: Effects of adenine nucleotides and caffeine. *Journal of Applied Physiology* 91 (5):2071–8.

Scerbo, F., G. Faulkner, A. Taylor, and S. Thomas. 2010. Effects of exercise on cravings to smoke: The role of exercise intensity and cortisol. *Journal of Sports Sciences* 28 (1):11–9. doi: 10.1080/02640410903390089.

Smits, P., L. Temme, and T. Thien. 1993. The cardiovascular interaction between caffeine and nicotine in humans. *Clinical Pharmacology and Therapeutics* 54 (2):194–204.

Spolarics, Z., G. J. Bagby, P. H. Pekala, C. Dobrescu, N. Skrepnik, and J. J. Spitzer. 1994. Acute alcohol administration attenuates insulin-mediated glucose use by skeletal muscle. *American Journal of Physiology* 267 (6 Pt 1):E886–91.

Spriet, L. L., D. A. MacLean, D. J. Dyck, E. Hultman, G. Cederblad, and T. E. Graham. 1992. Caffeine ingestion and muscle metabolism during prolonged exercise in humans. *American Journal of Physiology* 262 (6 Pt 1):E891–8.

Statland, B. E. and T. J. Demas. 1980. Serum caffeine half-lives. Healthy subjects vs. patients having alcoholic hepatic disease. *American Journal of Clinical Pathology* 73 (3):390–3.

Steadward, R. D. and M. Singh. 1975. The effects of smoking marijuana on physical performance. *Medicine and Science in Sports* 7 (4):309–11.

Stolerman, I. P. and M. J. Jarvis. 1995. The scientific case that nicotine is addictive. *Psychopharmacology* 117 (1):2–10; discussion 14–20.

Sturm, R. 2002. The effects of obesity, smoking, and drinking on medical problems and costs. *Health Affairs (Millwood)* 21 (2):245–53.

Taioli, E. 2008. Gene–environment interaction in tobacco-related cancers. *Carcinogenesis* 29 (8):1467–74.

Tarnopolsky, M. and C. Cupido. 2000. Caffeine potentiates low frequency skeletal muscle force in habitual and nonhabitual caffeine consumers. *Journal of Applied Physiology (Bethesda, MD.: 1985)* 89 (5):1719–24.

Tarnopolsky, M. A. 1994. Caffeine and endurance performance. *Sports Medicine* 18 (2):109–25.

Tashkin, D. P., B. J. Shapiro, Y. E. Lee, and C. E. Harper. 1975. Effects of smoked marijuana in experimentally induced asthma. *American Review of Respiratory Disease* 112 (3):377–86.

Tashkin, D. P., J. R. Soares, R. S. Hepler, B. J. Shapiro, and G. S. Rachelefsky. 1978. Cannabis, 1977. *Annals of Internal Medicine* 89 (4):539–49. doi: 10.7326/0003-4819-89-4-539.

Taylor, C., D. Higham, G. L. Close, and J. P. Morton. 2011. The effect of adding caffeine to postexercise carbohydrate feeding on subsequent high-intensity interval-running capacity compared with carbohydrate alone. *International Journal of Sport Nutrition and Exercise Metabolism* 21 (5):410–6.

Temple, J. L. 2009. Caffeine use in children: What we know, what we have left to learn, and why we should worry. *Neuroscience & Biobehavioral Reviews* 33 (6):793–806. doi: 10.1016/j.neubiorev.2009.01.001.

Thevis, M., T. Kuuranne, H. Geyer, and W. Schänzer. 2009. Annual banned-substance review: The Prohibited List 2008—Analytical approaches in human sports drug testing. *Drug Testing and Analysis* 1 (1):4–13. doi: 10.1002/dta.9.

Trounce, I., E. Byrne, and X. Dennett. 1990. Biochemical and morphological studies of skeletal muscle in experimental chronic alcoholic myopathy. *Acta Neurologica Scandinavica* 82 (6):386–91.

Tucha, O. and Lange, K. W. 2004. Effects of nicotine chewing gum on a real-life motor task: A kinematic analysis of handwriting movements in smokers and non-smokers. *Psychopharmacology (Berl)* 173:49–56.

Vachon, L., M. X. FitzGerald, N. H. Solliday, I. A. Gould, and E. A. Gaensler. 1973. Single-dose effects of marijuana smoke. Bronchial dynamics and respiratory-center sensitivity in normal subjects. *New England Journal of Medicine* 288 (19):985–9. doi: 10.1056/NEJM197305102881902.

Van Soeren, M. H., P. Sathasivam, L. L. Spriet, and T. E. Graham. 1993. Caffeine metabolism and epinephrine responses during exercise in users and nonusers. *Journal of Applied Physiology (Bethesda, MD.: 1985)* 75 (2):805–12.

Vella, L. D. and D. Cameron-Smith. 2010. Alcohol, athletic performance and recovery. *Nutrients* 2 (8):781–9.

Vila, L., A. Ferrando, J. Voces, C. Cabral de Oliveira, J. G. Prieto, and A. I. Alvarez. 2001. Effect of chronic ethanol ingestion and exercise training on skeletal muscle in rat. *Drug and Alcohol Dependence* 64 (1):27–33.

Vingren, J. L., D. W. Hill, H. Buddhadev, and A. Duplanty. 2013. Postresistance exercise ethanol ingestion and acute testosterone bioavailability. *Medicine & Science in Sports & Exercise* 45 (9):1825–32. doi: 10.1249/MSS.0b013e31828d3767.

Vingren, J. L., L. P. Koziris, S. E. Gordon, W. J. Kraemer, R. T. Turner, and K. C. Westerlind. 2005. Chronic alcohol intake, resistance training, and muscle androgen receptor content. *Medicine & Science in Sports & Exercise* 37 (11):1842–8.

WADA. 2012. World Anti-Doping Agency. The 2012 Monitoring Program. https://wada-main-prod.s3.amazonaws.com/resources/files/WADA_Monitoring_Program_2012_EN.pdf

WADA. 2016. World Anti-Doping Code International Standard-Prohibited List, January 2016. https://wada-main-prod.s3.amazonaws.com/resources/files/wada-2015-prohibited-list-en.pdf

Walker, J. F., L. C. Collins, P. P. Rowell, L. J. Goldsmith, R. J. Moffatt, and B. A. Stamford. 1999. The effect of smoking on energy expenditure and plasma catecholamine and nicotine levels during light physical activity. *Nicotine & Tobacco Research* 1 (4):365–70.

Weber, F., M. Anlauf, and R. D. Muller. 1989. Changes in muscle blood flow after smoking a cigarette determined by a new noninvasive method. *European Journal of Clinical Pharmacology* 37 (5):517–20.

West, R. J. and Jarvis, M. J. 1986. Effects of nicotine on finger tapping rate in nonsmokers. *Pharmacology Biochemistry and Behavior* 25:727–31.

Wiles, J. D., S. R. Bird, J. Hopkins, and M. Riley. 1992. Effect of caffeinated coffee on running speed, respiratory factors, blood lactate and perceived exertion during 1500-m treadmill running. *British Journal of Sports Medicine* 26 (2):116–20.

Winterfeldt, J. 2007. Die Welt. Ein bisschen Alkohol macht dich schneller. http://www.welt.de/sport/article1373824/Ein-bisschen-Alkohol-macht-dich-schneller.htm

Woolf, K., W. K. Bidwell, and A. G. Carlson. 2008. The effect of caffeine as an ergogenic aid in anaerobic exercise. *International Journal of Sport Nutrition and Exercise Metabolism* 18 (4):412–29.

Zimmermann, R., J. G. Strauss, G. Haemmerle, G. Schoiswohl, R. Birner-Gruenberger, M. Riederer et al. 2004. Fat mobilization in adipose tissue is promoted by adipose triglyceride lipase. *Science* 306 (5700):1383–6. doi: 10.1126/science.1100747.

9 Drugs, Steroids, and Youth

Andrew Jagim and Jonathan Mike

CONTENTS

Abstract	153
9.1 Introduction	154
9.2 Prevalence of Use	154
9.3 Reasons for Use	155
9.4 Other Related Drug Use	157
9.5 Prevention and Education	158
9.6 Management	158
9.7 Physiological Adaptations	159
9.7.1 Testosterone and Testosterone Analogs	159
9.7.2 Growth Hormone	161
9.8 Performance Benefits for Strength, Power, Endurance Athletes	162
9.9 Body Composition	164
9.10 Side Effects	164
9.10.1 Acute	164
9.10.2 Chronic	165
9.11 Legal Considerations and Testing	166
9.12 Conclusions	167
References	167

ABSTRACT

The use of elicit substances, in particular anabolic–androgenic steroids to improve performance, appears to be a practice that is gaining popularity in our society, especially among today's youth. Anabolic–androgenic steroids enhance strength, power, and endurance performance. However, performance is largely affected by many factors including the sport itself and sporting skill, training regimens, frequency of training, genetics, intensity, and environmental influences to name a few. Research has indicated increased use patterns among high school students, in particular male students, not only for the performance-enhancing benefits but also for increased self-esteem. Some of the acute side effects reported in male subjects in these studies include increased aggression, acne occurrence, increased body hair, and testicular atrophy. Use of such substances by women, children, and adolescents are of particular concern due to the addictive potential and how the substances impact the physiology of these types of individuals. Legal considerations and testing of anabolic–androgenic steroids are not cut and dry, which is further complicated by adequate and effective testing procedures as well as necessary funding to support widespread testing efforts. With regard to adolescents and sports, drug testing is largely punitive, with positive testing yielding significant penalties, including loss of player privileges, removal of both individual and team awards and championships, removal of scholarships, and potentially criminal punishment.

9.1 INTRODUCTION

The evolution of youth sports and fitness programs has placed a higher demand on young individuals to continually strive to improve themselves and compete at a higher level. Young athletes are pressured to look for ways to improve performance outside of the traditional practices of proper training and conditioning. The use of performance-enhancing substances, in particular anabolic–androgenic steroids to improve performance appears to be a practice that is gaining popularity in our society, especially among today's youth (Calfee and Fadale 2006, Castillo and Comstock 2007, Dodge and Jaccard 2006). It is important to first differentiate between performance-enhancing substances and anabolic–androgenic steroids as both terms are often used interchangeably and inappropriately. Too often when people hear the term "performance-enhancing substance," they assume one is talking about anabolic–androgenic steroids, "drugs," or some form of an illegal substance. When in reality, performance-enhancing substances can include a much broader class of constituents (Castillo and Comstock 2007). For example, ingested performance-enhancing substances can in fact include any ergogenic aid consumed by an athlete such as a glucose–electrolyte solution (i.e., Gatorade™ or Powerade™) during endurance activity, water ingestion to maintain hydration status, or a protein supplement to facilitate resistance-training adaptations and recovery, while other categories of performance-enhancing items could be more aerodynamic handlebars on a bicycle. As a category, various examples of performance-enhancing substances can include over-the-counter dietary supplements, vitamins, minerals, macronutrients, prohormones, caffeine, erythropoietin (EPO), or anabolic–androgenic steroids. Typically, performance-enhancing substances can be divided into three main categories: (1) Illegal substances that are not available without a prescription and banned by most if not all sports (i.e., anabolic steroids, hormone precursors, etc.); (2) Legally available substances that are banned by some but not all sports (i.e., caffeine in high doses, some herbal/botanical extracts, amino acids [banned by NCAA—National Collegiate Athletic Association], etc.); and (3) Legally available substances that are not banned by sports (i.e., most dietary supplements and food products) (Castillo and Comstock 2007). Therefore, anabolic–androgenic steroids are just a snapshot of a broader class of performance-enhancing substances that are sometimes taken by athletes of all ages. The remaining focus of this chapter will pertain to the first category, dealing with illegal performance-enhancing substances, specifically anabolic–androgenic steroids. Chapter 13 of this book will address use of dictary supplements by youth and adolescents and effectively capture portions of the other two categories of performance-enhancing substances. Additionally, it is recognized that use of other drugs such as EPO or blood doping practices are common in endurance sports, but fortunately this practice is quite uncommon in child and adolescent athlete populations and beyond the scope of this chapter.

9.2 PREVALENCE OF USE

Common anabolic–androgenic steroids are synthetic derivatives of the male hormone testosterone as well as growth hormone and when taken exogenously (orally or via intramuscular injection) increases body mass, fat-free mass, and strength along with concomitant decreases in fat mass (Bhasin et al. 1996, Evans 2004). A limited amount of research exists on the prevalence and direct effects of anabolic–androgenic steroid use in adolescents as the studies are difficult to complete due to privacy, ethical, and legal concerns (Yesalis et al. 2000). The majority of the completed studies are based on a self-report use, which can have underlying issues of accuracy and reliability. For example, a 1980 study found that only 1% of high school athletes had been surveyed (n = 295) for reported using of anabolic–androgenic steroids (Krowchuk et al. 1989). However, in 1988 as high as 6% of high school male seniors (n = 3403) across the country reported using of anabolic–androgenic steroids at one point during their athletic careers (Buckley et al. 1988). The prevalence of the use of anabolic–androgenic steroids was thought to have remained relatively stable during the late 1980s and early 1990s with prevalence rates of all high school students ranging from 0.9% to 1.2% (Johnston et al. 2013).

TABLE 9.1
Anabolic Steroid Use among U.S. Adolescents

Sample Population	Overall Prevalence (%)	References
3403 Male 12th graders	6.6	Buckley et al. (1988)
295 High school athletes	1.0	Krowchuk et al. (1989)
853 11th graders	11.1	Johnson et al. (1989)
3900 10th–12th graders	5.3	Whitehead et al. (1992)
810 7th graders	3.8	Radakovich et al. (1993)
6930 High school students	2.7	Tanner et al. (1995)
4722 Middle/high school students	2.5	Scott et al. (1996)
965 Middle school students	2.7	Faigenbaum et al. (1998)
1325 High school football players	6.3	Stilger and Yesalis (1999)

Source: Adapted from Castillo, E. M. and Comstock, R. D, *Pediatr. Clin. North Am.*, 54(4), 663–675, 2007; i–x. doi: 10.1016/j.pcl.2007.04.002. With permission.

However, the use of anabolic–androgenic steroids has seen an increase over the last 15 years. Survey data from the National Institute on Drug Abuse show that the annual use of anabolic–androgenic steroids among high school seniors in the United States has risen from 1.1% in 1992 to 2.5% in 2004 (Elin and Winters 2004). More recent evidence also suggests that anabolic–androgenic steroid use among adolescents may increase as a student progresses through high school, indicating that 6% of high school male 12th graders admitted to using androgens (Hoffman et al. 2008). The primary reason for this is unknown but it may be a result of the increased availability of such substances, the rise in their popularity seen in the world of professional sports and the young athletes' drive to excel athletically (Calfee and Fadale 2006, Castillo and Comstock 2007, Yesalis et al. 2000). Recently in 2007 it was estimated that up to 5%–10% of young males and approximately 3% of females were using anabolic–androgenic steroids (Kerr and Congeni 2007). Regardless of the time period or age group, it seems the majority of individuals who use anabolic–androgenic steroids are predominately male with prevalence rates in the range of 4%–6% as compared to 0.2%–2.9% of females (Dodge and Jaccard 2006). Nonetheless, in the early and mid-2000s, some investigators reported a greater frequency of androgen use among female adolescents have ranged from 2% (Miller et al. 2005) to 2.9% (Irving et al. 2002). Despite this reported data, more recent investigations have shown that increased frequency of androgen use between female adolescents may have been overstated or at least is declining (Dodge and Jaccard 2006, Hoffman et al. 2008).

Location may also have an impact on the prevalence of anabolic–androgenic steroid use. One report suggested that anabolic–androgenic steroid use in adolescents may be more prevalent in the south (3.46%) versus those living in the Midwest (3.0%), west (2.02%), or northeast (1.71%) (DuRant et al. 1995). According to some researchers, adolescents who use these drugs also appear to have below-averaged academic performance and are more susceptible to use recreational drugs (DuRant et al. 1995; Miller et al. 2005). What may come as a bit of a shock to some people is that certain studies have found evidence to suggest that individuals as young as middle school-age (12–14 years old) have used anabolic–androgenic steroids (Faigenbaum et al. 1998). In fact, it has been reported that 7% of adolescent anabolic–androgenic steroid users began using them at or before the age of 10 (Bahrke et al. 2000). Table 9.1 summarizes the prevalence of anabolic–androgenic steroid use in adolescents within the United States.

9.3 REASONS FOR USE

Several factors that may contribute to the use of anabolic–androgenic steroids include age, health behaviors, dietary habits, and physical activity (Castillo and Comstock 2007). It is estimated that two-thirds of the youth who use anabolic–androgenic steroids participate in sport(s), which is why it is often assumed to be one of the primary motivators for anabolic–androgenic steroid use as athletes believe it may help improve their performance (Calfee and Fadale 2006, Dodge and Jaccard 2006). One study involving high school students found that athletes were twice as likely to have reported using anabolic–androgenic steroids compared to nonathletes (Irving et al. 2002). As one might expect, the majority of high school athletes who report using steroids are those involved in strength and power sports. Researchers surveyed high school male seniors and found that 6.6% of the 3403 survey participants reported the use of anabolic–androgenic steroids; 67% of these were athletes and 44% of them were football players (Buckley et al. 1988). Interestingly enough, 30%–40% of adolescent anabolic–androgenic steroid users do not participate in school-sponsored sport, and are instead focused on body image (Castillo and Comstock 2007). Although there appears to be a positive relationship between sports participation and anabolic–androgenic steroid use, it should not be mistaken as a "cause and effect" relationship as the underlying cause for this phenomenon is unknown. Moreover, it is likely that such causes are somewhat individualized and otherwise multifactorial. One such theory is that the environment in which the athlete is surrounded may increase the exposure to more information related to anabolic–androgenic steroid use whether it is positive or negative (Dodge and Jaccard 2006). Research has indicated increased use patterns among high school students, particularly males (Pope et al. 2000) are not only for the performance-enhancing benefits but also for increased self-esteem (Cohane and Pope 2001, Pope et al. 2000). Interestingly, recent research has suggested that substance use, fighting, and sexual risk are actually better predictors of adolescent androgen use than participation in competitive sports (Miller et al. 2005). Evidence also exists on the use of anabolic steroids to narrow the gap of an individual's psychosocial experience(s) (Kanayama et al. 2003, Lantz et al. 2002). Furthermore, the prevalence of anabolic–androgenic steroid use by professional athletes, particularly at the elite and professional levels, continues to set a poor example for today's youth and may contribute to higher rates of use among youth who look up to these athletes and desire to perform at a similar level (Calfee and Fadale 2006). It is certainly worth mentioning that several sports idols who have been a part of record-breaking seasons and accomplishments have since been linked to anabolic–androgenic steroid use or other illegal performance-enhancing substances, which may be sending the wrong message to today's young athletes (Calfee and Fadale 2006). From a historical perspective it is widely understood that the modern introduction of anabolic–androgenic steroid use in sport began in the late 1950s and early 1960s. Although a broad and detailed history of anabolic–androgenic steroid exists, it is beyond the scope of this section to discuss these events, therefore, the reader is referred to the comprehensive review by Hoffman (2009). Despite the diverse history of anabolic–androgenic steroid use in sports, it is helpful to know that determination of anabolic–androgenic steroid usage in professional sports is often very challenging, given the restraint of the governing authorities of these sports to disclose accurate information regarding the banned performance-enhancing substances.

The development of select teams, travel teams, enhanced television, radio and internet coverage, and burgeoning pressures to succeed at the next level are likely contributing factors to anabolic–androgenic steroid use in youth as they look for ways to improve their performance and enhance the physical development of their bodies. Athletic scholarships at the collegiate level also increase the pressure placed upon younger athletes to do whatever they can to stand out among their peers and draw attention to their own athletic achievements. Outside of these reasons, significant financial incentives may exist that are many times coupled with signing bonuses and the large monetary contracts that athletes are able to secure when they begin their professional careers. The glamour, celebrity status, and substantial financial wealth all operate as pressure on a young athlete to do whatever it takes to gain a competitive edge (Calfee and Fadale 2006).

Another possible theory is a "win at all cost" mentality in which athletes do whatever it takes, legal or illegal, to be their best. This theory came about following a 1994 survey with Olympic athletes who were asked two questions, the first being, "If you were offered a banned performance-enhancing substance that guaranteed that you would win an Olympic medal and you could not be caught, would you take it?" A startling 195 out of 198 athletes who were surveyed responded in the affirmative. The second question was, "Would you take a banned performance-enhancing drug with a guarantee that you will not be caught and that you will win every competition for the next 5 years, but will then die from adverse effects of the substance?" Again, a startling majority (>50%) still responded in the affirmative (Bamberger and Yaeger 1997). Unfortunately, it may be the professional and world-class athletes or more accurately the celebrity status placed upon these individuals by society who are partially to blame for the high prevalence of anabolic–androgenic steroid use among adolescents. It appears as though achieving athletic success can be a very powerful motivator when it comes to using anabolic–androgenic steroids or other performance-enhancing substances that may or may not be good for one's overall health.

Whether or not sports are the primary driving force behind the justification of anabolic–androgenic steroid use, there does appear to be a growing number of individuals taking anabolic–androgenic steroids for aesthetic purposes as well, which is often the second-most reported reason for anabolic–androgenic steroid use (Kerr and Congeni 2007). Taylor et al. believes that some males may suffer from a psychological disorder referred to as "bigorexia," which is a body dysmorphic phenomenon in which one perceives oneself as smaller than they really are making them more desperate to look for ways to improve their muscularity (Taylor 1985). Other terms assigned to this phenomenon are the Adonis Complex, Reverse Anorexia, or Muscular Dysmorphia. Adolescents who are in the transition period of growth and development—entering puberty may suffer from this disorder, especially those who develop more slowly compared to some of their peers.

9.4 OTHER RELATED DRUG USE

Some people believe that the use of legal performance-enhancing substances may lead to the use of different categories of drugs—such as illegal or recreational substances—is similar to the Gateway Theory (Dodge and Jaccard 2006, Jessor 1991, Kandel et al. 2006). In fact, one study found that those who reported using legal performance-enhancing substances were 26 times more likely to use anabolic–androgenic steroids when compared to those who did not report using legal performance-enhancing substances (Dodge and Jaccard 2006). It should be noted that several legal performance-enhancing substances have been deemed safe and effective for young athletes to use and should not be looked upon negatively solely due to this association. With that being said, performance-enhancing substances are not limited to anabolic–androgenic steroids among adolescents. Adolescents have also reported using several other drugs and substances to improve their performance and/or appearance such as amphetamines, stimulants, steroid hormone precursors, proteins, amino acids, dehydroepiandrosterone (DHEA), EPO, growth hormones, diuretics, etc. (Yesalis et al. 2000). In 1992, a study found that 5% of 10th grade males reported using human growth hormone, a hormone purported to increase fat-free mass and one that has gained recent popularity in Major League Baseball (Rickert et al. 1992). A decade later, in 2002, it was reported that 4% of 475 high school athletes surveyed reported using androstenedione, which is a precursor to the male hormone testosterone (Reeder et al. 2002). As mentioned previously, the use of illegal performance-enhancing substances is not limited to synthetic hormones or other substances designed to stimulate muscle growth. Youth may also be interested in substances such as stimulants or weight loss products. In 2002, Kayton and associates surveyed 270 high school athletes and found that 12% of males and 26% of females reported using ephedrine, a type of stimulant (Kayton et al. 2002). Other related performance-enhancing substances and drug use may also be an issue; however, a full discussion on this topic is beyond the scope of this chapter and book. Considerations related specifically to dietary supplementation are covered more fully in Chapter 13 of this book.

9.5 PREVENTION AND EDUCATION

Prevention strategies typically fall into one of two categories: (1) new rules and policies regarding drug testing, or (2) educational initiatives (Calfee and Fadale 2006). After a 1995 Supreme Court ruling, random drug testing of high school athletes was deemed appropriate and not a violation of the Fourth Amendment (Calfee and Fadale 2006). However, since then the National Federation of State High School Associations has said that approximately 13% of all high schools subject athletes to drug testing with only 29% of those testing for anabolic–androgenic steroid use (Kerr and Congeni 2007). A common concern with drug testing is the financial burden it places on the state and individual school districts. As a result, schools have sought out other prevention strategies to deter adolescents away from anabolic–androgenic steroid use. Education is one of those strategies and has been seen as a valuable tool within certain community and athletic populations.

Once it became apparent that high school athletics had a problem with adolescents using anabolic–androgenic steroids, educational programs were developed in an attempt to prevent future anabolic–androgenic steroid use and decrease current participation (Yesalis 2000). Unfortunately, only a limited number of these educational programs have seen a success (Goldberg et al. 1991, Yesalis et al. 2000). Some researchers actually believe that educational programs that employ scare tactics designed to deter adolescents from using anabolic–androgenic steroids may have the opposite effect and leave the adolescents curious about using them or seeking out more information (Goldberg et al. 1991). Goldberg et al. (Goldberg, Elliot, Clarke, MacKinnon, Moe et al. 1996, Goldberg, Elliot, Clarke, MacKinnon, Zoref et al. 1996) have found some success in changing the perception of adolescents' viewpoints on using anabolic–androgenic steroids by instilling a program focused on education and team building classes, which emphasize the importance of nutrition, and proper strength-training practices rather than anabolic–androgenic steroid use. The program is referred to as the Adolescents Training and Learning to Avoid Steroids (ATLAS) program and consists of interactive classroom and strength-training sessions over a period of 7 weeks during which athletes participate in team building exercises and expand their knowledge of the dangers of anabolic–androgenic steroid use while developing strategies for alternative ways to improve performance, handle peer pressure, and make informed choices. Elliot et al. (2008) created a similar program, Athletes Targeting Healthy Exercise and Nutrition Alternatives (ATHENA), which has also been shown to reduce the use of diet pills, amphetamines, and anabolic–androgenic steroids in female athletes. Unfortunately, a disturbing trend has been observed over the past 14 years whereby only 55% of the youth viewed anabolic–androgenic steroid use as risky behavior, which may in fact constitute as another underlying problem in and of itself (Johnston et al. 2013). Further research needs to be done in this area so that effective educational and preventative measures can be implemented to help decrease anabolic–androgenic steroid use among adolescents.

9.6 MANAGEMENT

If a coach or parent suspects that a young adolescent may be using anabolic–androgenic steroid it may be a difficult topic to address. Further, how the situation is handled may have a significant impact on the treatment of the issue at hand and future implications. Unfortunately, no "How To" manual is available to parents and coaches on how to properly handle this situation. Although the situations are quite different, perhaps parents and coaches can adopt a similar strategy on how to manage this situation that is used by the coaches and the Strength and Conditioning professionals when they suspect their athletes might have an eating disorder. The National Strength and Conditioning Association recommends a four-step process on how to manage the situation (Baechle and Earle 2008). Step one consists of fact finding and making sure that you are picking up on certain cues that may suggest the adolescent is using anabolic–androgenic steroids. These cues may include rapid weight gain, increases in muscular strength and power, irritability, secretive behavior, and mood swings. It is important to pay attention to anything unusual and be sure to collect the facts in the event you do confront the individual the action is warranted. Step two is the process of actually confronting the individual. During this step it is important to involve the parents of the young individual and inform them of everything taking place. One should confront the individual in a calm and supportive manner so as to not scare off or intimidate the adolescent. Step three involves referring the individual to outside sources so that they may seek guidance or get help with their problem if need be. This outside source may be a family doctor, guidance counselor or therapist, or a qualified and trained individual who has experience working with these types of situations. Step four is following up. As one could imagine, this step involves the future monitoring of the young individual to ensure they have made the necessary adjustments to avoid anabolic–androgenic steroid use and continue to resort to healthier and safer alternatives. With that being said, the management of anabolic–androgenic steroid use among adolescents is especially difficult as the possession of these substances is illegal and therefore special care and judgment is needed. Whether or not law enforcement professionals and criminal proceedings need to be a part of the process are sometimes a matter of judgment, but in many situations the possession of an illegal substance on public school grounds can violate school district policies that force the hand of school administrators on whether or not to involve local authorities and press charges.

9.7 PHYSIOLOGICAL ADAPTATIONS

9.7.1 Testosterone and Testosterone Analogs

One of the most thought-provoking questions that have fascinated the fields of medicine, endocrinology, and exercise science is, "How do anabolic steroids work?" Although anabolic–androgenic steroids have been studied significantly in animal models, clinical populations, and in healthy humans, the identification of cellular mechanisms that fully explains their actions remains somewhat elusive. Therefore, based on both physiological and scientific evidence regarding anabolic–androgenic steroids, the involved mechanism of action is multifactorial in nature.

Considering testosterone is both a naturally occurring hormone, it can also be administered orally, by intramuscular injection, or transdermally by using gels or creams. However, it is important to highlight how testosterone concentrations change in the blood. Testosterone is often known as hydrophobic (having little or no affinity for water) and consequently does not readily dissolve in the blood. In fact, almost all testosterone in the circulation is bound to binding proteins that are hydrophilic (strong affinity for water) (Schwarz and Pohl 1992). A review of testosterone physiology indicates that the primary binding protein for testosterone is referred to as sex hormone-binding globulin or SHBG, which binds approximately 44%–60% of total serum testosterone (Vingren et al. 2010). Once secreted, testosterone travels through the circulation either free (i.e., free testosterone) or bound to a carrier protein. About 35%–38% of testosterone travels bound to albumin, with the remaining bound to the glycoprotein SHBG (Srinivas-Shankar and Wu 2006). Testosterone cannot be stored in the cells that produce it, which is in contrast to most peptide hormones, so the association with binding proteins can act as storage in the circulation. The bound testosterone can then be released to become free testosterone in order to enter the cell. It has been estimated that healthy men produce approximately 4.0–9.0 mg of testosterone per day with blood concentrations ranging from 300 to 1000 ng/dL, whereas females produce blood concentrations ranging from 15 to 65 ng/dL (Basaria et al. 2001, Bhasin et al. 2006).

Testosterone is primarily produced by the Leydig cells of the testes with a small quantity also coming from the adrenal cortex as well as peripheral conversion of androstenedione. Testosterone is one of the most potent naturally secreted anabolic–androgenic hormones and its biological effects include promotion of secondary male-sex characteristics, such as facial and body hair growth, nitrogen retention, as well as bone and muscle growth, in particular males. It is well established that young adolescent males experiencing puberty undergo substantial increases in the circulating levels of testosterone, which effectively works to drive the physical changes previously discussed (Vingren et al. 2010).

One of the most commonly used classes of anabolic–androgenic steroids are synthetic derivatives of testosterone and are commonly administered orally by intramuscular injection, or transdermally by using as gels or creams. Such derivatives and analogs of testosterone are well known to elicit their effects on the musculoskeletal system by increasing lean body mass, muscular strength, hypertrophy, and protein synthesis (Bhasin et al. 1996, 2001, Sinha-Hikim et al. 2002). From a mechanistic perspective, it is known that testosterone binds predominantly to androgen receptors found in the nuclei of skeletal muscle cells which activate the transcription of genes necessary for muscle growth (Bhasin et al. 1996, Kadi 2000, Sinha-Hikim et al. 2002). In addition to testosterone's ability to increase rates of protein synthesis through intracellular mechanisms, it also effectively works to offset the breakdown of muscle tissue. Overall what results is a heightened anabolic environment in the muscle that over a time translates into a greater ability to maintain a high level of intensity, higher volume of training, and improved recovery between training sessions (Laos and Metzl 2006).

A fundamental process of muscle growth is the activation, proliferation, and differentiation of muscle satellite cells as they play a vital part in the regulation of skeletal muscle growth and repair (Adams 2006, Hawke and Garry 2001) whereby their increased activity results in an increase in the number of myonuclei (Sinha-Hikim et al. 2003), which fundamentally expands the pool of genetic material that regulates the expression and development of various intramuscular components. Furthermore, testosterone-induced increases in skeletal muscle mass are associated with hypertrophy of both type I and type II fibers (Sinha-Hikim et al. 2002) in addition to changes in pennation angle and possibly fascicle length (Blazevich and Giorgi 2001). A final, intriguing point of discussion regarding testosterone use in humans is the potential for it to stimulate hyperplasia (an increase in the number of muscle fibers) (Hartgens and Kuipers 2004, Kadi 2008) in addition to the previously discussed mechanistic changes that heighten hypertrophic responses. Collectively, these findings reiterate and emphasize the multiple levels of hypertrophy expression seen in conjunction with anabolic–androgenic steroid use.

Considering the strong association between strength and fast twitch muscle fibers, previous and even recent evidence reports anabolic–androgenic steroids certainly affects both type II (fast twitch) muscle fibers and type I (slow twitch) fibers (Kadi 2008, Sinha-Hikim et al. 2002, Yu et al. 2014). Interestingly, studies indicate that the largest difference in muscle fiber size between anabolic–androgenic steroid users and nonusers was observed in type I muscle fibers of the vastus lateralis (Hartgens et al. 1996) and the trapezius muscle (Kadi et al. 1999) as a result of long-term anabolic–androgenic steroid self-administration. Similar outcomes are present in the human (Kadi 2000, Kadi et al. 1999) and animal (Fontana et al. 2013) literature. For example, Hartgens (2002) demonstrated that poly-drug regimens for 8 weeks increased muscle fiber size of the deltoid muscle in strength athletes, with the greatest effect being on the type II fibers, which experienced a 15% rate of growth. However, the authors noted that administration of intramuscular nandrolone decanoate (200 mg/week) for 8 weeks had no effect on the size of deltoid muscle fibers (Hartgens et al. 2002). The effects of anabolic–androgenic steroids on skeletal muscle mass are dose-dependent and involve upregulation of gene transcription and synthesis of messenger RNA. In this respect, Sinha-Hikim et al. (2002) performed muscle biopsies of the vastus lateralis and found that administration of testosterone in 300 and 600 mg doses increased the cross-sectional areas of type I muscle fibers and fiber number, while type II motor units were only enlarged after the 600 mg administration regimen in eugonadal males. Interestingly, it was also reported that lower doses of testosterone (e.g., 25, 50, and 125 mg/week) had no effects on muscle fiber cross-sectional areas (Sinha-Hikim et al. 2002). Based on the studies, it was found that the anabolic–androgenic steroid administration did increase muscle mass, however, it seemed that the increase occurred in a dose-dependent manner, but independent of the regimen used (single drug vs. multiple-drug regimen). Finally, although anabolic–androgenic steroids and changes in muscle fiber types have been thoroughly studied, the effects of anabolic–androgenic steroid dosage on skeletal muscles over several years are lacking in the literature (Table 9.2).

TABLE 9.2
General Effects of Testosterone and Androgens
- Increases lean body mass
- Increases cardiac tissue size
- Decreases body fat percentage
- Increases isometric and dynamic muscle strength and power
- Enhances recovery ability between within and between training sessions
- Increases protein synthesis, accretion, and nitrogen retention (and likely anti-catabolic properties)
- Increases muscle cross-sectional area
- Increases erythropoiesis, hemoglobin, and hematocrit
- Enhanced vasodilation (blood flow)
- Increases bone mineral content and density
- Increases lipolysis (fat breakdown) and low-density lipoproteins and decreases high-density lipoproteins
- Enhances neural conduction, neurotransmitter discharge, and myelination

Source: Modified from Hoffman, J. R. et al. *J. Strength Cond. Res.*, 23(5 Suppl), S1–59. doi: 10.1519/JSC.0b013e31819df2e6.

9.7.2 Growth Hormone

Growth hormone (also referred to as somatotropin) is a polypeptide hormone considered to have both anabolic and catabolic actions. In this respect, growth hormone acts as a repartitioning agent to induce fat metabolism toward mobilization of triglycerides while also stimulating cellular uptake of amino acids and their incorporation into various proteins, including muscle (Vierck et al. 2000). At the tissue level, growth hormone is most widely recognized for its impact on bone and muscle. Inside bone, growth hormone instigates longitudinal bone growth by actions at the epiphysis and differentiation of the osteoblasts (bone building cells). Within skeletal muscle, growth hormone works by increasing myonuclear number and facilitating the synthesis of myoblasts, creating potential for the development of a muscle fiber (Sotiropoulos et al. 2006).

Growth hormone is secreted by the anterior pituitary gland and released in a pulsatile fashion, with the greatest nonexercise secretions induced during sleep. The largest concentration occurs about an hour after the onset of sleep, with smaller peaks occurring during the rest of the sleep cycle. Growth hormone levels spike after the performance of various types of exercise, particularly those that are of higher intensity and involve large amounts of muscle (Kraemer and Ratamess 2005). For example, McCall and investigators in 1999 reported that exercise-induced increases in growth hormone are highly correlated to both type I and type II muscle fiber hypertrophy (McCall et al. 1999). Further, it is proposed that a transient growth hormone increase may lead to an enhanced interaction with muscle cell receptors, facilitating fiber recovery and stimulating a hypertrophic response (Ojasto and Hakkinen 2009).

Mechanistically, growth hormone elicits muscle anabolism and mediates hypertrophic adaptations through the releasing action of insulin-like growth factor-1, or IGF-1 (Velloso 2008). However, some researchers debate this theory and postulate the hypertrophic effects of growth hormone and IGF-1 are cumulative (Sotiropoulos et al. 2006). Secretion of growth hormone is regulated by numerous factors, including growth hormone-releasing factor, sleep, exercise, L-dopa (precursor to dopamine), and arginine (Williams and Branch 2000). The half-life of growth hormone is short but it does stimulate the release of somatomedins, a group of hormones that promote cell growth in response to stimulation by growth hormone (Williams and Branch 2000). Although complex and beyond the intended scope of this section, the effect of growth hormone signaling and its impact on skeletal muscle physiology and muscle hypertrophy appears to lie in its ability to indirectly stimulate various cellular communication pathway (i.e., mammalian target of rapomyosin or mTOR) via formation of molecules and receptors creating a cascade of events activating the Janus/signal transducer and activator of transcription (JAK/STAT) pathway. It is within these complex pathways that resistance exercise stimulates muscle fiber contractions and stimulates responses that subsequently activate satellite cells. These various signals stimulate transcription and translation and, over a time, assists in facilitating muscle hypertrophy (Hoffman et al. 2009, Schoenfeld 2013a,b).

Numerous factors also affect the regulation of growth hormone, which include deep sleep, exercise, various forms of stress, hypoglycemia, nutritional intake, some amino acids, and some pharmacologic agents. Variables that can induce an inhibitory effect of growth hormone include a heavy emphasis of a carbohydrate-rich diet and several pharmacologic agents (i.e., beta-2 adrenergic agonists) (Hoffman et al. 2009). An attractive feature of growth hormone use particularly for athletes is its direct actions on amino acid transport in muscle tissue leading to increased protein synthesis and nitrogen balance, coupled with increased fat mobilization through lipolysis (fat breakdown). From a clinical perspective, these effects can be exhibited in the longer term by a reduction in body fat and a decrease in the fat cell size and lipid content.

9.8 PERFORMANCE BENEFITS FOR STRENGTH, POWER, ENDURANCE ATHLETES

As highlighted previously, reasons for using anabolic–androgenic steroids are typically focused upon strength, power, and muscle mass development. Indeed, several early studies that investigated anabolic–androgenic steroid administration on experienced resistance-trained athletes reported significant strength and body-mass gains (Blazevich and Giorgi 2001, Stamford and Moffatt 1974, van Marken Lichtenbelt et al. 2004, Ward 1973) as well as a threefold difference in the accretion of lean body mass (van Marken Lichtenbelt et al. 2004). These findings are particularly striking when one considers the well-known reductions in these adaptations that occur with greater levels of training background. When a cross-sectional comparison is made, users of anabolic–androgenic steroids exhibit a 2–3 times greater ability to increase strength when compared to similar athletes not currently using anabolic–androgenic steroids (Blazevich and Giorgi 2001). A review on anabolic–androgenic steroids in athletes revealed that strength improvements range from approximately 5% to 20% over baseline levels, depending on the administered dose and regimen (Hartgens and Kuipers 2004). In fact, reports show that the anabolic effects of anabolic–androgenic steroids are indeed dose-dependent (Bhasin et al. 2001, Sinha-Hikim et al. 2002) and that resistance training coupled with anabolic–androgenic steroid use promotes greater increases in muscle hypertrophy and strength than are achieved with either intervention alone (Bhasin et al. 1996).

With regards to power output, short-term administration of anabolic–androgenic steroids has been shown to increase power output levels. Rogerson et al. (2007) examined the effect of short-term use of testosterone enanthate on muscular strength and power in healthy young men. The two objectives of this study were to (a) establishing injection of 3.5 mg/kg testosterone enanthate once per week could increase muscular strength and cycling sprint performance in 3–6 weeks; and (b) whether the World Anti-Doping Agency (WADA) imposed urinary testosterone/estrogen (T/E) ratio of 4:1 could identify all subjects being administered 3.5 mg/kg testosterone enanthate. Sixteen healthy young men were match-paired and randomly assigned in a double-blind manner to either a testosterone enanthate or a placebo group. All subjects performed a structured heavy resistance training program while receiving either testosterone enanthate (3.5 mg/kg) or saline injections once weekly for 6 weeks. One-repetition maximum (1RM) strength measures and 10-s cycle sprint performance were monitored at the pre- (baseline), mid- (week 3), and post- (week 6) time points. Body mass and the urinary T/E ratio were measured at the pre- (week 0) and post- (week 6) time points. When compared with baseline, 1RM bench press strength and total work during the cycle sprint increased significantly at week 3 and week 6 in the testosterone enanthate group, but not in the placebo group. Body mass at week 6 was significantly greater compared to baseline in the testosterone enanthate group versus placebo. Despite the clear ergogenic effects of testosterone enanthate in as little as 3 weeks, 4 of the 9 subjects in the testosterone enanthate group (~44%) did not test positive to testosterone under current WADA urinary T/E ratio criteria.

To further illustrate these findings, a series of well-controlled studies by Bhasin and colleagues investigated the effects of exogenous testosterone enanthate administration, with and without a strength-training program, on muscle tissue in males with healthy testes (Bhasin et al. 1996). Through the use of magnetic resonance imaging (MRI) measurements they observed that 10 weeks of testosterone administration (600 mg/week) led to increases in cross-sectional area of the triceps brachii and quadriceps muscles. Moreover, the gains in muscle mass were larger when testosterone administration was coupled with a resistance-training program resulting in approximately 15% greater areas of the triceps and quadriceps muscles. One interesting feature about this study was that the group that was administered testosterone experienced a significantly greater increase in fat-free mass (+6.1 kg) in the triceps and quadriceps regions when compared to any other. They also experienced the greatest increase in bench press (+22%) and back squat performance (+38%) compared to the other groups. These data are striking considering that the placebo and exercise group only experienced a 21% increase in back squat performance while the group that received no drug treatment and no exercise experienced a 19% increases in the back squat. Notably, no side effects were reported in the treatment group (Srinivas-Shankar and Wu 2006) providing clear evidence that moderate doses of exogenous testosterone use stimulate considerable improvement in fat-free mass, strength, and hypertrophy when combined with rigorous strength-training program in the absence of deleterious side effects.

In a similar study by Bhasin et al. (2001), different dosages of testosterone enanthate (25, 50, 125, 300, and 600 mg/week) for 10 weeks were administered to nonexercising volunteers. It was found that the effects on thigh muscle volume and quadriceps muscle volume were highly dose-dependent. No other related work has been completed and ethically it is challenging to further study higher doses and for longer periods of time due to the known detrimental outcomes that result from higher doses. At this point, it is tempting to speculate that the physiological and clinical effects of using anabolic–androgenic steroids is misunderstood and grossly underestimated when one considers the large doses, multiple drugs, and training regimens commonly reported by the anabolic–androgenic steroid users as effective. While this may be true, it is important to highlight that the incidence and severity of adverse effects from anabolic–androgenic steroid use goes up markedly with higher doses of these agents.

Recently, in endurance sports like cycling, running, and triathlons, some athletes anonymously reported the use of anabolic steroids (testosterone and nandrolone) as effective exogenous aids to recover more rapidly following intense physical efforts (Hartgens and Kuipers 2004). Although dosages vary considerably, swimmers and runners administer anabolic–androgenic steroids to be able to perform their frequent, high-intensity, long-duration sessions without physical breakdown. The drugs most often linked to endurance events, such as the Tour de France, are those related to blood doping, which is essentially a method(s) of enhancing the number of red blood cells in the body, and administration of EPO, a drug that stimulates increased production of red blood cells. Various blood doping methods exist but the fundamental basis involves extracting an individual's own blood (i.e., 1–4 units) several weeks before a competition and freezing it. The red blood cells are then reinfused back into the body within a week of the competition, leading to an elevated hemoglobin (and hematocrit) level in the blood, providing increased oxygen delivery capacity, which translates into increased endurance performance and reduced fatigue. While the overall scope of anabolic–androgenic steroids on endurance capabilities are less researched compared to strength and power, there have been many reports that have shown improvement (Birkeland et al. 2000, Ekblom 1996, Loughton and Ruhling 1977, Van Zyl et al. 1995, Williams and Branch 2000), while others have not indicated an ergogenic outcome (Baume et al. 2006). Most pointedly and related to the use of anabolic–androgenic steroids by child and adolescent athletes, much less evidence exists to indicate that these types of drugs and approaches (for enhancement of endurance performance) are being used in child and youth populations.

Ergogenic outcomes linked to anabolic–androgenic steroid use are well established in areas related to both strength and power and endurance performance as well as improvements in muscle mass. However, perspective is needed as ergogenic outcomes are largely affected by many factors including the sport itself, sporting skill, training regimens, frequency of training, genetics, intensity, and environmental influences, for example. Certainly, anabolic–androgenic steroid use can assist in recovery and facilitate a greater overall training load, which ultimately can drive ergogenic outcomes and enhanced physiological adaptations, but a key point remains that many other factors contribute ultimately go on to positively impact performance.

9.9 BODY COMPOSITION

Studies have shown that anabolic steroids are linked with a reduction in body fat, and even significant improvements in body composition when combined with resistance training, both in young athletes and the elderly (Hartgens et al. 2001a, van Marken Lichtenbelt et al. 2004). In a systematic review by Bhasin et al. (2006) of mostly healthy, androgen-deficient men, testosterone therapy was associated with significant gains in fat-free mass and maximal voluntary strength and a significant decrease in whole-body fat mass.

Improvements in body composition (i.e., body fat reduction) from anabolic–androgenic steroid use is likely due to their ability to increase lean body mass. van Marken Lichtenbelt et al. (2004) demonstrated that the effects of anabolic–androgenic steroids on lean body mass could be attributed to real muscle growth, since no alterations of hydration status of lean body mass could be observed. In addition, Forbes et al. (1992) also studied the effects of testosterone on healthy subjects, and in addition, they studied the effects of these agents on these subjects after the drug was stopped. These authors found that testosterone enanthate administration led to a progressive increase in lean body mass and a decrease in body fat. They also found that body composition reverted slowly toward normal when the injections were stopped but that the effects of the drug lingered for some time. They concluded that testosterone is a powerful anabolic agent that can have profound and lasting effects on body composition. Interestingly, after anabolic–androgenic withdrawal the alterations in body composition fade away slowly, but may be partially sustained for time periods up to 3 months (Hartgens et al. 2001a,b, Kuipers et al. 1991). Further, the impact of anabolic–androgenic steroids on body composition also appear to be largely dose-dependent (Bhasin et al. 2001, Hartgens et al. 2001a,b) in addition to instigating regional differences in lean body-mass gains (Hartgens et al. 2001a,b, Kadi 2000, Kadi et al. 2000, Kuipers et al. 1991).

9.10 SIDE EFFECTS

9.10.1 Acute

The application of and physician involvement in a majority of drugs, regardless of how they are used, have known side effects, and anabolic–androgenic steroids are no exception. Examining the side effects and health risk of anabolic steroids is challenging. This is mainly due to the overall ban of these drugs by various governmental and sporting agencies, and because most well-designed and controlled studies are not able (or intended) to examine the utility of anabolic–androgenic steroid use in applications related to healthy adults. That being said, commonly reported acute side effects in male subjects include increased sexual drive (Strauss et al. 1983, Yesalis and Bahrke 2002, Yesalis et al. 1988), occurrence of acne, increased body hair (Yesalis and Bahrke 2002, Yesalis et al. 1988), testicular atrophy, and patterns of altering mood states.

Dangers and concerns abound when anabolic–androgenic steroids are being used and abused by any individual. However, greater levels of concern are present when the situation moves toward anabolic–androgenic steroid use in women, children, and adolescents. It is well known that women are masculinized when sufficient quantities of anabolic–androgenic steroids are used, which can go on to negatively impact normal physiological and endocrinological function within women. Examples of these changes include deepening of voice, enlargement of clitoris, widening of upper torso, decreased breast size, menstrual irregularities, and male pattern baldness (Calfee and Fadale 2006, Derman 1995, Evans 2004, Hartgens and Kuipers 2004). It is worth mentioning that many of these side effects are quite similar to those found in males who abuse anabolic–androgenic steroids. Similar concerns reside with children and adolescents. For example, studies indicate that prepubescent boys and girls may be at greater risk of premature epiphyseal fusion, which may result in reduced adult height (Casavant et al. 2007, vandenBerg et al. 2007) from any abuse of anabolic–androgenic steroids. It is important to highlight that many therapeutic applications exist for androgens and growth hormone in children, a topic that goes well beyond the scope of this chapter. Certainly, these uses should be under the care of a licensed healthcare provider. As a brief example, previous research has determined whether oxandrolone (a testosterone analog) administration for 1 year after a burn reverses muscle and bone loss in hypermetabolic pediatric burn patients. They found that long-term administration of oxandrolone safely improves lean body mass, as well as bone mineral content and density, in severely burned children (Murphy et al. 2004). Children with burns greater than 40% total body surface area were enrolled into a randomized controlled trial to receive oxandrolone as a long-term anabolic agent. All patients received similar clinical care. Subjects were studied at discharge (95% healed) and at 6, 9, and 12 months after the burn, after the treatment with 0.1 mg/kg oxandrolone or placebo. It was found that lean body mass was significantly greater with oxandrolone at 6, 9, and 12 months after the burn and bone mineral content at 12 months. Much debate remains surrounding the efficacy of short-term use of various anabolic–androgenic steroids in other clinical situations such as the potential for beneficial effects in immobilized patients, healthy older men, healthy middle-aged men, space travel, patients with cancer-related disease, and many other chronic diseases where significant muscle wasting occurs.

9.10.2 Chronic

Overall, long-term health risks associated with supra-physiological anabolic–androgenic steroid use are not well established. Some evidence exists to indicate that chronic anabolic–androgenic steroid users, including those who administer more than one drug concurrently may have increased risk for cardiovascular disease. Many of the cardiovascular effects associated with anabolic steroid use are decreased high-density lipoprotein (HDL), increased total and low-density lipoprotein (LDL) cholesterol, increased triglycerides, elevated blood pressure, and increased risk of thrombosis. However, it is important to note that the magnitude of the effect likely differs upon the consumption of specific drugs(s), their dosages and the duration of use at the said dosages. Further, each individual reacts differently and there is large inter-individual variation and how it interacts with an individual's own genetics. Some of the potential adverse complications have been overstated and most of the harmful effects are largely dependent upon the dose, cycles, type of drug, and impact of the drug, thus creating a challenge of the precise effects on each person, specific regimen or each drug(s). In addition, numerous case reports exist of sudden death among power athletes who were abusing anabolic–androgenic steroids (Dhar et al. 2005, Dickerman et al. 1996, Di Paolo et al. 2007, Fineschi et al. 2001, 2007, Hausmann et al. 1998, Sullivan et al. 1998). However, these case reports are largely anecdotal, and a cause and effect relationship between anabolic–androgenic steroid use and the risk of sudden death is far from definitive, but does represent a significant area of concern.

One of the more pressing issues with anabolic–androgenic steroid use is that of the behavioral effects, in what many refer to as "roid rage." This has attracted significant attention over the years and has even created media hysteria. Despite the notion this behavioral characteristic is largely anecdotal, numerous scientific placebo-controlled trials of testosterone have shown inconsistent changes in anger scores or measures of aggressive behaviors (Daly et al. 2003, Kouri et al. 1995,

Pope et al. 2000, Tricker et al. 1996). A wide variety of factors may have attributed to the lack of consistency across studies, including variation among instruments used to measure aggressive behavior and lack of sensitivity of self-reporting questionnaires to detect small, but significant, changes in aggression.

In fact, a study by Wang et al. (1996) who used testosterone replacement in healthy androgen-deficient men has reported improved positive aspects of mood and attenuate negative aspects of mood. While this specific topic of androgens and aggressive behavior is certainly warranted, it is important to mention that only a small number of subjects (<5%) in controlled trials have demonstrated noticeable increases in aggression measures with a large majority of individuals taking supra-physiologic doses of testosterone. The majority of participants show little or no change (Daly et al. 2003, Kouri et al. 1995, Pope et al. 2000, Tricker et al. 1996, Yesalis et al. 2000).

9.11 LEGAL CONSIDERATIONS AND TESTING

It was the Anabolic Steroid Control Act of 1990 that reclassified androgens as a schedule III substance, essentially making it a crime to use these drugs for nonmedical purposes. In 2004, an amended version of the Anabolic Steroid Control Act was passed that modified the definition of androgens to include 26 additional compounds that comprised designer androgens, such as tetrahydrogestrinone (THG, aka The Clear), and several prohormones whereby the most popular has been androstenedione and its many analogs. Although considered a scheduled III substance, anabolic–androgenic steroids are banned and tested for by the International Olympic Committee and most American sporting organizations, including the NCAA, National Football League (NFL), and National Basketball Association (NBA). Major League Baseball has become more stringent in recent years and recently implemented in-season blood tests to detect human growth hormone. To date, the better part of the twenty-first century has been marred with investigations, lawsuits, and congressional hearings on the topic of illegal use of anabolic–androgenic steroids by these athletes. Possession alone of any schedule III substance including androgens is punishable by up to a year in prison and/or a fine of $1000. However, if an individual has any related (or potentially unrelated) previous convictions and are caught with anabolic–androgenic steroids or committed another crime and the substances themselves are found, they could potentially face greater punishment including imprisonment for at least 15 days and up to 2 years with a minimum fine of $2500.

It is important to mention that the legal consideration and testing of anabolic–androgenic steroids are not cut and dry; in fact, the process is wrought with challenges and difficulties regarding the adequacy, effectiveness, and accuracy of the testing process. For example, considerable variation can occur among normal results and the testing process including procurement and maintenance of necessary equipment is exorbitantly expensive and this does not even include the legal ramifications of being found positive and/or being the clinical laboratory that conducted the test and provide result. Finally and equally problematic is that newer versions of drugs are developed rapidly each year and they can go seemingly undetected for years.

With regards to adolescents and sports, drug testing is largely punitive, with a positive test yielding significant penalties, including loss of player privileges, removal of awards and championships, removal of scholarships, and of course legal and criminal proceedings. Surprisingly, these intended deterrents have little to no effect on most adolescents (Gomez, American Academy of Pediatrics Committee on Sports, and Fitness 2005). In terms of testing, although urine tests are quite common, they are limited in their ability to detect certain outcomes. For example, a negative outcome could mean that the individual indeed is not using any drugs, but it could also mean that the test was not strong enough to detect necessary threshold levels to classify it as a positive test. Furthermore, numerous diuretics are a common method of decreasing urinary concentration of these drugs (which in and of themselves present dangers, particularly in athletes competing and training in hot and humid environments). Unfortunately, these tests, and the more effective methods of testing are not very cost-effective, and even associative deficiencies with detection create a challenging atmosphere of widespread testing, thus making it less practical. Simply, currently there is no cost-effective means of identifying adolescents who use anabolic–androgenic steroids or any other large group of athletes for that matter. As an example, Texas has been and is still currently conducting random drug testing (both recreational drugs and anabolic–androgenic steroids) of high school athletes. It is important that continued debate exists whether or not this expense has been justified. Based on the current literature, extensive educational programs such as ATLAS or ATHENA seem to be the most effective means of preventing steroid use among adolescents (Elliot et al. 2004, Goldberg, Elliot, Clarke, MacKinnon, Zoref, et al. 1996).

9.12 CONCLUSIONS

The use of anabolic–androgenic steroids appears to be a continuing problem with today's youth. This problem is especially of interest with regard to youth sports, as athletes appear to be twice as likely to experiment with anabolic–androgenic steroids compared to their nonathlete peers. The increasing media exposure of professional athletes who have been associated with these substances sets a poor example to today's young athletes. The development of select teams and higher demands placed upon athletes may also serve as reasons for anabolic–androgenic steroid use. Outside of sports, adolescents may also experiment with androgenic–anabolic steroids for aesthetic purposes or to improve self-esteem. Regardless of the reason for use, it is important to educate adolescents on the dangers of androgenic–anabolic steroid use and the negative impact it can have on one's health.

REFERENCES

Adams, G. R. 2006. Satellite cell proliferation and skeletal muscle hypertrophy. *Appl Physiol Nutr Metab* 31 (6):782–90. doi: h06-053 [pii]10.1139/h06-053.

Baechle, T., and R. Earle. 2008. *Essentials of Strength Training and Conditioning*, 3rd ed. Champagne, IL: Human Kinetics.

Bahrke, M. S., C. E. Yesalis, A. N. Kopstein, and J. A. Stephens. 2000. Risk factors associated with anabolic-androgenic steroid use among adolescents. *Sports Med* 29 (6):397–405.

Bamberger, M. and D. Yaeger. 1997. Over the edge: Special report. *Sports Illustrated*, 86, 64.

Basaria, S., J. T. Wahlstrom, and A. S. Dobs. 2001. Clinical review 138: Anabolic-androgenic steroid therapy in the treatment of chronic diseases. *J Clin Endocrinol Metab* 86 (11):5108–17. doi: 10.1210/jcem.86.11.7983.

Baume, N., Y. O. Schumacher, P. E. Sottas, C. Bagutti, M. Cauderay, P. Mangin, and M. Saugy. 2006. Effect of multiple oral doses of androgenic anabolic steroids on endurance performance and serum indices of physical stress in healthy male subjects. *Eur J Appl Physiol* 98 (4):329–40. doi: 10.1007/s00421-006-0271-0.

Bhasin, S., O. M. Calof, T. W. Storer, M. L. Lee, N. A. Mazer, R. Jasuja, V. M. Montori, W. Gao, and J. T. Dalton. 2006. Drug insight: Testosterone and selective androgen receptor modulators as anabolic therapies for chronic illness and aging. *Nat Clin Pract Endocrinol Metab* 2 (3):146–59. doi: 10.1038/ncpendmet0120.

Bhasin, S., G. R. Cunningham, F. J. Hayes, A. M. Matsumoto, P. J. Snyder, R. S. Swerdloff, and V. M. Montori. 2006. Testosterone therapy in adult men with androgen deficiency syndromes: An endocrine society clinical practice guideline. *J Clin Endocrinol Metab* 91 (6):1995–2010. doi: 10.1210/jc.2005-2847.

Bhasin, S., T. W. Storer, N. Berman, C. Callegari, B. Clevenger, J. Phillips, T. J. Bunnell, R. Tricker, A. Shirazi, and R. Casaburi. 1996. The effects of supraphysiologic doses of testosterone on muscle size and strength in normal men. *N Engl J Med* 335 (1):1–7. doi: 10.1056/NEJM199607043350101.

Bhasin, S., L. Woodhouse, R. Casaburi et al. 2001. Testosterone dose–response relationships in healthy young men. *Am J Physiol Endocrinol Metab* 281 (6):E1172–81.

Birkeland, K. I., J. Stray-Gundersen, P. Hemmersbach, J. Hallen, E. Haug, and R. Bahr. 2000. Effect of rhEPO administration on serum levels of sTfR and cycling performance. *Med Sci Sports Exercise* 32 (7):1238–43.

Blazevich, A. J. and A. Giorgi. 2001. Effect of testosterone administration and weight training on muscle architecture. *Med Sci Sports Exercise* 33 (10):1688–93.

Buckley, W. E., C. E. Yesalis, 3rd, K. E. Friedl, W. A. Anderson, A. L. Streit, and J. E. Wright. 1988. Estimated prevalence of anabolic steroid use among male high school seniors. *JAMA* 260 (23):3441–5.

Calfee, R. and P. Fadale. 2006. Popular ergogenic drugs and supplements in young athletes. *Pediatrics* 117 (3):e577–89. doi: 10.1542/peds.2005-1429.

Casavant, M. J., K. Blake, J. Griffith, A. Yates, and L. M. Copley. 2007. Consequences of use of anabolic androgenic steroids. *Pediatr Clin North Am* 54 (4):677–90; x. doi: 10.1016/j.pcl.2007.04.001.

Castillo, E. M. and R. D. Comstock. 2007. Prevalence of use of performance-enhancing substances among United States adolescents. *Pediatr Clin North Am* 54 (4):663–75; ix–x. doi: 10.1016/j.pcl.2007.04.002.

Cohane, G. H. and H. G. Pope, Jr. 2001. Body image in boys: A review of the literature. *Int J Eat Disord* 29 (4):373–9.

Daly, R. C., T. P. Su, P. J. Schmidt, M. Pagliaro, D. Pickar, and D. R. Rubinow. 2003. Neuroendocrine and behavioral effects of high-dose anabolic steroid administration in male normal volunteers. *Psychoneuroendocrinology* 28 (3):317–31.

Derman, R. J. 1995. Effects of sex steroids on women's health: Implications for practitioners. *Am J Med* 98 (1A):137S–43S.

Dhar, R., C. W. Stout, M. S. Link, M. K. Homoud, J. Weinstock, and N. A. Estes, 3rd. 2005. Cardiovascular toxicities of performance-enhancing substances in sports. *Mayo Clin Proc* 80 (10):1307–15. doi: 10.4065/80.10.1307.

Di Paolo, M., M. Agozzino, C. Toni, A. B. Luciani, L. Molendini, M. Scaglione, F. Inzani, M. Pasotti, F. Buzzi, and E. Arbustini. 2007. Sudden anabolic steroid abuse-related death in athletes. *Int J Cardiol* 114 (1):114–7. doi: 10.1016/j.ijcard.2005.11.033.

Dickerman, R. D., W. J. McConathy, F. Schaller, and N. Y. Zachariah. 1996. Cardiovascular complications and anabolic steroids. *Eur Heart J* 17 (12):1912.

Dodge, T. L. and J. J. Jaccard. 2006. The effect of high school sports participation on the use of performance-enhancing substances in young adulthood. *J Adolesc Health* 39 (3):367–73. doi: 10.1016/j.jadohealth.2005.12.025.

DuRant, R. H., L. G. Escobedo, and G. W. Heath. 1995. Anabolic-steroid use, strength training, and multiple drug use among adolescents in the United States. *Pediatrics* 96 (1 Pt 1):23–8.

Ekblom, B. 1996. Blood doping and erythropoietin. The effects of variation in hemoglobin concentration and other related factors on physical performance. *Am J Sports Med* 24 (6 Suppl):S40–2.

Elin, R. J. and S. J. Winters. 2004. Current controversies in testosterone testing: Aging and obesity. *Clin Lab Med* 24 (1):119–39. doi: 10.1016/j.cll.2004.01.010.

Elliot, D. L., L. Goldberg, E. L. Moe, C. A. Defrancesco, M. B. Durham, and H. Hix-Small. 2004. Preventing substance use and disordered eating: Initial outcomes of the ATHENA (Athletes Targeting Healthy Exercise and Nutrition Alternatives) program. *Arch Pediatr Adolesc Med* 158 (11):1043–9. doi: 10.1001/archpedi.158.11.1043.

Elliot, D. L., L. Goldberg, E. L. Moe, C. A. Defrancesco, M. B. Durham, W. McGinnis, and C. Lockwood. 2008. Long-term outcomes of the ATHENA (Athletes Targeting Healthy Exercise & Nutrition Alternatives) program for female high school athletes. *J Alcohol Drug Educ* 52 (2):73–92.

Evans, N. A. 2004. Current concepts in anabolic-androgenic steroids. *Am J Sports Med* 32 (2):534–42.

Faigenbaum, A. D., L. D. Zaichkowsky, D. E. Gardner, and L. J. Micheli. 1998. Anabolic steroid use by male and female middle school students. *Pediatrics* 101 (5):E6.

Fineschi, V., G. Baroldi, F. Monciotti, L. Paglicci Reattelli, and E. Turillazzi. 2001. Anabolic steroid abuse and cardiac sudden death: A pathologic study. *Arch Pathol Lab Med* 125 (2):253–5. doi: 10.1043/0003-9985(2001)125 <0253:ASAACS> 2.0.CO;2.

Fineschi, V., I. Riezzo, F. Centini, E. Silingardi, M. Licata, G. Beduschi, and S. B. Karch. 2007. Sudden cardiac death during anabolic steroid abuse: Morphologic and toxicologic findings in two fatal cases of bodybuilders. *Int J Legal Med* 121 (1):48–53. doi: 10.1007/s00414-005-0055-9.

Fontana, K., G. E. Campos, R. S. Staron, and M. A. da Cruz-Hofling. 2013. Effects of anabolic steroids and high-intensity aerobic exercise on skeletal muscle of transgenic mice. *PLoS One* 8 (11):e80909. doi: 10.1371/journal.pone.0080909.

Forbes, G. B., C. R. Porta, B. E. Herr, and R. C. Griggs. 1992. Sequence of changes in body composition induced by testosterone and reversal of changes after drug is stopped. *JAMA* 267 (3):397–9.

Goldberg, L., D. Elliot, G. N. Clarke, D. P. MacKinnon, E. Moe, L. Zoref, C. Green, S. L. Wolf, E. Greffrath, D. J. Miller, and A. Lapin. 1996. Effects of a multidimensional anabolic steroid prevention intervention. The Adolescents Training and Learning to Avoid Steroids (ATLAS) Program. *JAMA* 276 (19):1555–62.

Goldberg, L., D. L. Elliot, G. N. Clarke, D. P. MacKinnon, L. Zoref, E. Moe, C. Green, and S. L. Wolf. 1996. The Adolescents Training and Learning to Avoid Steroids (ATLAS) prevention program. Background and results of a model intervention. *Arch Pediatr Adolesc Med* 150 (7):713–21.

Goldberg, L., Elliot, D., Clake, G. et al. 1991. Anabolic steroid education and adolescents: Do scare tactics work? *Pediatrics* 87:283–6.

Gomez, J. Medicine American Academy of Pediatrics Committee on Sports and Fitness. 2005. Use of performance-enhancing substances. *Pediatrics* 115 (4):1103–6. doi: 10.1542/peds.2005-0085.

Hartgens, F. and H. Kuipers. 2004. Effects of androgenic-anabolic steroids in athletes. *Sports Med* 34 (8):513–54.

Hartgens, F., H. Kuipers, J. A. Wijnen, and H. A. Keizer. 1996. Body composition, cardiovascular risk factors and liver function in long-term androgenic-anabolic steroids using bodybuilders three months after drug withdrawal. *Int J Sports Med* 17 (6):429–33. doi: 10.1055/s-2007-972873.

Hartgens, F., W. D. van Marken Lichtenbelt, S. Ebbing, N. Vollaard, G. Rietjens, and H. Kuipers. 2001a. Androgenic-anabolic steroid-induced body changes in strength athletes. *Phys Sportsmed* 29 (1):49–65. doi: 10.3810/psm.2001.01.316.

Hartgens, F., W. D. Van Marken Lichtenbelt, S. Ebbing, N. Vollaard, G. Rietjens, and H. Kuipers. 2001b. Body composition and anthropometry in bodybuilders: Regional changes due to nandrolone decanoate administration. *Int J Sports Med* 22 (3):235–41. doi: 10.1055/s-2001-18679.

Hartgens, F., H. van Straaten, S. Fideldij, G. Rietjens, H. A. Keizer, and H. Kuipers. 2002. Misuse of androgenic-anabolic steroids and human deltoid muscle fibers: Differences between polydrug regimens and single drug administration. *Eur J Appl Physiol* 86 (3):233–9.

Hausmann, R., S. Hammer, and P. Betz. 1998. Performance enhancing drugs (doping agents) and sudden death—A case report and review of the literature. *Int J Legal Med* 111 (5):261–4.

Hawke, T. J., and D. J. Garry. 2001. Myogenic satellite cells: Physiology to molecular biology. *J Appl Physiol (1985)* 91 (2):534–51.

Hoffman, J. R., A. D. Faigenbaum, N. A. Ratamess, R. Ross, J. Kang, and G. Tenenbaum. 2008. Nutritional supplementation and anabolic steroid use in adolescents. *Med Sci Sports Exercise* 40 (1):15–24. doi: 10.1249/mss.0b013e31815a5181.

Hoffman, J. R., W. J. Kraemer, S. Bhasin, T. Storer, N. A. Ratamess, G. G. Haff, D. S. Willoughby, and A. D. Rogol. 2009. Position stand on androgen and human growth hormone use. *J Strength Cond Res* 23 (5 Suppl):S1–59. doi: 10.1519/JSC.0b013e31819df2e6.

Irving, L. M., M. Wall, D. Neumark-Sztainer, and M. Story. 2002. Steroid use among adolescents: Findings from Project EAT. *J Adolesc Health* 30 (4):243–52.

Jessor, R. 1991. Risk behavior in adolescence: A psychosocial framework for understanding and action. *J Adolesc Health* 12 (8):597–605.

Johnson, M. D., M. S. Jay, B. Shoup, and V. I. Rickert. 1989. Anabolic steroid use by male adolescents. *Pediatrics* 83 (6):921–4.

Johnston, L. D., P. M. O'Malley, R. A. Miech, J. G. Bachman, and L. E. Schulenberg. 2015. Monitoring the future national survey results on drug use: 1975–2014. Overview, key findings on adolescent drug use. Ann Arbor: Institute for Social Research, The University of Michigan.

Kadi, F. 2000. Adaptation of human skeletal muscle to training and anabolic steroids. *Acta Physiol Scand Suppl* 646:1–52.

Kadi, F. 2008. Cellular and molecular mechanisms responsible for the action of testosterone on human skeletal muscle. A basis for illegal performance enhancement. *Br J Pharmacol* 154 (3):522–8. doi: 10.1038/bjp.2008.118.

Kadi, F., P. Bonnerud, A. Eriksson, and L. E. Thornell. 2000. The expression of androgen receptors in human neck and limb muscles: Effects of training and self-administration of androgenic-anabolic steroids. *Histochem Cell Biol* 113 (1):25–9.

Kadi, F., A. Eriksson, S. Holmner, G. S. Butler-Browne, and L. E. Thornell. 1999. Cellular adaptation of the trapezius muscle in strength-trained athletes. *Histochem Cell Biol* 111 (3):189–95.

Kadi, F., A. Eriksson, S. Holmner, and L. E. Thornell. 1999. Effects of anabolic steroids on the muscle cells of strength-trained athletes. *Med Sci Sports Exercise* 31 (11):1528–34.

Kanayama, G., H. G. Pope, G. Cohane, and J. I. Hudson. 2003. Risk factors for anabolic-androgenic steroid use among weightlifters: A case-control study. *Drug Alcohol Depend* 71 (1):77–86.

Kandel, D. B., K. Yamaguchi, and L. C. Klein. 2006. Testing the gateway hypothesis. *Addiction* 101 (4):470–2; discussion 474-6. doi: 10.1111/j.1360-0443.2006.01426.x.

Kayton, S., Cullen, R. W., Memken, J. A. et al. 2002. Supplement and ergogenic aid use by competitive male and female high school athletes. *Med Sci Sports Exercise* 34 (5):193.

Kerr, J. M. and J. A. Congeni. 2007. Anabolic-androgenic steroids: Use and abuse in pediatric patients. *Pediatr Clin North Am* 54 (4):771–85, xii. doi: 10.1016/j.pcl.2007.04.010.

Kouri, E. M., S. E. Lukas, H. G. Pope, Jr., and P. S. Oliva. 1995. Increased aggressive responding in male volunteers following the administration of gradually increasing doses of testosterone cypionate. *Drug Alcohol Depend* 40 (1):73–9.

Kraemer, W. J. and N. A. Ratamess. 2005. Hormonal responses and adaptations to resistance exercise and training. *Sports Med* 35 (4):339–61. doi: 3544 [pii].

Krowchuk, D. P., T. M. Anglin, D. B. Goodfellow, T. Stancin, P. Williams, and G. D. Zimet. 1989. High school athletes and the use of ergogenic aid. *Am J Dis Child* 143 (4):486–9.

Kuipers, H., J. A. Wijnen, F. Hartgens, and S. M. Willems. 1991. Influence of anabolic steroids on body composition, blood pressure, lipid profile and liver functions in body builders. *Int J Sports Med* 12 (4):413–8. doi: 10.1055/s-2007-1024704.

Lantz, C. D., D. J. Rhea, and A. E. Cornelius. 2002. Muscle dysmorphia in elite-level power lifters and bodybuilders: A test of differences within a conceptual model. *J Strength Cond Res* 16 (4):649–55.

Laos, C. and J. D. Metzl. 2006. Performance-enhancing drug use in young athletes. *Adolesc Med Clin* 17 (3):719–31; abstract xii. doi: 10.1016/j.admecli.2006.06.011.

Loughton, S. J. and R. O. Ruhling. 1977. Human strength and endurance responses to anabolic steroid and training. *J Sports Med Phys Fitness* 17 (3):285–96.

McCall, G. E., W. C. Byrnes, S. J. Fleck, A. Dickinson, and W. J. Kraemer. 1999. Acute and chronic hormonal responses to resistance training designed to promote muscle hypertrophy. *Can J Appl Physiol* 24 (1):96–107.

Miller, K. E., J. H. Hoffman, G. M. Barnes, D. Sabo, M. J. Melnick, and M. P. Farrell. 2005. Adolescent anabolic steroid use, gender, physical activity, and other problem behaviors. *Subst Use Misuse* 40 (11):1637–57. doi: 10.1080/10826080500222727.

Murphy, K. D., S. Thomas, R. P. Mlcak, D. L. Chinkes, G. L. Klein, and D. N. Herndon. 2004. Effects of long-term oxandrolone administration in severely burned children. *Surgery* 136 (2):219–24. doi: 10.1016/j.surg.2004.04.022.

Ojasto, T. and K. Hakkinen. 2009. Effects of different accentuated eccentric loads on acute neuromuscular, growth hormone, and blood lactate responses during a hypertrophic protocol. *J Strength Cond Res* 23 (3):946–53. doi: 10.1519/JSC.0b013e3181a2b22f.

Pope, H. G., Jr., A. J. Gruber, B. Mangweth, B. Bureau, C. deCol, R. Jouvent, and J. I. Hudson. 2000. Body image perception among men in three countries. *Am J Psychiatry* 157 (8):1297–301.

Pope, H. G. and G. Kanayama. 2000. Abuse of anabolic steroids. *Pharm News* 7:13–20.

Pope, H. G., Jr., E. M. Kouri, and J. I. Hudson. 2000. Effects of supraphysiologic doses of testosterone on mood and aggression in normal men: A randomized controlled trial. *Arch Gen Psychiatry* 57 (2):133–40; discussion 155-6.

Radakovich, J., P. Broderick, and G. Pickell. 1993. Rate of anabolic-androgenic steroid use among students in junior high school. *J Am Board Fam Pract* 6 (4):341–5.

Reeder, B. M., A. Rai, D. R. Patel et al. 2002. The prevalence of nutritional supplement use among high school students: A pilot study. *Med Sci Sports Exercise* 34 (5):193.

Rickert, V. I., C. Pawlak-Morello, V. Sheppard, and M. S. Jay. 1992. Human growth hormone: A new substance of abuse among adolescents? *Clin Pediatr* (Philadelphia) 31 (12):723–6.

Rogerson, S., R. P. Weatherby, G. B. Deakin, R. A. Meir, R. A. Coutts, S. Zhou, and S. M. Marshall-Gradisnik. 2007. The effect of short-term use of testosterone enanthate on muscular strength and power in healthy young men. *J Strength Cond Res* 21 (2):354–61. doi: 10.1519/R-18385.1.

Schoenfeld, B. J. 2013a. Postexercise hypertrophic adaptations: A reexamination of the hormone hypothesis and its applicability to resistance training program design. *J Strength Cond Res* 27 (6):1720–30. doi: 10.1519/JSC.0b013e31828ddd53.

Schoenfeld, B. J. 2013b. Potential mechanisms for a role of metabolic stress in hypertrophic adaptations to resistance training. *Sports Med* 43 (3):179–94. doi: 10.1007/s40279-013-0017-1.

Schwarz, S. and P. Pohl. 1992. Steroid hormones and steroid hormone binding globulins in cerebrospinal fluid studied in individuals with intact and with disturbed blood-cerebrospinal fluid barrier. *Neuroendocrinology* 55 (2):174–82.

Scott, D. M., J. C. Wagner, and T. W. Barlow. 1996. Anabolic steroid use among adolescents in Nebraska schools. *Am J Health Syst Pharm* 53 (17):2068–72.

Sinha-Hikim, I., J. Artaza, L. Woodhouse, N. Gonzalez-Cadavid, A. B. Singh, M. I. Lee, T. W. Storer, R. Casaburi, R. Shen, and S. Bhasin. 2002. Testosterone-induced increase in muscle size in healthy young men is associated with muscle fiber hypertrophy. *Am J Physiol Endocrinol Metab* 283 (1):E154–64. doi: 10.1152/ajpendo.00502.2001.

Sinha-Hikim, I., S. M. Roth, M. I. Lee, and S. Bhasin. 2003. Testosterone-induced muscle hypertrophy is associated with an increase in satellite cell number in healthy, young men. *Am J Physiol Endocrinol Metab* 285 (1):E197–205. doi: 10.1152/ajpendo.00370.2002.

Sotiropoulos, A., M. Ohanna, C. Kedzia, R. K. Menon, J. J. Kopchick, P. A. Kelly, and M. Pende. 2006. Growth hormone promotes skeletal muscle cell fusion independent of insulin-like growth factor 1 upregulation. *Proc Natl Acad Sci U S A* 103 (19):7315–20. doi: 10.1073/pnas.0510033103.

Srinivas-Shankar, U. and F. C. W. Wu. 2006. Drug insight: Testosterone preparations. *Nat Clin Pract Urol* 3:653–65.

Stamford, B. A. and R. Moffatt. 1974. Anabolic steroid: Effectiveness as an ergogenic aid to experienced weight trainers. *J Sports Med Phys Fitness* 14 (3):191–7.

Stilger, V. G. and C. E. Yesalis. 1999. Anabolic-androgenic steroid use among high school football players. *J Community Health* 24 (2):131–45.

Strauss, R. H., J. E. Wright, G. A. M. Finerman et al. 1983. Side effects of anabolic steroids in weight trained men. *Phys Sportsmed* 87–96.

Sullivan, M. L., C. M. Martinez, P. Gennis, and E. J. Gallagher. 1998. The cardiac toxicity of anabolic steroids. *Prog Cardiovasc Dis* 41 (1):1–15.

Tanner, S. M., D. W. Miller, and C. Alongi. 1995. Anabolic steroid use by adolescents: Prevalence, motives, and knowledge of risks. *Clin J Sport Med* 5 (2):108–15.

Taylor, W. N. 1985. *Hormonal Manipulation: A New Era of Monstrous Athletes*. McFarland: Jefferson.

Tricker, R., R. Casaburi, T. W. Storer, B. Clevenger, N. Berman, A. Shirazi, and S. Bhasin. 1996. The effects of supraphysiological doses of testosterone on angry behavior in healthy eugonadal men—A clinical research center study. *J Clin Endocrinol Metab* 81 (10):3754–8. doi: 10.1210/jcem.81.10.8855834.

van Marken Lichtenbelt, W. D., F. Hartgens, N. B. Vollaard, S. Ebbing, and H. Kuipers. 2004. Bodybuilders' body composition: Effect of nandrolone decanoate. *Med Sci Sports Exercise* 36 (3):484–9.

Van Zyl, C. G., T. D. Noakes, and M. I. Lambert. 1995. Anabolic-androgenic steroid increases running endurance in rats. *Med Sci Sports Exercise* 27 (10):1385–9.

vandenBerg, P., D. Neumark-Sztainer, G. Cafri, and M. Wall. 2007. Steroid use among adolescents: Longitudinal findings from Project EAT. *Pediatrics* 119 (3):476–86. doi: 10.1542/peds.2006-2529.

Velloso, C. P. 2008. Regulation of muscle mass by growth hormone and IGF-I. *Br J Pharmacol* 154 (3):557–68. doi: 10.1038/bjp.2008.153.

Vierck, J., B. O'Reilly, K. Hossner, J. Antonio, K. Byrne, L. Bucci, and M. Dodson. 2000. Satellite cell regulation following myotrauma caused by resistance exercise. *Cell Biol Int* 24 (5):263–72. doi: 10.1006/cbir.2000.0499 S1065-6995(00)90499-2 [pii].

Vingren, J. L., W. J. Kraemer, N. A. Ratamess, J. M. Anderson, J. S. Volek, and C.M. Maresh. 2010. Testosterone physiology in resistance exercise and training: The up-stream regulatory elements. *Sports Med* 40 (12):1037–53. doi: 10.2165/11536910-000000000-00000.

Wang, C., G. Alexander, N. Berman, B. Salehian, T. Davidson, V. McDonald, B. Steiner, L. Hull, C. Callegari, and R. S. Swerdloff. 1996. Testosterone replacement therapy improves mood in hypogonadal men—A clinical research center study. *J Clin Endocrinol Metab* 81 (10):3578–83. doi: 10.1210/jcem.81.10.8855804.

Ward, P. 1973. The effect of an anabolic steroid on strength and lean body mass. *Med Sci Sports* 5 (4):277–82.

Whitehead, R., S. Chillag, and D. Elliott. 1992. Anabolic steroid use among adolescents in a rural state. *J Fam Pract* 35 (4):401–5.

Williams, M. H. and J. D. Branch. 2000. Ergogenic aids for improved performance. In: Garrett WE, Kirkendall DT, eds. *Exercise and Sport Science*. Philadelphia, PA: Lippincott, Williams and Wilkins, pp. 373–84.

Yesalis, C. E. and M. S. Bahrke. 2002. Anabolic-androgenic steroids and related substances. *Curr Sports Med Rep* 1 (4):246–52.

Yesalis, C. E., M. S. Bahrke, A. N. Kopstein et al. 2000. Incidence of anabolic steroid use: A discussion of methodological issues. In: Yesalis CE, ed. *Anabolic Steroids in Sport and Exercise*, 2nd ed. Champaign, IL: Human Kinetics.

Yesalis, C. E., S. P. Courson, and J. Wright. 2000. History of anabolic steroid use in sport and exercise. In: Yesalis CE, ed. *Anabolic Steroids in Sport and Exercise*, 2nd ed. Champaign, IL: Human Kinetics.

Yesalis, C. E., R. T. Herrick, and R. T. Buckley. 1988. Self-reported use of anabolic-androgenic steroids by elite power lifters. *Phys Sportsmed* 16:90–100.

Yu, J. G., P. Bonnerud, A. Eriksson, P. S. Stal, Y. Tegner, and C. Malm. 2014. Effects of long term supplementation of anabolic androgen steroids on human skeletal muscle. *PLoS One* 9 (9):e105330. doi: 10.1371/journal.pone.0105330.

10 Clinical Considerations for the Child and Adolescent Athlete

Jessika Brown, Elizabeth Yakes Jimenez, Carole A. Conn, and Christine M. Mermier

CONTENTS

Abstract	174
10.1 Clinical Considerations	174
10.2 Type 1 Diabetes	174
10.2.1 Exercise Physiology and T1D	174
10.2.2 Assessment	175
10.2.3 Medical Diagnosis	175
10.2.4 Nutrition Diagnosis	175
10.2.5 Medical Interventions	176
10.2.6 Nutrition Interventions	177
10.2.7 Monitoring and Evaluation	179
10.2.8 Your Responsibilities	179
10.2.9 Case Study	179
10.3 Type 2 Diabetes	180
10.3.1 Exercise and T2D	180
10.3.2 Assessment	180
10.3.3 Medical Diagnosis	181
10.3.4 Nutritional Diagnosis	181
10.3.5 Medical Intervention	182
10.3.6 Nutrition Interventions	182
10.3.7 Monitoring and Evaluation	183
10.3.8 Your Responsibilities	184
10.3.9 Case Study	184
10.4 Eating Disorders	184
10.4.1 Exercise and Eating Disorders	184
10.4.2 Assessment	185
10.4.3 Medical Diagnosis	186
10.4.4 Nutrition Diagnosis	187
10.4.5 Medical Interventions	187
10.4.6 Nutrition Interventions	187
10.4.7 Monitoring and Evaluation	188
10.4.8 Your Responsibilities	188
10.4.9 Case Study	189
10.5 Conclusions	189
References	189

ABSTRACT

A number of clinical considerations may exist for health and fitness practitioners, coaches, school nurses, dietitians, or medical providers. This chapter focuses upon the three most prevalent clinical considerations for a child and youth population involved in sport participation. For each considerations, this chapter offers advice and recommendations surrounding the underlying pathology, commons means to assess the presence or development of the underlying condition. Further, each section extends this discussion to include feedback related to necessary diagnosis and interventions. Finally, ways to evaluate and a highlighting of expected responsibilities are included along with case studies to help guide the reader through any of these situations. In all circumstances, individuals without appropriate education and training are first advised to consult with such individuals to ensure key prudent steps are taken to ensure safety and to help promote a positive outcome.

10.1 CLINICAL CONSIDERATIONS

A thorough nutrition assessment is critical to determine the interventions necessary for child and adolescent athletes with special clinical considerations, and for monitoring and evaluating progress toward clinical and athletic goals. As young athletes are at a vulnerable stage in the lifespan, optimal nutrient intake is essential to support healthy growth and development. Certain clinical considerations and specialized meal plans may need to be addressed to maximize the health status of the child, limit potential harm to the athlete's growth, and promote safe exercise. Diagnoses, such as type 1 diabetes (T1D) or type 2 diabetes (T2D), involve alterations in glycemic control, impacting energy utilization. Eating disorders and associated nutrient deficits can increase risk of malnutrition and impair healthy growth and development [1]. Such clinical instances not only jeopardize athletic performance, but can also cause medical instability resulting in health risks and consequences. This chapter will discuss common clinical considerations healthcare providers must be aware of when working with child and adolescent athletes.

10.2 TYPE 1 DIABETES

T1D, formerly known as "juvenile-onset diabetes" or "insulin-dependent diabetes," is an autoimmune disease involving destruction of the pancreatic beta cells resulting in a lack of insulin production [2]. Insulin is the hormone responsible for moving glucose into the cells for energy. Exogenous insulin therapy has opened many doors in the treatment and management of T1D. Elite athletes with T1D, such as swimmer Gary Hall Jr, former NBA player Adam Morrison, and NFL quarterback Jay Cutler, serve as inspiration and demonstrate that individuals with T1D can excel in athletics with proper management [3]. Furthermore, the benefits of exercise for individuals with T1D include improved fitness level and overall well-being, and long-term weight control [2]. While athletic participation is both safe and beneficial for those with T1D, precautions must be taken to reduce risk of certain complications. This section will discuss disease pathophysiology and best practices when working with athletes with T1D.

10.2.1 Exercise Physiology and T1D

A young athlete with T1D requires support, as insulin therapy and physical activity both play a crucial role in glycemic control. During exercise, the body utilizes fuel from various energy sources, primarily serum glucose and stored glycogen in the liver and muscles. When energy needs are increased during exercise, glycogenolysis releases glucose from liver glycogen into the blood. Energy needs are also met through gluconeogenesis, a metabolic process that provides glucose to the blood through the creation of new glucose molecules from noncarbohydrate substrates such as glycerol, amino acids, and lactate. Fatty acids are also released and oxidized by muscles to provide additional energy.

Exercise causes the body to release hormones to initiate this process, resulting in elevated blood sugar to meet increased energy demands during exercise. Normally, these higher blood sugar levels are monitored by the pancreas, which responds by increasing insulin secretion to move glucose into the body's cells [4]. This process occurs seamlessly in a nondiabetic athlete, who automatically responds to the increased energy needs during exercise by increasing gluconeogenesis to meet muscle demands for glucose [2,5,6]. Following this process, the nondiabetic athlete's pancreas adjusts insulin secretion to move serum glucose into the cells for energy utilization. The athlete with T1D must rely on an exogenous insulin injection to respond to the hyperglycemia (high blood sugar) caused by exercise in order to maintain glycemic control. Failure to appropriately monitor blood sugar and insulin needs while exercising can result in initial hyperglycemia, signaling the need for insulin.

If the consequent insulin injection is inappropriate, there is then a risk of hypoglycemia, or low blood sugar [7]. The contraction of muscles during exercise can enhance uptake of glucose in muscles by way of a second mechanism independent of insulin causing athletes with T1D to require individualized insulin therapy to maintain glycemic control given the elevated risk of hypoglycemia. Endurance exercise also increases the risk of hypoglycemia due to the increased release of counter-regulatory hormones to supply energy for longer duration exercises [5]. The risk of hypoglycemia can persist for 6–15 h after endurance exercise due to elevated energy expenditure and loss of glycogen [2,8]. Balancing food intake, physical activity, and adjusting insulin dosage can be a challenge, but is attainable for the athlete with T1D.

10.2.2 Assessment

T1D occurs in about 5% of individuals with diabetes [9]. Onset in children and adolescents can be abrupt, while onset in adults may progress more slowly [2]. Rapid onset is often characterized by unexplained weight loss, polyuria (excessive urination), polydipsia (excessive thirst), and hyperglycemia [4]. Prolonged hyperglycemia can result in ketosis, a condition in which the body utilizes fat as a fuel source, and in the process produces elevated ketone bodies in the blood. High concentrations of ketone bodies acidifies the blood, causing a condition known as ketoacidosis, which can lead to a coma or death if untreated. A hallmark of ketoacidosis is fruity or sweet-smelling breath [4]. Ketosis can result in low energy available for metabolism, which often manifests as unexplained weight loss. Unlike T2D, most individuals with T1D fall within ideal body weight range (for children and adolescents, between the 5th and 85th percentile on age-appropriate growth charts) [10]. Therefore, analysis of unexplained weight loss and growth changes is important for assessing T1D in children and adolescents. Growth changes or unexplained weight loss demonstrated by dropping across percentiles on height-for-age growth charts, weight-for-age growth charts, or BMI-for-age growth charts can be warning signs of T1D or other medical problems and require further medical evaluation (Figure 10.1).

10.2.3 Medical Diagnosis

T1D is predominately diagnosed early in life. Diagnosis is made by a physician in an individual with elevated blood glucose levels [2]. Table 10.1 outlines the various laboratory tests used to screen for and diagnose T1D [4].

10.2.4 Nutrition Diagnosis

Nutrition diagnosis is made by a registered dietitian and will influence dietary interventions. Example nutrition diagnoses that may present in T1D are outlined, but not limited to, those listed in Table 10.2. Dietitians working with athletes with T1D may review the signs and symptoms from the medical and dietary assessment to prioritize nutrition diagnosis and provide recommendations accordingly.

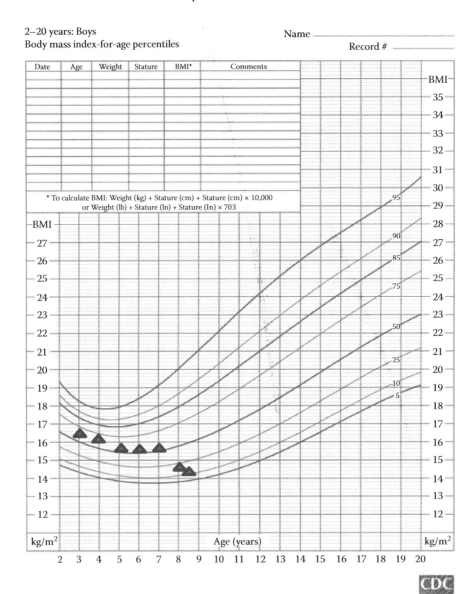

FIGURE 10.1 Outline of a sudden change in growth trend that may indicate metabolic changes such as T1D and indicate further medical evaluation. This example shows an 8-year-old male whose BMI plotted along the 50th percentile from ages 3 to 7, then drops drastically around age 8. (Adapted from Centers for Disease Control and Prevention, National Center for Health Statistics. CDC growth charts: United States. http://www.cdc.gov/growthcharts/. May 30, 2000.)

10.2.5 Medical Interventions

Insulin therapy is necessary for all individuals with T1D. To normalize metabolism in individuals with T1D, exogenous insulin is crafted with an identical amino acid structure and activity comparable to endogenously produced insulin [7]. Various types of insulin offer varying onset, peak, and duration of action, such as rapid-acting, short-acting, basal, and long-acting insulin [9]. In children and adolescents, 50%–65% of insulin needs are met with basal insulin doses and the remaining needs are provided from rapid- or short-acting insulin to prevent hyperglycemia after eating [2].

TABLE 10.1
Laboratory Tests Used to Screen T1D and T2D Mellitus

Test	Description	Reference Ranges
Hemoglobin A1C	This is nonfasting blood test that estimates blood sugars over a 2–3-month period	<5.7% normal 5.7%–6.5% prediabetes >6.5% diabetes
Fasting plasma glucose	This a blood sugar test after an 8-h fast where an individual has nothing to eat or drink	<100 mg/dL normal 100–126 mg/dL prediabetes >126 mg/dL diabetes
Oral glucose tolerance test	This is a test after an 8-h fast in which an individual has blood sugar tested before and 2 h after drinking a glucose-based sweet beverage. This test shows how an individual processes glucose	<140 mg/dL normal 140–200 mg/dL prediabetes >200 mg/dL diabetes

Note: A positive diagnosis for diabetes is commonly indicated when two of the three laboratory tests yield values beyond the provided reference ranges [4,9].

TABLE 10.2
Nutrition Diagnoses for T1D

- Altered nutrition-related laboratory values
- Unintended weight loss
- Inconsistent carbohydrate intake
- Food- and nutrition-related knowledge deficit
- Not ready for diet/lifestyle change
- Inability or lack of desire to manage self-care
- Impaired ability to prepare foods/meals

Source: Adapted from Dietetics, A.o.N.a., *International Dietetics and Nutrition Terminology (IDNT) Reference Manual: Standardized Language for the Nutrition Care Process*, 4th ed. 2012. Chicago, IL: Academy of Nutrition and Dietetics.

Insulin administration can take place via injections and/or pump therapy. An insulin pump, or continuous subcutaneous insulin infusion (CSII), is an apparatus that is inserted into subcutaneous tissue to allow for close monitoring of blood sugar and convenient insulin injection. A CSII remains attached to the individual at all times with insulin cartridges, and may be located at the stomach, hips, outer thigh, buttocks, or back of the arm. Think of CSII as an external pancreas, releasing basal insulin continuously and providing the option for insulin correction injections as needed. With or without an insulin pump, the individual must increase or decrease insulin dosage depending on glycemic control. Athletes should work closely with a physician and certified diabetes educator to generate an appropriate basal insulin dosage, discuss consistent carbohydrate intake, and determine a carbohydrate to insulin correction ratio [5,7,9].

10.2.6 Nutrition Interventions

Nutrition interventions for T1D involve carbohydrate-specific recommendations. Table 10.3 outlines the Academy of Nutrition and Dietetics guidelines when working with T1D [11].

Carbohydrate recommendations for athletes range from 50% to 60% of total energy needs [12]. Recommendations do not differ for athletes with T1D; however, maintaining the consistency and timing of carbohydrate intake is imperative as insulin needs are calculated based on carbohydrate intake [5].

TABLE 10.3
The Academy of Nutrition and Dietetics T1D Evidence-Based Practice Guidelines

- Individuals receiving standard insulin doses should have consistent carbohydrate intake to maximize glycemic control
- Insulin-to-carbohydrate ratios should be individually determined by a diabetes educator for all who utilize insulin pump therapy. Insulin should be adjusted based on meals and snacks using this ratio

Source: Adapted from Dietetics, A.o.N.a., Evidence Analysis Library: Diabetes 1 and 2 Evidence Analysis Project. 2013 (cited October 16, 2013). Available at: http://andevidencelibrary.com/topic.cfm?cat=1615.

Eating or drinking foods with carbohydrates before exercise increases the risk of hyperglycemia, while lack of carbohydrate intake after exercise increases the risk of hypoglycemia. Consuming a carbohydrate-rich snack before and during exercise without providing insulin correction may result in hyperglycemia [5]. Greater carbohydrate intake or "carbohydrate loading" before exercise has been shown to decrease sports performance for athletes with T1D and is not recommended [5]. High-intensity sports, such as sprinting, may initially cause hyperglycemia, and therefore, carbohydrate intake during this type of exercise is not warranted. However, there may be a risk of hypoglycemia immediately and up to 15 h after exercise [2,5]. Blood sugar readings taken from an athlete's finger or big toe after exercise can determine serum glucose level and indicate insulin and carbohydrate needs. Treatment guidelines for hypoglycemia are as follows: administer 5–15 g of carbohydrate; wait 10–15 min; provide an additional 5–15 g of carbohydrates if athlete is still hypoglycemic and symptoms persist [2]. Table 10.4 outlines examples of snacks that provide appropriate carbohydrate amounts. Prevention of postexercise hypoglycemia should be a priority by consuming carbohydrates as a snack and/or at the meal consumed after exercise. This can also be accomplished by including an additional bedtime snack to fully replenish glycogen stores.

TABLE 10.4
Recognizing and Treating Hypoglycemia

Signs and Symptoms of Hypoglycemia

- Fatigue
- Dizziness and lightheadedness
- Shakiness
- Hunger or nausea
- Unexplained sweating, chills, or clamminess
- Headache
- Blurred or impaired vision
- Current blood sugar reading below 70 mg/dL

Treatment Recommendations

- Provide 15 g of carbohydrate
- Wait 10–15 min
- Repeat if hypoglycemic symptoms persist

Recommended Snacks to Have "On Hand" to Counteract Hypoglycemia

(Read food labels to determine carbohydrate concentrations)

- Hard candies, small sugar candies such as Starburst or Skittles
- Packaged fruit snacks
- 4 oz juice or 4–8 oz of sports beverage
- 1 tablespoon of honey

Other nutritional complications may present in children and adolescents with T1D. Celiac disease is an autoimmune disease that occurs in people who possess a genetic susceptibility to the protein gliadin (found in gluten), leading to an inflammatory gut reaction when the protein is ingested [13]. This disease occurs in 1%–16% of individuals with T1D [10]. The Academy of Nutrition and Dietetics recommends screening all individuals with T1D for celiac disease and rescreening children or adolescents that demonstrate growth stunting or failure, unexplained weight loss, or chronic diarrhea [9]. Another concern is the increasing incidence of "diabulimia," a term used to describe individuals with T1D who omit, reduce, or manipulate insulin dosages in efforts to manage weight [14]. Individuals with T1D demonstrate increased risk behaviors and frequency of eating disorders compared to the general population [15]. Diabulimia is not a formal diagnosis; however, it is a growing concern, particularly among female adolescents with T1D [14–16]. Symptoms of diabulimia include frequent urination with ketones in urine, increased thirst, elevated blood sugars (>250 but <600 mg/dL), dehydration, weight loss, muscle atrophy, and edema [14]. Extreme and long-term consequences include permanent kidney damage, blindness, neuropathy, high cholesterol, and osteoporosis [14]. Should an athlete present with signs and symptoms of celiac disease or "diabulimia," practitioners should recommend further medical assessment.

10.2.7 Monitoring and Evaluation

Athletes with T1D should monitor blood sugar regularly in order to optimally manage glucose control according to type and length of exercise, and provide exogenous insulin accordingly. Regular checkups with a primary care physician should occur to review hemoglobin A_{1c} and blood sugar readings over the last several months. One challenge young athletes with T1D face is ever-changing schedules that may limit food availability or intake. Sporadic events and activities may cause an athlete to miss a snack or meal, which can lead to hypoglycemia. Individuals working with athletes can assist athletes with T1D by ensuring consistent and appropriate food intake and encouraging regular blood sugar testing.

10.2.8 Your Responsibilities

Working with athletes with T1D requires vigilance and understanding of the disease. Managing blood glucose levels during practices and games and preventing hypoglycemia are challenges. Knowing how to identify and treat hypoglycemia is essential when working with this population and preventing postexercise hypoglycemia is a priority. Consistent carbohydrate intake and periodic monitoring of blood sugars should be supported. The athlete should be encouraged to consume 1.0–1.5 g carbohydrate/kg of body weight at 2-h intervals up to 6 h beginning immediately after exercise [12]. For example, a 100-lb (45.5-kg) athlete would maximize glycogen replenishment by consuming 46–55 g of carbohydrates with individualized insulin injection immediately after exercise, followed by 46–55 g of carbohydrates with individualized insulin injection at 2, 4, and 6 h after exercise to total 184–220 g of carbohydrates consumed within 6 h after exercise. Examples of snacks and meal items that offer 46–55 g of carbohydrates include a large whole-wheat bagel, an 8 oz glass of chocolate milk with 1 bran muffin, 1 large sweet potato, 1 cup cooked rice or quinoa, 1 1/2 cups of cooked pasta, or a banana with 1 tbsp of peanut butter and 1 tbsp of honey. Those who work with an athlete with T1D should provide time and access to nutritious, high-carbohydrate foods immediately after exercise to maximize glycogen replenishment and prevent hypoglycemia. Ultimately, this will support healthy growth and development, as well as maximize athletic potential in the athlete with T1D.

10.2.9 Case Study

Patrick is a 15-year-old male basketball player with T1D. He has an insulin pump and works closely with his physician to monitor his insulin needs and blood sugar readings. He consistently eats three meals and three snacks per day. He normally eats a carbohydrate-based snack 1 h before practice. One day at practice, you notice Patrick is moving a little slower than usual and his free throws are falling shy of the basket (which is abnormal for him). As you watch him practice, you also notice his hands are shaky. You overhear other teammates discussing how the entire team left school early to go to a homecoming event that involved a high-energy dance practice. You begin to wonder if Patrick was able to have his afternoon snack.

1. What are the signs that Patrick is demonstrating that may indicate hypoglycemia?
2. What would you recommend Patrick do?
3. If Patrick has low blood sugar, what would you recommend he eat?

10.3 TYPE 2 DIABETES

There has been an alarming increase in T2D in the pediatric population. A 33% increase in T2D among children and adolescents over the past 20 years parallels the increase in childhood obesity [17,18]. This concomitant increase prioritizes weight management as a key factor in the treatment of pediatric T2D [17,19]. Many healthcare providers may recommend organized physical activities as a way for children to acquire healthy habits that will aid in losing weight and maintaining weight loss. Therefore, coaches and other physical activity professionals may encounter more children and adolescents with T2D than they have in the past. While a great deal of pediatric diabetes education is designed for T1D and focuses primarily on insulin therapy and hypoglycemia, T2D calls for alternative treatments and interventions. Practitioners should recognize the difference between the two diseases and understand the varying modes of treatment to best support the child or adolescent athlete with T2D.

T2D differs from T1D in that it is not an autoimmune disease resulting in lack of insulin production from pancreatic beta cells. Instead, T2D is a progressive disease in which insulin resistance, not absence of insulin, leads to poor glycemic control [4]. Insulin resistance, a condition in which muscle, fat, and liver cells do not respond to insulin, results in hyperglycemia [4]. This condition is not the result of a lack of insulin, therefore the body responds to the hyperglycemic state by continuing to secrete more insulin resulting in hyperinsulinemia. Initial treatment for T2D usually consists of lifestyle changes to promote weight loss: a healthy diet and increased physical activity. Over time, oral medications and injected insulin may be necessary to manage hyperglycemia. This section will discuss important considerations when working with athletes with T2D, including disease progression, lifestyle interventions, and weight management strategies.

10.3.1 Exercise and T2D

Regular exercise is key to managing T2D [20]. The World Health Organization (WHO) recommends that the pediatric population participate in at least 60 min of physical activity daily [20]. Children and adolescents with T2D will benefit from organized athletics to meet activity recommendations. In particular, progressive resistance training has been shown to be effective in improving insulin sensitivity in both adults and children [21]. Since approximately 85% of glucose uptake occurs directly in the skeletal muscle, activating and strengthening muscle mass is strongly associated with improved glycemic control [21,22]. Many organized sports, such as track and football, offer forms of resistance exercise as a part of regular training programs. Understanding the importance of exercise in the management of T2D makes it clear that a diagnosis of T2D should encourage, rather than deter, children and adolescents from participating in organized and lifelong sport activities.

10.3.2 Assessment

Practitioners should be aware of risk factors and warning signs associated with T2D. Risk factors for T2D include a strong family history of the disease, excess body fat, and a sedentary lifestyle

[17,23]. Insulin resistance is the hallmark of T2D and is often present in those with acanthosis nigricans, a skin condition in which dark pigmentation appears in body creases and areas such as the armpits, groin, and neck [4,9,24]. Other signs of hyperglycemia include frequent thirst and excessive urination. Children and adolescents who demonstrate signs or have associated risk factors for T2D should be referred to a primary care physician for further medical assessment.

Pediatric assessment may include anthropometric, biochemical, and dietary assessment. Anthropometric assessment, such as measuring height and weight to determine body mass index (BMI) percentile on age- and gender-specific growth charts as a proxy for excess body fat, is a good indicator of T2D risk [2]. Individuals who plot above the 85th percentile may possess elevated levels of body fat [25]. While high BMI-for-age percentiles are a strong indicator of risk in nonathletic individuals, further assessment may be necessary to determine risk in athletic individuals who may have a high BMI as a result of increased lean body mass. For athletes, it may be necessary to use more direct means to assess risk, such as waist circumference or body fat analysis as determined by skin folds or bioelectric impedance. In general, this anthropometric assessment should be completed and assessed in a medical setting.

Biochemical assessment reviewed by a physician will ultimately determine diagnosis of T2D and is outlined in Section 10.3.3. Measurement of lipid profile and blood pressure is indicated for children diagnosed with T2D, due to the association between metabolic syndrome, hypertension, and insulin resistance [13]. Dietary assessment is also critical to direct the treatment and management of T2D, and may be carried out by a registered dietitian with the intention of determining energy intake, energy expenditure, and possible micronutrients of concern.

10.3.3 MEDICAL DIAGNOSIS

Table 10.1 outlines each biochemical marker of diabetes and diagnostic criteria. It is important to consider that although biochemical markers diagnose T2D, signs and symptoms may present differently, depending on the disease's level of progression. Individuals can be asymptomatic in the initial stages of the disease due to compensatory mechanisms. Table 10.5 outlines the American Diabetes Association criteria for screening asymptomatic children for T2D.

10.3.4 NUTRITIONAL DIAGNOSIS

Nutrition diagnosis is made by a registered dietitian and can direct dietary treatment and weight management interventions. Examples of nutrition diagnoses are outlined in Table 10.6; other diagnoses may also be appropriate. Altered nutritional laboratory values can influence the development and macronutrient distribution of the meal plan. Excessive carbohydrate intake is diagnosed in

---

TABLE 10.5
Academy of Nutrition and Dietetics Criteria for Screening Asymptomatic Children for T2D

- Overweight as defined by those who fall above the 85th percentile on age-appropriate growth charts with two of the following risk factors:
    - First or second degree relative with history of T2D
    - Of the following ethnic descent: Native American, African American, Asian American, Latino, or Pacific Islander
    - Signs of insulin resistance: Acanthosis nigricans, hypertension, dyslipidemia, polycystic ovarian syndrome, or small-for-gestational age at birth
    - Maternal history of diabetes (type 2 or gestational diabetes)

Source: Adapted from Executive summary: Standards of medical care in diabetes—2013. *Diabetes Care,* 2013. 36(Suppl 1): p. S4–S10. PMID: 23264424.

TABLE 10.6
Nutrition Diagnosis in Individuals with T2D

- Altered nutrition-related laboratory values
- Excessive carbohydrate intake
- Inconsistent carbohydrate intake
- Inappropriate intake of fats
- Food- and nutrition-related knowledge deficit
- Inability or lack of desire to manage self-care
- Impaired ability to prepare foods/meals

Source: Adapted from Dietetics, A.o.N.a., *International Dietetics and Nutrition Terminology (IDNT) Reference Manual: Standardized Language for the Nutrition Care Process*, 4th ed. 2012. Chicago, IL: Academy of Nutrition and Dietetics.

individuals who consume carbohydrates beyond needs as evidenced by hyperglycemia [26]. Simple carbohydrates such as sugar-sweetened beverages and candy can have especially profound effects on blood glucose and are commonly provided as snacks at athletic events and fundraisers. Excessive fat intake can result from frequent intake of foods such as chips, candy, and French fries, which are also staples at school events. A nutrition diagnosis of inappropriate fat intake may be prioritized in the presence of metabolic syndrome, due to increased risk of heart disease [13]. Specific nutrition diagnoses can help to direct individualized nutrition interventions.

10.3.5 Medical Intervention

Pharmacological therapy in combination with diet and exercise interventions are recommended for the general pediatric population with T2D compared to using lifestyle interventions alone [27]. This is because diet and exercise interventions alone may be less effective due to low adherence in the general pediatric population [23]. However, athletes may have additional motivation to manage their illness through diet and exercise interventions. Pediatric individuals with T2D are at increased risk for complications due to longer exposure to the disease; therefore, aggressive intervention is warranted in order to preserve long-term health [19]. The American Academy of Pediatrics recommends insulin therapy for youth who present with ketosis, and Metformin as the primary mode of therapy in newly diagnosed individuals [23]. Metformin is a medication that improves insulin sensitivity and decreases hepatic glucose production [2]. A physician and certified diabetes educator may work closely with the athlete to monitor medication efficacy.

10.3.6 Nutrition Interventions

Nutrition intervention for T2D includes nutrition education at the time of diagnosis, and as a method of ongoing support. Nutrition education is essential for adherence to management of T2D and long-term healthy lifestyle habits. The American Academy of Pediatrics and the Academy of Nutrition and Dietetics' Pediatric Weight Management Evidence-Based Nutrition Practice Guidelines outline specific nutrition interventions listed in Table 10.7 [23,28].

Weight management may be recommended for children and adolescents who demonstrate an elevated BMI with comorbidities such as T2D [25]. Calorie-restricted, nutrient-dense diets should be offered to those who would benefit from weight loss in conjunction with lifestyle interventions such as exercise recommendations and possible medication [28]. Nutrition education should focus on the practice of consuming three meals and planned snacks to promote a healthy weight. Meal plans can be provided by a registered dietitian with individualized macronutrient recommendations based on

TABLE 10.7
Academy of Nutrition and Dietetics Pediatric Weight Management Guidelines

- Diets 900–1200 cal/day in ages 6–12*
- No less than 1200 cal/day in ages 13–18*
- Short-term (often 10 weeks) protein-sparing, ketogenic diet in children greater than 120% of ideal body weight or with serious medical complications

Nutrition education to promote healthy eating patterns including the following:

- Three meals with planned snacks per day
- Not consuming meals or snacks while watching television or on the computer
- Reducing portion sizes (use of smaller plates, bowls, and cups)
- Leaving small amounts of food on the plate
- Limiting caloric beverages (with the exception of milk)
- Increasing consumption of fruits and vegetables
- Limiting intake of high-fat foods
- Limiting intake of high-sugar foods
- Reducing food consumed from fast food establishments

Source: Adapted from Copeland, K.C. et al., *Pediatrics*, 131(2), 364–82, 2013; Dietetics, A.o.N.a., Recommendations summary: Pediatric weight management (PWM) using protein sparing modified fast diets for pediatric weight loss. 2013 (cited October 16, 2013). Available at: http://andevidencelibrary.com/topic.cfm?cat=3010.
Note: Restricted diets with the intention of weight loss should be included with other lifestyle modifications, including exercise interventions and possibly medications.

nutrition diagnosis. For example, if an individual is diagnosed with excessive carbohydrate intake, the registered dietitian may recommend a meal plan with adjusted carbohydrate intake between 45% and 55% of total calories. If an individual presents with excessive fat intake, the registered dietitian may provide nutrition education focusing on dietary sources of fat and limiting foods such as French fries, donuts, chips, fast food, and other high-fat items.

Portion control is another priority in weight management, considering the increasing portion sizes in typical American foods. Reducing plate or bowl size is one method of practicing portion control and can be used as an education modality. It is important to consider that making substantial dietary changes can be overwhelming, considering the influence of social eating, media, and cultural norms on food intake. Therefore, family involvement is crucial when educating the athlete with T2D on appropriate food intake to ensure environmental support [23]. Furthermore, all pediatric athletes can benefit from consuming less high-fat and high-sugar snacks in the diet. Coaches can encourage healthy snacks such as fruits, vegetables, whole-grain crackers with cheese, popcorn, or water in place of high-fat, high-sugar snacks such as chips, cookies, and fruit drinks. Encouraging healthy eating habits for all children and adolescents can provide a more supportive environment for those who must make these changes as a result of a medical diagnosis.

10.3.7 Monitoring and Evaluation

Monitoring the athlete with T2D requires regular follow-up to monitor glycemic control, medication efficacy, and adherence to lifestyle interventions. Regular monitoring is critical, as the consequences of untreated T2D include increased risk of cardiovascular disease and diabetic ketoacidosis [23]. The American Academy of Pediatrics recommends monitoring hemoglobin A_{1c} every 3 months until glycemic control is attained, as demonstrated by a hemoglobin A_{1c} of 7% or less, and then monitoring biannually [23]. Newly diagnosed children and adolescents should monitor serum blood sugar before all meals and at bedtime until glycemic control is reached [23].

10.3.8 YOUR RESPONSIBILITIES

Coaches, athletic trainers, and pediatric practitioners have a unique role in supporting healthy lifestyles in the pediatric population. Reinforcement of healthy eating habits and appropriate exercise will encourage effective management of T2D, and weight management can be a side effect of a healthy lifestyle. It is important that the emphasis of T2D management remains focused on lifestyle changes, as opposed to weight loss alone. Undue pressure and focus on weight can have adverse effects, such as poor body image and increased risk of eating disorders. To support long-term health, those working with the T2D population should place emphasis on cultivating a healthy diet and exercise lifestyle, rather than focusing on weight and body fat alone.

10.3.9 CASE STUDY

Tyler is a 17-year-old defensive lineman on the high school football team. He is 6 ft tall and weighs 200 lb. His BMI of 27.1 is above the 85th percentile on the BMI-for-age growth chart. He wants to remain "big" for football purposes, but you are worried as he appears to be chronically thirsty, needs frequent bathroom breaks at practice, and he has a dark discoloration around his neck. You begin to notice his snacks consist of the following: candy bar and energy drink before practice, 24 oz sports beverage during practice, and a protein bar with two packages of fruit snacks immediately after practice. You also notice that Tyler consumes large regular sodas at most team gatherings, and talks a great deal about the need for "carb loading."

1. Does Tyler demonstrate any warning signs of T2D? If so, what are they?
2. Is Tyler overweight or obese? How do you know? Would you recommend any further anthropometric evaluation? If so, why?
3. How would you handle Tyler's food intake? Do you have any suggestions for him?

10.4 EATING DISORDERS

While athletic participation offers a multitude of benefits, athletes also demonstrate significantly higher rates of eating disorders compared to the general population [29,30]. In particular, females participating in judged sports or sports that require minimal clothing demonstrate higher risk of eating disorders compared to other sports [31,32]. Males are not excluded from this clinical consideration, as up to 95% of males have reported body dissatisfaction in a survey of adult males [33]. Considering the elevated risk of eating disorders in athletes, it is imperative that practitioners working with pediatric athletes are able to screen for eating disorders and refer to appropriate clinicians.

10.4.1 EXERCISE AND EATING DISORDERS

Exercise has many physical and psychological benefits, but participation should be carefully evaluated when working with athletes with eating disorders. Excessive exercise is defined as exercise that interferes with other valuable activities, occurs at inappropriate or inconvenient times or settings, or continues despite injury or other inhibiting conditions and may cause harm or prevent recovery [34]. Such exercise can be used as a form of purging in individuals with eating disorders.

On the other hand, research supports exercise as a viable treatment method for individuals with depression and anxiety disorders [35–37]. Considering that both depression and anxiety disorders are common comorbidities in individuals with all types of eating disorders, exercise therapy may also benefit individuals with eating disorders [38]. A study that evaluated the recovery markers of bulimic women after 8 weeks of psychotherapy alone, nutrition therapy alone, and psychotherapy combined with exercise, found that bulimia symptoms were most improved at the 8-week and 16-week follow-up evaluations when exercise was included in the therapy process [37].

Studies suggest physical activity increases tolerance to everyday stress triggers among those with eating disorders [37]. Mental health benefits were most often seen with 30–60 min of moderate-intensity activities and low frequency (3 days/week), and no difference was found when frequency was increased to 5 days/week in depressed patients [38,39].

The psychological benefits of exercise may occur from as little as 20 min of light activity two times per week, and socially driven activities may augment the mental benefits [40]. However, it is a delicate balance to recommend exercise participation in clients who are actively engaging in eating disorder behaviors. As such, practitioners should seek medical clearance to ensure the athlete's safety. For athletes with a normal BMI, exercise is usually appropriate. For athletes with a low BMI (<18.5) or those who fall below the 5th percentile on age- and gender-specific BMI growth charts, exercise should be limited until weight gain is achieved [41]. Medical markers that contraindicate exercise participation include amenorrhea in females, an abnormal electrocardiograph reading, low blood pressure, low resting heart rate, imbalanced electrolytes, elevated liver enzymes, elevated cholesterol, and low prealbumin [41]. Resumption of menses is an indicator that the female athlete is within ideal body weight range and exercise participation is likely safe. Exercise recommendations should be agreed upon between exercise professionals and eating disorder specialists, as the benefits associated with exercise need to be balanced against the medical risks.

10.4.2 Assessment

Being aware of eating disorder symptoms is the first step in working to support athletes who may be at risk. Symptoms of an eating disorder may present as physical, anthropometric, and/or food behavior changes. Warning signs such as sudden weight changes, isolation, references to feeling "fat," or changes in eating habits should cue screening for an eating disorder. For example, vegetarian or vegan diets may be an indicator of an eating disorder. The Academy of Nutrition and Dietetics states that well-planned vegetarian diets can provide adequate nutrition to support growth and development for children and adolescents; however, this dietary change must come with careful attention and education [42]. Although not always the case, some intentions for switching to a vegetarian or vegan diet may derive from the desire to restrict calories [12]. Screening questions about eating patterns and body image can be useful in noting any disordered eating behaviors. The American Academy of Pediatrics recommends the SCOFF questionnaire as a framework for screening children and adolescents for eating disorders [1,43].

Anthropometric, biochemical, and psychological assessment are necessary when an eating disorder is suspected. Weight, height, and BMI should be routinely checked by health professionals and plotted on growth charts, noting any sudden or unusual changes in growth [43]. For example, if an athlete has attended yearly physicals for many years and has demonstrated a growth trend along the 25th percentile for BMI-for-age, then suddenly presents with a BMI along the 5th percentile, this may be a red flag for an eating disorder. Such sudden or abnormal changes warrant further monitoring and assessment. Some athletes manifest their eating disorder with weight loss, while others may show growth failure without weight loss and even demonstrate a "normal" BMI [44]. Calorie restriction or micronutrient deficiency can stunt linear growth without changing weight, which can also be a red flag for an eating disorder. This is important to recognize, as eating disorder behaviors can be present without physical signs and symptoms, such as weight loss or gain.

Low energy availability is a distinct symptom that presents in individuals with or at risk for an eating disorder. Energy availability is the amount of energy available for metabolism, based on total calories consumed after subtracting calories burned from exercise [45,46]. For example, if an athlete with an eating disorder consumes 800 kcal/day and burns 400 kcal/day at cross-country practice, energy availability for metabolic needs would total an insufficient amount of 400 kcal/day. Energy availability can be assessed by completing a dietary and exercise analysis and estimating total energy intake and total energy burn. Research suggests energy availability should be greater than 45 kcal/kg of lean body mass to support healthy growth and development [45,46].

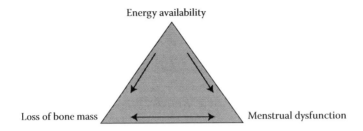

FIGURE 10.2 The female athlete triad.

Female athletes with low energy availability may consequently exhibit menstrual dysfunction and low bone mineral density [45]. This triad of symptoms is outlined in Figure 10.2 and is referred to as the female athlete triad. The female athlete triad is commonly observed among patients with an eating disorder. The triad includes a spectrum of menstrual dysfunction including the following: oligomenorrhea, menstrual cycles lasting longer than 35 days; amenorrhea, absence of a period for 3 months or longer; and primary amenorrhea, delay in menarche onset beyond 15 or 16 years of age [45,46]. Menstrual dysfunction may be the first symptom recognized in the triad, and can indicate the need for additional medical assessment.

10.4.3 Medical Diagnosis

The fifth edition of the *Diagnostic and Statistical Manual of Mental Disorders* (DSM-V) outlines four categories of eating disorders with specific criteria [35]. Table 10.8 outlines each disorder and its respective hallmark symptoms. Beyond eating disorders, muscular dysmorphia is also a concern, particularly in males. This is a psychiatric condition characterized by extreme efforts to reach a level of muscularity that is associated with body image distortion [47]. If concerned, it is appropriate to ask the athlete if he/she notices anything abnormal about his/her eating patterns and behaviors. Questions regarding body image can also provide insight. If there is concern about an eating

TABLE 10.8
Considerations for Recommending Assessment for an Eating Disorder

Binge Eating Disorder
- Recurring episodes of eating an amount of food that is more than most people would eat in a short period of time
- Feelings of lack of control present when eating large amounts of food
- Bingeing occurs at least once per week over a 3-month period
- Often, but not always, presents with a normal or elevated BMI

Anorexia Nervosa
- Severe calorie restriction
- Distorted body image
- Excessive dieting and/or calorie restriction that leads to severe weight loss
- Significantly low body weight demonstrated by low BMI or changes in growth curve

Bulimia Nervosa
- Bingeing episodes and the use of a compensatory mechanism that occurs at least once per week for 3 months
- Compensatory mechanisms may include but are not limited to the following: Vomiting, exercise "purging," and the use of laxatives
- BMI is not an effective indicator
- Other specified feeding and eating disorders
- Demonstrates disordered eating patterns such as food restriction, purging, chewing and spitting food, bingeing, etc.

TABLE 10.9
Nutrition Diagnoses for Individuals with Eating Disorders

- Inadequate oral intake
- Excessive oral intake
- Inadequate fluid intake
- Malnutrition
- Food- and nutrition-related knowledge deficit
- Disordered eating patterns

Source: Adapted from Dietetics, A.o.N.a., *International Dietetics and Nutrition Terminology (IDNT) Reference Manual: Standardized Language for the Nutrition Care Process*, 4th ed. 2012. Chicago, IL: Academy of Nutrition and Dietetics.

disorder, recommending further assessment from a primary care physician or mental healthcare provider is warranted. Treatment of each disorder requires a team of eating disorder specialists and a multidisciplinary treatment approach. Symptoms that may require immediate medical attention include dizziness, fainting, chest tightness or pain, blood found in vomit or stool, prolonged constipation or diarrhea, and/or the inability to keep food contents in stomach after eating.

10.4.4 Nutrition Diagnosis

Nutrition diagnosis in individuals with eating disorders focuses on medical stability and normalization of eating patterns. Table 10.9 outlines potential nutrition diagnoses in athletes with eating disorders. Nutrition diagnosis can assist in determining if exercise is an appropriate part of treatment for the individual athlete.

10.4.5 Medical Interventions

Medical interventions for all types of eating disorders should include a physician to monitor medical stability, and a mental healthcare provider to treat the underlying cause of the disorder. Family-based therapy or the "Maudsley" method is widely accepted as an evidenced-based intervention for children and adolescents with eating disorders [48]. This is a three-phase treatment strategy that begins by instructing the parents or guardians to take full responsibility, with the help of a clinician, of the child/adolescent's meal plans until weight is restored within a healthy range. Phases two and three work to gradually reintroduce food control back into the hands of the child or adolescent based on detailed guidelines and milestones accomplished in treatment. Each step is outlined in detail by a healthcare provider and discussed with the family before being implemented in the home. The "Maudsley" method, although evidence based, may not be appropriate for all clients and the recommendation to use this approach should come from a skilled team of eating disorder specialists [1].

10.4.6 Nutrition Interventions

The primary nutrition intervention in working with athletes who have eating disorders is to balance energy intake with energy expenditure and ensure adequate micronutrient intake in efforts to restore adequate growth and development [46]. Thorough assessment of caloric intake by a registered dietitian can determine energy availability. Studies reveal up to 45 kcal/kg of fat free mass to be the most effective balance of energy availability in children and adolescents [46,49].

Paying close attention to energy intake can also bring to light any micronutrient concerns. Micronutrients such as iron, calcium, vitamins C, B12, and E, zinc, and magnesium all play a key role in metabolic pathways that are in higher demand during exercise [12]. Iron is of specific concern as it is responsible for the generation of oxygen-carrying proteins within the body. Low iron stores may have long-term neurological effects and should be addressed quickly and prevented when possible [1]. Iron deficiency anemia may develop if iron needs are increased and/or intake is limited; this is commonly observed in vegetarians or vegans with a poorly planned diet [42]. In addition, vegetarians and vegans may be at increased risk of low iron status because the iron available in plants is not as bioavailable as animal sources of iron. Signs of iron deficiency include weakness and fatigue, heart palpitations, sensitivity to cold temperatures, and loss of appetite [12].

10.4.7 Monitoring and Evaluation

Monitoring the athlete with an eating disorder includes ensuring that the patient follows up with a physician to ensure medical stability, attends therapy sessions as directed by a mental healthcare provider, and adheres to an appropriate meal plan. A multidisciplinary team made up of eating disorder specialists is ideal in working with this population. The International Association for Eating Disordered Professionals is a credentialing organization that certifies eating disorder specialists who are most qualified to work with these young athletes. Monitoring every 1–2 weeks may be necessary in the initial stages of the disorder [1]. In females, monitoring symptoms of the female athlete triad, specifically menstruation, can be used to determine adequate energy availability [45].

10.4.8 Your Responsibilities

Practitioners working with youth athletes need to be aware of eating disorder risks and encourage a healthy lifestyle. Table 10.10 suggests ways to promote a healthy relationship with food. If an athlete demonstrates signs of an eating disorder, recommendations for further medical assessment and pausing athletic participation may be necessary. Ceasing athletic activities until a thorough assessment is completed and the safety of the athlete has been established is crucial, as exercising may worsen eating disorder consequences [41]. For example, exercising with low energy availability increases risk for bone fractures and stunted growth; in females, it may also cause hormonal imbalances leading to irregular menses [46]. Minimizing medical complications, positively balancing energy expenditure for optimal growth, and addressing underlying psychological triggers for an eating disorder are the primary responsibilities when working with individuals with eating disorders [1,46,49]. During this time, sport participation may or may not be appropriate. Only when energy and micronutrient needs are met and the athlete is no longer at medical risk can an exercise regimen be reintroduced.

TABLE 10.10
How to Promote a Healthy Relationship with Food

Not Recommended	Recommended
Comments regarding weight, body shape, in a positive or negative manner	Emphasize what an individual's body is capable of rather than how it appears
Weighing athletes and recommending body weight based on BMI	Only weigh children and adolescents at medical checkups and allow discussion of BMI to be offered by medical professionals
Discussing and endorsing popular diets especially any diets that eliminate food groups	Note any changes in eating habits and/or elimination of food groups. If an athlete presents with such a change, refer to a specialist for evaluation of motives and maintenance of optimal nutrient intake
Labeling foods as "good" or "bad"	Discuss foods as a source of fuel and recommend ways to maximize athletic performance

10.4.9 CASE STUDY

Charly is a 17-year-old female soccer player who recently lost 15 lb in a 2-month period. Her current weight is 91 lb and her height is 62 in. Charly has never had a menstrual period. She plays high school soccer, which includes 5 days of 2 h practices in addition to weekly games. Charly's parents report that her decision to become a vegetarian 2 months ago has led to a decline in eating with the family. Charly's soccer coach is concerned as her performance has worsened, and she has gone from being a starting forward to little playing time. Charly's coach also reports that she has become more reserved over the last 2 months and calls the high school athletic trainer for support.

1. Does Charly demonstrate any eating disorder symptoms and/or red flags? If yes, what are they?
2. What does Charly's menstrual history reveal?
3. If you were the high school athletic trainer, what would you recommend to Charly and her family?

10.5 CONCLUSIONS

Any individual working with the child and adolescent population carries a responsibility of understanding how to best support the athlete's growth and development in addition to athletic goals. The clinical considerations outlined in this chapter target conditions that are common in the pediatric population. Dietitians working directly with this population play an integral role as a member of the healthcare team, in particular in cases of youth athletes with diabetes and/or eating disorders. Thorough understanding and support of these considerations will ultimately assist the athlete in maintaining long-term well-being and enhanced athletic performance.

REFERENCES

1. Rosen, D.S. and American Academy of Pediatrics Committee on Adolescence. Identification and management of eating disorders in children and adolescents. *Pediatrics*, 2010. 126(6): p. 1240–53.
2. Educators, A.A.o.D., *Diabetes in the Life Cycle and Research*. 4th ed. Vol. 4. 2001, Chicago, IL: American Association of Diabetes Educators. 278pp.
3. Gallen, I.W., A. Redgrave, and S. Redgrave, Olympic diabetes. *Clin Med*, 2003. 3(4): p. 333–7.
4. Educators, A.A.o.D., *Diabetes and Complications*. in: ed. M.J. Franz, 4th ed, Vol. 1. 2001, Chicago, IL: American Association of Diabetes Educators. 232pp.
5. Gallen, I.W., C. Hume, and A. Lumb, Fuelling the athlete with type 1 diabetes. *Diabetes Obes Metab*, 2011. 13(2): p. 130–6.
6. Jegdic, V., Z. Roncevic, and V. Skrabic, Physical fitness in children with type 1 diabetes measured with six-minute walk test. *Int J Endocrinol*, 2013. 2013: p. 190454.
7. Draznin, M.B., Managing the adolescent athlete with type 1 diabetes mellitus. *Pediatr Clin North Am*, 2010. 57(3): p. 829–37.
8. MacDonald, M.J., Postexercise late-onset hypoglycemia in insulin-dependent diabetic patients. *Diabetes Care*, 1987. 10(5): p. 584–8.
9. Executive summary: Standards of medical care in diabetes—2013. *Diabetes Care*, 2013. 36(Suppl 1): p. S4–S10. PMID: 23264424.
10. Silverstein, J. et al., Care of children and adolescents with type 1 diabetes: A statement of the American Diabetes Association. *Diabetes Care*, 2005. 28(1): p. 186–212.
11. Dietetics, A.o.N.a., Evidence Analysis Library: Diabetes 1 and 2 Evidence Analysis Project. 2013 (cited October 16, 2013). Available at: http://andevidencelibrary.com/topic.cfm?cat=1615.
12. Rodriguez, N.R. et al., Position of the American Dietetic Association, Dietitians of Canada, and the American College of Sports Medicine: Nutrition and athletic performance. *J Am Diet Assoc*, 2009. 109(3): p. 509–27.
13. Academy of Nutrition and Dietetics. Nutrition Care Manual. Available at: https://www.nutritioncaremanual.org/.
14. Ruth-Sahd, L.A., M. Schneider, and B. Haagen, Diabulimia: What it is and how to recognize it in critical care. *Dimens Crit Care Nurs*, 2009. 28(4): p. 147–53; quiz 154–5.

15. Philippi, S.T. et al., Risk behaviors for eating disorder in adolescents and adults with type 1 diabetes. *Rev Bras Psiquiatr*, 2013. 35(2): p. 150–6.
16. Larranaga, A., M.F. Docet, and R.V. Garcia-Mayor, Disordered eating behaviors in type 1 diabetic patients. *World J Diabetes*, 2011. 2(11): p. 189–95.
17. Peterson, K. et al., Management of type 2 diabetes in youth: An update. *Am Fam Physician*, 2007. 76(5): p. 658–64.
18. Prevention, C.f.D.C.a., National Diabetes Fact Sheet. General information and national estimates on diabetes in the United States, 2011 (cited October 16, 2013). Available at: http://www.cdc.gov/diabetes/pubs/pdf/ndfs_2011.pdf.
19. Willi, S.M. et al., Treatment of type 2 diabetes in childhood using a very-low-calorie diet. *Diabetes Care*, 2004. 27(2): p. 348–53.
20. Ellery, C.V., H.A. Weiler, and T.J. Hazell, Physical activity assessment tools for use in overweight and obese children. *Int J Obes (Lond)*, 2013. 38: p. 1–10.
21. Lee, S. and Y. Kim, Effects of exercise alone on insulin sensitivity and glucose tolerance in obese youth. *Diabetes Metab J*, 2013. 37(4): p. 225–32.
22. DeFronzo, R.A. et al., Effects of insulin on peripheral and splanchnic glucose metabolism in noninsulin-dependent (type II) diabetes mellitus. *J Clin Invest*, 1985. 76(1): p. 149–55.
23. Copeland, K.C. et al., Management of newly diagnosed type 2 diabetes mellitus (T2DM) in children and adolescents. *Pediatrics*, 2013. 131(2): p. 364–82.
24. Wilson, V., Type 2 diabetes: An epidemic in children. *Nurs Child Young People*, 2013. 25(2): p. 14–7.
25. Barlow, S.E. and C. Expert, Expert committee recommendations regarding the prevention, assessment, and treatment of child and adolescent overweight and obesity: Summary report. *Pediatrics*, 2007. 120(Suppl 4): p. S164–92.
26. Dietetics, A.o.N.a., *International Dietetics and Nutrition Terminology (IDNT) Reference Manual: Standardized Language for the Nutrition Care Process*, 4th ed. 2012. Chicago, IL: Academy of Nutrition and Dietetics.
27. Rosenbloom, A.L. et al., ISPAD Clinical Practice Consensus Guidelines 2006–2007. Type 2 diabetes mellitus in the child and adolescent. *Pediatr Diabetes*, 2008. 9(5): p. 512–26.
28. Dietetics, A.o.N.a., Recommendations summary: Pediatric weight management (PWM) using protein sparing modified fast diets for pediatric weight loss. 2013 (cited October 16, 2013). Available at: http://andevidencelibrary.com/topic.cfm?cat=3010.
29. Sundgot-Borgen, J. and M.K. Torstveit, Prevalence of eating disorders in elite athletes is higher than in the general population. *Clin J Sport Med*, 2004. 14(1): p. 25–32.
30. Sundgot-Borgen, J., M.K. Torstveit, and F. Skarderud, Eating disorders among athletes. *Tidsskr Nor Laegeforen*, 2004. 124(16): p. 2126–9.
31. Lombardo, C. et al., Body dissatisfaction among pre-adolescent girls is predicted by their involvement in aesthetic sports and by personal characteristics of their mothers. *Eat Weight Disord*, 2012. 17(2): p. e116–27.
32. Torres-McGehee, T.M. et al., Eating disorder risk and the role of clothing in collegiate cheerleaders' body images. *J Athl Train*, 2012. 47(5): p. 541–8.
33. Murray, S.B. et al., A comparison of eating, exercise, shape, and weight related symptomatology in males with muscle dysmorphia and anorexia nervosa. *Body Image*, 2012. 9(2): p. 193–200.
34. American Psychiatric Association. *Diagnostic and Statistical Manual of Mental Disorders.* 5th ed. 2013, Washington, DC: American Psychiatric Publishing.
35. Kaye, W.H. et al., Comorbidity of anxiety disorders with anorexia and bulimia nervosa. *Am J Psychiatr*, 2004. 161(12): p. 2215–21.
36. Mond, J.M. et al., An update on the definition of "excessive exercise" in eating disorders research. *Int J Eat Disord*, 2006. 39(2): p. 147–53.
37. Sundgot-Borgen, J. et al., The effect of exercise, cognitive therapy, and nutritional counseling in treating bulimia nervosa. *Med Sci Sports Exercise*, 2002. 34(2): p. 190–5.
38. Strohle, A., Physical activity, exercise, depression and anxiety disorders. *J Neural Transm*, 2009. 116(6): p. 777–84.
39. Silveira, H. et al., Physical exercise and clinically depressed patients: A systematic review and meta-analysis. *Neuropsychobiology*, 2013. 67(2): p. 61–8.
40. Callaghan, P., Exercise: A neglected intervention in mental health care? *J Psychiatr Ment Health Nurs*, 2004. 11(4): p. 476–83.
41. Herrin, M., *Nutrition Counseling in the Treatment of Eating Disorders.* 2003, New York, NY: Brunner-Routledge.

42. Craig, W.J., A.R. Mangels, and American Dietetic Association, Position of the American Dietetic Association: Vegetarian diets. *J Am Diet Assoc*, 2009. 109(7): p. 1266–82.
43. Morgan, J.F., F. Reid, and J.H. Lacey, The SCOFF questionnaire: Assessment of a new screening tool for eating disorders. *Br Med J*, 1999. 319(7223): p. 1467–8.
44. Modan-Moses, D. et al., Linear growth and final height characteristics in adolescent females with anorexia nervosa. *PLoS One*, 2012. 7(9): p. e45504.
45. Nattiv, A. et al., American College of Sports Medicine position stand. The female athlete triad. *Med Sci Sports Exercise*, 2007. 39(10): p. 1867–82.
46. Barrack, M., Low energy availability: Recognizing and addressing an intentional versus inadvertent energy deficit, in: *Sports, Cardiovascular, and Wellness Nutrition: SCAN'S PULSE 2011.* 30(2): p. 11–14.
47. Murray, S.B. et al., Muscle dysmorphia and the DSM-V conundrum: Where does it belong? A review paper. *Int J Eat Disord*, 2010. 43(6): p. 483–91.
48. Findlay, S. et al., Family-based treatment of children and adolescents with anorexia nervosa: Guidelines for the community physician. *Paediatr Child Health*, 2010. 15(1): p. 31–40.
49. Hoch, A.Z. et al., Prevalence of the female athlete triad in high school athletes and sedentary students. *Clin J Sport Med*, 2009. 19(5): p. 421–8.

11 Nutrition and the Overweight Athlete

Elizabeth Fox

CONTENTS

Abstract 193
11.1 Introduction 193
11.2 Nutritional Interventions 194
    11.2.1 Energy Balance 194
    11.2.2 Macronutrient Needs 194
11.3 Diets for Weight Loss in Youth 196
11.4 Other Weight-Loss Remedies 197
    11.4.1 Medications 197
    11.4.2 Bariatric Surgery 197
11.5 Guidelines for Healthy Weight Control/Loss Practices 198
11.6 Psychological Considerations 198
11.7 Resources for Parents and Health Educators 199
References 200

ABSTRACT

This chapter discusses nutritional and psychological considerations for an overweight or obese athlete attempting to lose weight. Information for creating a supportive and healthy environment for weight loss is described in detail for coaches, trainers, parents, and health professionals. Accurate determination of energy and macronutrient balance is the first step to ensure slow and sustained weight loss without negatively impacting growth and development or performance. The use of medications or bariatric surgery in obese adolescent youth is discussed, as well as inappropriate methods for weight loss, such as fad diets, supplements, or fluid and food restriction. Healthy eating tips to encourage weight loss in adolescent athletes and resources for parents and healthcare educators are provided.

11.1 INTRODUCTION

Over the past 30 years, there has been a twofold increase in obesity rates in children aged 2–5 years, and a threefold increase in children aged 6–11 years and adolescents 12–19 years (Ogden et al. 2012). Currently, obesity prevalence increases from early childhood (8.4% of 2–5-year-olds) to early adolescence (17.7% of 6–11-year-olds) (Ogden et al. 2014), and risk for overweight or obesity increases into adulthood for children who are overweight or obese as youth (Ferraro et al. 2003).

Physical inactivity and unhealthy eating behaviors are the two modifiable risk factors that play a dominant role in the development of obesity in this population. In 2013, only 36.6% of male high school students and 17.7% of female high school students in the United States met the Department of Health and Human Services recommendation for 60 minutes of physical activity per day (Centers for Disease Control and Prevention 2013). Additionally, high saturated fat intake (Tippet and Cypel 1997), and low fruit and vegetable consumption (Lin et al. 2001) contribute to calorie and nutrient insufficiencies in children and adolescents.

Coaches, parents, and healthcare practitioners (nurses, dietitians, and pediatricians) must be educated on how to provide a supportive environment for weight loss that still maintains normal growth and development in youth athletes. In order to appropriately and safely address weight loss in child (6–11 years) and adolescent (12–19 years) athletes, evidence-based recommendations and comprehensive nutritional services must be provided, and should include nutrition, exercise, and psychological interventions. This chapter will discuss the nutritional and psychological components for healthy weight loss in youth. For more information regarding physical activity recommendations for weight loss, see Chapter 14.

11.2 NUTRITIONAL INTERVENTIONS

11.2.1 ENERGY BALANCE

An individual's weight, regardless of age, gender, and physical activity, is determined by his or her energy balance: calories consumed (intake) versus calories expended (output). When intake exceeds output, weight gain occurs; when intake is less than output, weight loss occurs; and when intake equals output, an individual will maintain weight. While this concept seems simple in nature, there are a number of factors that influence a young athlete's intake and expenditure.

The current estimated energy requirement (EER) for males 9–13 years of age is 2279 kcal, and for 14–18-year-old males, the EER is 3152 kcal (National Academies Press 2006). Similarly, the EER for 9–13-year-old females is 2071 kcal and 2368 kcal for 14–18-year-old females (National Academies Press 2006). This calorie level is based on an "active" person, of reference height and weight, and may not be applicable for all young persons, in particular, athletes. When possible, indirect calorimetry should be used to measure resting energy expenditure (REE) and multiplied by an appropriate activity factor. If indirect calorimetry is not available, the Harris Benedict equation (Henes et al. 2013), Molnar and the Institutes of Medicine for Obese Youth (IOM-OY) predictive equation (Molnar et al. 1995, National Academies Press 2006, Trumbo et al. 2002), or the IOM for children and Schofield equation for the pediatric population (regardless of obesity status) should be used to estimate calorie needs (Schofield 1985, Trumbo et al. 2002). Weight loss should be a gradual process, with a starting goal of losing 5%–10% of initial body weight (De Miguel-Etayo et al. 2013). For a comparison of common predictive equations used in obese youth, see Table 11.1 (Henes et al. 2013).

Fad diets and other inappropriate weight-loss methods are becoming more and more prevalent in a child's or adolescent's attempt to lose weight. Calorie restriction for weight loss has been recently studied in obese adolescents. Very low calorie diets (≤1000 kcal/day) in severely obese youth have been evaluated by the Academy's Evidence Analysis Library on Pediatric Weight Management and the Expert Committee on the treatment of childhood and adolescent overweight and obesity. While short-term (6–12 months) weight loss has been documented, a slowed growth velocity has also been found (Suskind et al. 2000), and therefore, because of limited evidence, this diet approach should only be used for a short-term (10 weeks) intervention, under the supervision of a multidisciplinary healthcare team (Academy of Nutrition and Dietetics 2007). Other fad diets, medications, and weight-loss surgery will be discussed in Section 11.4.

11.2.2 MACRONUTRIENT NEEDS

It is critical to provide a balanced intake of carbohydrate, protein, and fat when an adolescent athlete is in negative energy balance for weight loss. The acceptable macronutrient distribution range (AMDR) for 9–18-year-olds is currently 45%–65% carbohydrate, 10%–30% protein, and 25%–35% fat (Trumbo et al. 2002). For youth athletes, approximately 55%–65% of calories should come from carbohydrate, 15%–20% from protein, and 20%–30% from fat (American Academy of Pediatrics, Committee on Nutrition 2004, Steen and Berning 1992).

TABLE 11.1
Common Predictive Equations in Obese Youth

Gender	Age	Predictive Equation for REE (kcal/day)	References
Male	3–10	19.6(wt) + 1.033(ht) + 414.9	Schofield (1985)
Female	3–10	16.8(wt) + 1.618(ht) + 371.3	
Male	10–18	16.25(wt) + 1.373(ht) + 515.5	
Female	10–18	8.37(wt) + 4.65(ht) + 200	
Male	3–10	22.7(wt) + 495	World Health Organization (1985)
Female	3–10	22.5(wt) + 499	
Male	10–18	17.5(wt) + 651	
Female	10–18	12.2(wt) + 74	
Male	All	420 − 35.5(age) + 418.9(ht in meters) + 16.7(wt)	Institute for Medicine of the National Academies, Food and Nutrition Board (2005)
Female	All	516 − 26.8(age) + 347(ht in meters) + 12.4(wt)	
Male	All	50.9(wt) + 25.3(ht) − 50.3(age) + 26.9	Molnar (1995)
Female	All	51.2(wt) + 24.5(ht) − 207.5(age) + 1629.8	
Male	All	54.96(wt) + 1816.23(ht) + 892.68(sex[a])	Lazzer (2006)
Female	All	− 115.93(age) + 1484.5	
Male	All	66.47 + 13.75(wt) + 5(ht) − 6.8(age)	Harris and Benedict (1918)
Female	All	665 + 9.6(wt) + 1.8(ht) − 4.7(age)	
Male	All	10(wt) + 6.3(ht) − 5 × age − 5	Mifflin (1990)
Female	All	10(wt) + 6.3(ht) − 5 × age − 161	
		Predictive Equations for TEE	
Male	All	114 − (50.9 × age) + PA × (19.5 × wt + 1161 × ht in meters)	Institute for Medicine of the National Academies, Food and Nutrition Board (2005)
Female	All	389 − (41.2 × age) + PA × (15 × wt + 701.6 × ht in meters)	
Male	3–8	88.5 − 61.9(age) + PA × (26.7 × wt + 903 × ht in meters) + 20 kcal	Institute for Medicine of the National Academies, Food and Nutrition Board (2005)
Female	3–8	135.3 − 30.8(age) + PA × (10 × wt + 934 × ht in meters) + 20 kcal	
Male	9–18	88.5 − 61.9(age) + PA × (26.7 × wt + 903 × ht in meters) + 25 kcal	
Female	9–18	135.3 − 30.8(age) + PA × (10 × wt + 934 × ht in meters) + 25 kcal	

Note: wt = kg, ht = cm, age = years.
[a] Sex: males = 1, females = 0.

How do we modify this for young athletes attempting to lose weight? There is no single dietary approach that will provide greater weight loss in adolescents (Armeno et al. 2011, Gow et al. 2014). However, research shows that long-term, low-fat diets consistently reduce blood lipids, glucose, and blood pressure, as well as lead to long-term weight loss (Gow et al. 2014). Furthermore, studies have found that a low glycemic index diet produces a significant weight loss in adolescents (Diaz et al. 2010, Ebbeling et al. 2003, Kirk et al. 2012, Spieth et al. 2000) and the two studies that included a follow up reported a sustained weight loss (Ebbeling et al. 2003, Kirk et al. 2012).

Ultimately, slow and sustained weight loss in adolescent athletes can be achieved with a modest restriction in calories (while still providing sufficient energy for normal growth and development) and a macronutrient intake balanced to resemble the guidelines provided above. Specific energy requirements and macronutrient levels should be determined on an individual level, with the guidance of a registered dietitian (RD).

11.3 DIETS FOR WEIGHT LOSS IN YOUTH

As children enter adolescence, significant changes in height, weight, and body fat can trigger the use of dieting or other inappropriate methods for weight loss, which have been shown to compromise nutritional status (Guest et al. 2010), influence feelings of depression and low self-esteem (Neumark-Sztainer and Hannan 2000), lead to the development of eating disorders (Patton et al. 1999), and promote weight gain (Lowe et al. 2013). One nationwide survey discovered that 11.8% of high school students attempted fasting for at least 24 hours, 4.3% had tried laxatives or vomiting, and 5.9% had taken diet pills, powders, or liquids intended for weight loss (Centers for Disease Control and Prevention 2013). No child or adolescent should attempt any such approach to weight loss without first consulting a medical professional. Table 11.2 lists the negative health and performance consequences that can occur with such weight-loss strategies (Beals 2004, Sundgot-Borgen et al. 2013).

TABLE 11.2
Health and Performance Consequences of Various Extreme Weight Control Behaviors

Weight Control and Behavior	Physiological Effects and Health Consequences	Effect on Performance
Fasting or starvation	Energy and nutrient deficiency, glycogen depletion, loss of lean body mass, a decrease in metabolic rate, and reduced bone mineral density.	Poor exercise performance due to general weakness, reduced ability to cope with pressure, decreased muscle force, and increased susceptibility for disease and injuries.
Diet pills	Typically function by suppressing appetite and may cause a slight increase in metabolic rate. May induce rapid heart rate, anxiety, nervousness, inability to sleep, and dehydration. Any weight loss is quickly regained once use is discontinued.	Indirectly results in poor performance and may be classified as doping.
Laxatives or enemas	Weight loss is primarily water and any weight loss is regained once use is discontinued. Dehydration, electrolyte imbalances, constipation, cathartic colon, and steatorrhea (excessive fat in the feces) are common.	May affect concentration and hydration status. May be addictive and athlete can develop resistance, thus requiring larger and larger doses to produce the same effect.
Diuretics	Weight loss is primarily water and any weight loss is quickly regained once use is discontinued. Dehydration and electrolyte imbalances are not uncommon.	Poor performance and classified as doping.
Self-induced vomiting	Large body water losses can lead to dehydration and electrolyte imbalances. Gastrointestinal problems, including oesophagitis, oesophageal perforation, and oesophageal ulcers, may occur.	May lead to electrolyte imbalance. Largely ineffective in promoting weight (body fat) loss.
Saunas	Dehydration and electrolyte imbalances can occur in extreme cases.	Weight loss is primarily water and any weight loss is quickly regained once fluids are replaced.
Excessive exercise	If combined with low energy availability, it will increase risk of staleness, chronic fatigue, illness, overuse, injury, and menstrual dysfunction.	Experience the effect of lack of recovery.

Source: Adapted from Beals, K.A., *Disordered Eating among Athletes: A Comprehensive Guide for Health Professionals*, Human Kinetics, Champaign, IL. et al. 2004; *Br J Sports Med*, 47(16), 1012–22, 2013, doi: 10.1136/bjsports-2013-092966.

TABLE 11.3
Healthy Eating Tips to Encourage Weight Loss in Adolescent Athletes

- Eat a balance breakfast, including protein, fiber, and fruit.
- Plan ahead and bring snacks to school and for after-school activities. Each snack should contain protein and carbohydrate (whole wheat, fruit).
- Prepare meals at home and limit calories consumed eating out.
- Include adolescents in grocery shopping and meal preparation.
- Limit simple carbohydrates (sugars, sweets).
- Incorporate different colors, textures, and temperatures in meals and snacks.
- If you do not consume 1.5–2.5 cups of fruits and vegetables per day, a multivitamin supplement may be necessary.
- Keep food positive! Focus on maximizing foods for fueling performance, rather than focusing on removal of unhealthy foods.
- Drink plenty of fluids. Individual fluid needs can be calculated, especially for endurance and weight category athletes.
- Bring your lunch to school. Include protein, fiber, fruit, and vegetables.

Source: Adapted from Information adapted from Gravelle, B. L. and M. Broyles. *Am J Ther* 22 (2):159–66, 2015. doi: 10.1097/MJT.0b013e318293b0c4.

In order to decrease the prevalence of unhealthy weight-loss practices in young athletes, it is important to consider the major external influences on eating behaviors and food choices. Neumark-Sztainer and colleagues (Neumark-Sztainer et al. 1999) analyzed adolescent focus groups, and found taste and appeal, followed by time and convenience as the largest influences on food choices. Furthermore, adolescents responded they would be more likely to choose healthier foods if they appeared and tasted better, were convenient, and "cool" (Neumark-Sztainer et al. 1999). Simple dietary strategies for parents and adolescents to reduce caloric intake, while balancing nutrient intake are highlighted in Table 11.3.

11.4 OTHER WEIGHT-LOSS REMEDIES

11.4.1 Medications

Orlistat (Xenical) is currently the only prescription weight-loss medication approved by the Federal Drug Administration (FDA) for use in obese adolescents 12 years and older (Food and Drug Administration 2003, Gravelle and Broyles 2015). By reducing fat absorption, Orlistat has been shown to significantly decrease body mass index (BMI) at 1 year (Chanoine et al. 2005). While evidence-based guidelines regarding the specific use of Orlistat in adolescents are currently undetermined, factors to consider when determining the use of medication include the presence of comorbidities and continued weight gain (Rogovik and Goldman 2011). Reported side effects include gastrointestinal distress, fatty or oily stools, fatty leakage, and fecal urgency (Chanoine et al. 2005). However, these side effects were more common when dietary fat consumption was greater than 30% of calories (Chanoine et al. 2005). Therefore, drug therapy should only be used in conjunction with medical and nutritional treatment.

11.4.2 Bariatric Surgery

Surgical treatment for adolescent obesity has become more prevalent and has shown to consistently produce long-term clinically significant weight loss in those who did not see results with medically supervised treatment (diet and exercise) for at least 6 months (Michalsky et al. 2012). The BMI threshold requirements for bariatric surgery in adolescents have recently changed and are now supported by the American Society for Metabolic and Bariatric Surgery (Michalsky et al. 2012): adolescents with a BMI > 35 with serious comorbidities or a BMI ≥ 40 with less severe comorbidities (Pratt et al. 2009). Additional requirements for surgery include having reached skeletal and sexual maturity, demonstration of ability to adhere to nutritional guidelines postoperation, and evaluation of family support and motivation (Inge et al. 2004). Nutritional management before and after bariatric surgery requires a multidisciplinary team approach in order to sustain weight loss and reduce the risk of complications.

11.5 GUIDELINES FOR HEALTHY WEIGHT CONTROL/LOSS PRACTICES

Youth athletes attempting to lose weight or "make weight" for performance should do so in the off-season, to ensure that caloric restriction and exercise energy expenditure are adequate to support optimal performance and growth and development. Guidelines have been established for those athletes attempting to lose weight, as inappropriate methods for weight control are popular in this age group (as discussed earlier) (American Academy of Pediatrics, Committee on Adolescence 2003, American Academy of Pediatrics, Committee on Sports Medicine and Fitness 2005):

- Weight loss should not exceed 1.5% of an athlete's body weight per week (American Academy of Pediatrics, Committee on Adolescence 2003).
- Fluid or food restriction should not be attempted.
- Male high school athletes must have a minimum body fat of 7% (American Academy of Pediatrics, Committee on Sports Medicine and Fitness 2005).
- Female athletes must consume enough calories and nutrients to support menstruation (American Academy of Pediatrics, Committee on Sports Medicine and Fitness 2005).
- Physicians must be educated on appropriate weight-loss methods, as well as take part in the education of athletes, families, coaches, trainers, and school administrators (American Academy of Pediatrics, Committee on Sports Medicine and Fitness 2005).
- In weight classification sports, athletes' body composition should be assessed 1–2 times per year.
- A weight-loss plan for weight-control practice should never be used before the 9th grade (American Academy of Pediatrics, Committee on Sports Medicine and Fitness 2005).

Weight-loss goals should be determined on an individual basis, but should never exceed 2 pounds per week (Spear et al. 2007). Body composition analysis (see Chapter 2) will aid in tracking fat and fat-free mass changes with changes in body weight. Table 11.4 lists weight recommendations based on age and BMI percentile (Spear et al. 2007).

11.6 PSYCHOLOGICAL CONSIDERATIONS

In addition to the plethora of health problems associated with obesity, psychosocial struggles, including low self-esteem and depression, are also higher in adolescents with obesity (Atlantis and Ball 2008, Dierk et al. 2006, Wardle and Cooke 2005). Obese adolescents often exhibit more risk factors for traditional bullying (Wardle and Cooke 2005) and cyber-victimization (Kautiainen et al. 2005, Storch and Ledley 2005). This was found to be a significant result in a recent study, which also determined that adolescents with obesity had lower quality of life and motivation for physical activity, as well as higher levels of emotional coping or avoidance of healthy lifestyles compared to nonvictimized controls (DeSmet et al. 2014).

The behavioral and environmental influences on dietary habits, including emotional and external eating, and dietary restraint (Braet et al. 2008, van Strien et al. 2009), must be included in the assessment and management of weight loss for a young athlete. Behavioral therapy (self-monitoring of eating behaviors and influences on behavior) and cognitive therapy (connecting

TABLE 11.4
Weight Recommendations According to Age and BMI Percentile

Age	Target
2–5 years	
BMI of 85–94th percentile	Weight maintenance until BMI of <85th percentile or slowing of weight gain, as indicated by downward deflection in BMI curve.
BMI of ≥95th percentile	Weight maintenance until BMI of <85th percentile; however, if weight loss occurs with healthy, adequate-energy diet, then it should not exceed 1 lb/mo. If greater loss is noted, then patient should be monitored for causes of excessive weight loss.
BMI of >21 kg/m^2 (rare, very high)	Gradual weight loss, not to exceed 1 lb/mo. If greater loss occurs, then patient should be monitored for causes of excessive weight loss.
6–11 years	
BMI of 85–94th percentile	Weight maintenance until BMI of <85th percentile or slowing of weight gain, as indicated by downward deflection in BMI curve.
BMI of 95–98th percentile	Weight maintenance until BMI of <85th percentile or gradual weight loss of ~1 lb/mo. If greater loss is noted, then patient should be monitored for causes of excessive weight loss.
BMI of ≥99th percentile	Weight loss not to exceed average of 2 lb/week. If greater loss is noted, then patient should be monitored for causes of excessive weight loss.
12–18 years	
BMI of 85–94th percentile	Weight maintenance until BMI of <85th percentile or slowing of weight gain, as indicated by downward deflection in BMI curve.
BMI of 95–98th percentile	Weight loss until BMI of <85th percentile, no more than average of 2 lb/week. If greater loss is noted, then patient should be monitored for causes of excessive weight loss.
BMI of ≥99th percentile	Weight loss not to exceed average of 2 lb/week. If greater loss is noted, then patient should be monitored for causes of excessive weight loss.

emotions and feelings with behavior for development and maintenance of healthy weight loss) are two interrelated approaches that have been shown to be effective for weight loss (De Miguel-Etayo et al. 2013). These behavioral-based interventions can be completed as group or individual counseling sessions and typically include family members when working with young children (Whitlock et al. 2010). Parental self-efficacy and motivation to promote healthy eating behaviors are two critical factors to include in obesity treatment (Iniguez et al. 2014). Additionally, peer support for healthy eating behaviors, in particular, from peers concurrently attempting to lose weight, has been shown to be effective (Thoits 1995), as peer relationships are a major influence on behaviors at this age.

11.7 RESOURCES FOR PARENTS AND HEALTH EDUCATORS

- My Plate Kid's Place (http://www.choosemyplate.gov/kids/)
- Kids Health (http://www.kidshealth.org)
- Weight Management for Youth (http://www.nutrition.gov/youthweight)
- Healthy Youth Childhood Obesity (http://www.cdc.gov/healthyyouth/obesity)
- We Can! (http://www.nhlbi.nih.gov/health/public/heart/obesity/wecan)
- SmallStep Kids (http://familyfirst.com/smallsteps-gov.html)
- Kidnetic (http://www.kidnetic.com)

REFERENCES

Academy of Nutrition and Dietetics. 2007. Evidence-Based Nutrition Practice Guidelines. Pediatric Weight Management.
American Academy of Pediatrics, Committee on Adolescence. 2003. Identifying and treating eating disorders. *Pediatrics* 111 (1):204–11.
American Academy of Pediatrics, Committee on Nutrition. 2004. Sports nutrition. In *Pediatric Nutrition Handbook*, edited by R.E. Kleinman, 155–66. Elk Grove Village, IL: American Academy of Pediatrics.
American Academy of Pediatrics, Committee on Sports Medicine and Fitness. 2005. Promotion of healthy weight-control practices in young athletes. *Pediatrics* 116 (6):1557–64. doi: 10.1542/peds.2005-2314.
Armeno, M. L., A. G. Krochik, and C. S. Mazza. 2011. Evaluation of two dietary treatments in obese hyperinsulinemic adolescents. *J Pediatr Endocrinol Metab* 24 (9–10):715–22.
Atlantis, E. and K. Ball. 2008. Association between weight perception and psychological distress. *Int J Obes (Lond)* 32 (4):715–21. doi: 10.1038/sj.ijo.0803762.
Beals, K. A. 2004. *Disordered Eating among Athletes: A Comprehensive Guide for Health Professionals*. Champaign, IL: Human Kinetics.
Braet, C., L. Claus, L. Goossens, E. Moens, L. Van Vlierberghe, and B. Soetens. 2008. Differences in eating style between overweight and normal-weight youngsters. *J Health Psychol* 13 (6):733–43. doi: 10.1177/1359105308093850.
Centers for Disease Control and Prevention. 2013. Youth risk behavior Surveillance—United States. *Morb Mortal Wkly Rep* 63 (SS-4):1–131.
Chanoine, J. P., S. Hampl, C. Jensen, M. Boldrin, and J. Hauptman. 2005. Effect of orlistat on weight and body composition in obese adolescents: A randomized controlled trial. *JAMA* 293 (23):2873–83. doi: 10.1001/jama.293.23.2873.
De Miguel-Etayo, P., G. Bueno, J. M. Garagorri, and L. A. Moreno. 2013. Interventions for treating obesity in children. *World Rev Nutr Diet* 108:98–106. doi: 10.1159/000351493.
DeSmet, A., B. Deforche, A. Hublet, A. Tanghe, E. Stremersch, and I. De Bourdeaudhuij. 2014. Traditional and cyberbullying victimization as correlates of psychosocial distress and barriers to a healthy lifestyle among severely obese adolescents—A matched case-control study on prevalence and results from a cross-sectional study. *BMC Public Health* 14:224. doi: 10.1186/1471-2458-14-224.
Diaz, R. G., J. Esparza-Romero, S. Y. Moya-Camarena, A. E. Robles-Sardin, and M. E. Valencia. 2010. Lifestyle intervention in primary care settings improves obesity parameters among Mexican youth. *J Am Diet Assoc* 110 (2):285–90. doi: 10.1016/j.jada.2009.10.042.
Dierk, J. M., M. Conradt, E. Rauh, P. Schlumberger, J. Hebebrand, and W. Rief. 2006. What determines well-being in obesity? Associations with BMI, social skills, and social support. *J Psychosom Res* 60 (3):219–27. doi: 10.1016/j.jpsychores.2005.06.083.
Ebbeling, C. B., M. M. Leidig, K. B. Sinclair, J. P. Hangen, and D. S. Ludwig. 2003. A reduced-glycemic load diet in the treatment of adolescent obesity. *Arch Pediatr Adolesc Med* 157 (8):773–9. doi: 10.1001/archpedi.157.8.773.
Ferraro, K. F., R. J. Thorpe, Jr., and J. A. Wilkinson. 2003. The life course of severe obesity: Does childhood overweight matter? *J Gerontol B Psychol Sci Soc Sci* 58 (2):S110–9.
Food and Drug Administration. 2003. (HFD-510). Clinical review for NDA 20–766/S018. http://www.fda.gov/downloads/Drugs/DevelopmentApprovalProcess/DevelopmentResources/UCM163348.pdf. Accessed July 12, 2014.
Gow, M. L., M. Ho, T. L. Burrows, L. A. Baur, L. Stewart, M. J. Hutchesson, C. T. Cowell, C. E. Collins, and S. P. Garnett. 2014. Impact of dietary macronutrient distribution on BMI and cardiometabolic outcomes in overweight and obese children and adolescents: A systematic review. *Nutr Rev* 72 (7):453–70. doi: 10.1111/nure.12111.
Gravelle, B. L. and M. Broyles. 2015. Interventions of weight reduction and prevention in children and adolescents: Update. *Am J Ther* 22 (2):159–66. doi: 10.1097/MJT.0b013e318293b0c4.
Guest, J., A. Bilgin, R. Pearce, S. Baines, C. Zeuschner, C. L. Rossignol-Grant, M. J. Morris, and R. Grant. 2010. Evidence for under-nutrition in adolescent females using routine dieting practices. *Asia Pac J Clin Nutr* 19 (4):526–33.
Harris, J. A. and F. G. Benedict. 1918. A biometric study of human basal metabolism. *Proc Natl Acad Sci USA* 4 (12):370–3.

Henes, S. T., D. M. Cummings, R. C. Hickner, J. A. Houmard, K. M. Kolasa, S. Lazorick, and D. N. Collier. 2013. Comparison of predictive equations and measured resting energy expenditure among obese youth attending a pediatric healthy weight clinic: One size does not fit all. *Nutr Clin Pract* 28 (5):617–24. doi: 10.1177/0884533613497237.

Inge, T. H., N. F. Krebs, V. F. Garcia, J. A. Skelton, K. S. Guice, R. S. Strauss, C. T. Albanese et al. 2004. Bariatric surgery for severely overweight adolescents: Concerns and recommendations. *Pediatrics* 114 (1):217–23.

Iniguez, I. R., J. Yap, and D. R. Mager. 2014. Parental perceptions regarding lifestyle interventions for obese children and adolescents with nonalcoholic fatty liver disease. *Paediatr Child Health* 19 (5):e24–9.

IOM for Obese Children. 2005. Institute for Medicine of the National Academies, Food and Nutrition Board. Dietary Reference Intakes for Energy, Carbohydrate, Fiber, Fat, Fatty Acids, Cholesterol, Protein, and Amino Acids. Washington DC: The National Academies Press. http://www.nap.edu/openbook.php?record_id=10490&page=107. Accessed May 3, 2013.

Kautiainen, S., L. Koivusilta, T. Lintonen, S. M. Virtanen, and A. Rimpela. 2005. Use of information and communication technology and prevalence of overweight and obesity among adolescents. *Int J Obes (Lond)* 29 (8):925–33. doi: 10.1038/sj.ijo.0802994.

Kirk, S., B. Brehm, B. E. Saelens, J. G. Woo, E. Kissel, D. D'Alessio, C. Bolling, and S. R. Daniels. 2012. Role of carbohydrate modification in weight management among obese children: A randomized clinical trial. *J Pediatr* 161 (2):320–7e1. doi: 10.1016/j.jpeds.2012.01.041.

Lazzer, S., F. Agosti, A. De Col, and A. Sartorio. 2006. Development of cross-validation of prediction equations for estimating energy expenditure in severely obese Caucasian children and adolescents. *Br J Nutr* 96 (5):973–9.

Lin, B. H., J. Guthrie, and E. Frazeo. 2001. American children's diets not making the grade. *Food Rev* 24 (2):8–17.

Lowe, M. R., S. D. Doshi, S. N. Katterman, and E. H. Feig. 2013. Dieting and restrained eating as prospective predictors of weight gain. *Front Psychol* 4:577. doi: 10.3389/fpsyg.2013.00577.

Michalsky, M., K. Reichard, T. Inge, J. Pratt, C. Lenders, and American Society for Metabolic and Bariatric Surgery. 2012. ASMBS pediatric committee best practice guidelines. *Surg Obes Relat Dis* 8 (1):1–7. doi: 10.1016/j.soard.2011.09.009.

Mifflin, M. D., S. T. St. Jeor, L. A. Hill, B. J. Scott, S. A. Daugherty, and Y. O. Koh. 1990. A new predictive equation for resting energy expenditure in healthy individuals. *Am J Clin Nutr* 51:241–7.

Molnar, D., S. Jeges, E. Erhardt, and Y. Schutz. 1995. Measured and predicted resting metabolic rate in obese and nonobese adolescents. *J Pediatr* 127 (4):571–7.

National Academies Press. 2006. *Dietary Reference Intakes: The Essential Guide to Nutrient Requirements.* Washington, DC.

Neumark-Sztainer, D., and P. J. Hannan. 2000. Weight-related behaviors among adolescent girls and boys: Results from a national survey. *Arch Pediatr Adolesc Med* 154 (6):569–77.

Neumark-Sztainer, D. M. Story, C. Perry, and M. A. Casey. 1999. Factors influencing food choices of adolescents: Findings from focus-group discussions with adolescents. *J Am Diet Assoc* 99 (8):929–37. doi: 10.1016/S0002-8223(99)00222-9.

Ogden, C. L., M. D. Carroll, B. K. Kit, and K. M. Flegal. 2012. Prevalence of obesity and trends in body mass index among US children and adolescents, 1999–2010. *JAMA* 307 (5):483–90. doi: 10.1001/jama.2012.40.

Ogden, C. L., M. D. Carroll, B. K. Kit, and K. M. Flegal. 2014. Prevalence of childhood and adult obesity in the United States, 2011–2012. *JAMA* 311 (8):806–14. doi: 10.1001/jama.2014.732.

Patton, G. C., R. Selzer, C. Coffey, J. B. Carlin, and R. Wolfe. 1999. Onset of adolescent eating disorders: Population based cohort study over 3 years. *BMJ* 318 (7186):765–8.

Pratt, J. S., C. M. Lenders, E. A. Dionne, A. G. Hoppin, G. L. Hsu, T. H. Inge, D. F. Lawlor, M. F. Marino, A. F. Meyers, J. L. Rosenblum, and V. M. Sanchez. 2009. Best practice updates for pediatric/adolescent weight loss surgery. *Obesity (Silver Spring)* 17 (5):901–10. doi: 10.1038/oby.2008.577.

Rogovik, A. L. and R. D. Goldman. 2011. Pharmacologic treatment of pediatric obesity. *Can Fam Physician* 57 (2):195–7.

Schofield, W. N. 1985. Predicting basal metabolic rate, new standards and review of previous work. *Hum Nutr Clin Nutr* 39 (Suppl 1):5–41.

Spear, B. A., S. E. Barlow, C. Ervin, D. S. Ludwig, B. E. Saelens, K. E. Schetzina, and E. M. Taveras. 2007. Recommendations for treatment of child and adolescent overweight and obesity. *Pediatrics* 120 (Suppl 4):S254–88. doi: 10.1542/peds.2007-2329F.

Spieth, L. E., J. D. Harnish, C. M. Lenders, L. B. Raezer, M. A. Pereira, S. J. Hangen, and D. S. Ludwig. 2000. A low-glycemic index diet in the treatment of pediatric obesity. *Arch Pediatr Adolesc Med* 154 (9):947–51.

Steen, S. N. and J.R. Berning. 1992. Sound nutrition for the athlete. In *Eating, Body Weight, and Performance in Athletes: Disorders of Modern Society*, edited by K. D. Brownell, J. Rodin and H. J. Wilmore, 293–314. Philadelphia, PA: Lea & Febiger.

Storch, E. A. and D. R. Ledley. 2005. Peer victimization and psychosocial adjustment in children: Current knowledge and future directions. *Clin Pediatr (Phila)* 44 (1):29–38.

Sundgot-Borgen, J., N. L. Meyer, T. G. Lohman, T. R. Ackland, R. J. Maughan, A. D. Stewart, and W. Muller. 2013. How to minimise the health risks to athletes who compete in weight-sensitive sports review and position statement on behalf of the Ad Hoc Research Working Group on Body Composition, Health and Performance, under the auspices of the IOC Medical Commission. *Br J Sports Med* 47 (16):1012–22. doi: 10.1136/bjsports-2013-092966.

Suskind, R. M., U. Blecker, J. N. Udall, Jr., T. K. von Almen, H. D. Schumacher, L. Carlisle, and M. S. Sothern. 2000. Recent advances in the treatment of childhood obesity. *Pediatr Diabetes* 1 (1):23–33. doi: 10.1034/j.1399-5448.2000.010105.x.

Thoits, P. A. 1995. Stress, coping, and social support processes: Where are we? What next? *J Health Soc Behav* Spec No:53–79.

Trumbo, P., S. Schlicker, A. A. Yates, M. Poos, and Food, and The National Academies Nutrition Board of the Institute of Medicine. 2002. Dietary reference intakes for energy, carbohydrate, fiber, fat, fatty acids, cholesterol, protein and amino acids. *J Am Diet Assoc* 102 (11):1621–30.

Tippet, K. S. and Y. S. Cypel, eds. 1997. Design and Operation: The Continuing Survey of Food Intakes by Individuals and the Diet and Health Knowledge Survey, 1994–96. U.S. Department of Agriculture, Agricultural Research Service, Nationwide Food Surveys Report No. 96-1, 197pp.

van Strien, T., C. P. Herman, and M. W. Verheijden. 2009. Eating style, overeating, and overweight in a representative Dutch sample. Does external eating play a role? *Appetite* 52 (2):380–7. doi: 10.1016/j.appet.2008.11.010.

Wardle, J. and L. Cooke. 2005. The impact of obesity on psychological well-being. *Best Pract Res Clin Endocrinol Metab* 19 (3):421–40. doi: 10.1016/j.beem.2005.04.006.

Whitlock, E. P., E. A. O'Connor, S. B. Williams, T. L. Beil, and K. W. Lutz. 2010. Effectiveness of weight management interventions in children: A targeted systematic review for the USPSTF. *Pediatrics* 125 (2):e396–418. doi: 10.1542/peds.2009-1955.

World Health Organization. 1985. Energy and protein requirements. Report of a joint FAO/WHO/UNU Expert Consultation. *World Health Organ Tech Rep Ser* 724:1–206.

12 Nutrition and the Weight-Conscious Athlete

Roger A. Vaughan and Christine M. Mermier

CONTENTS

Abstract	203
12.1 Introduction	204
12.2 Body Composition and Weight Management	204
12.3 Weight Management	204
12.3.1 Common Unsafe Weight Management Practices	204
12.3.2 Benefits of Exercise	205
12.3.3 Proper Exercise Prescription	205
12.3.4 Dehydration and Weight Management	206
12.3.5 Effects of Dehydration on Performance	206
12.3.6 Excessive Caloric Restriction	206
12.3.7 High Protein Intake	207
12.3.7.1 Benefits of High Protein Intake	207
12.3.7.2 Safety of High-Protein Diets	207
12.4 Disordered Eating and Weight Management	209
12.5 Assessing Successful Weight Change	209
12.6 General Nutritional Recommendations for Athletes	210
12.6.1 Dietary Guidelines	210
12.6.2 Predicted and Measured Energy Needs	210
12.6.3 Difficult Nutrients for Athletes	211
12.7 Maintaining Body Composition and Weight with Diet and Exercise	211
12.8 General Recommendations for the Weight-Conscious Athlete	211
12.8.1 Nutrition for Weight Modification	212
12.8.1.1 Principles of Weight Gain	213
12.8.1.2 Principles of Weight Loss	213
12.8.2 Exercise and Nutritional Timing	213
12.8.3 Nutrition during Exercise	214
12.8.4 Nutrition for Postexercise Recovery	214
References	214

ABSTRACT

Body weight and composition are important determinants of exercise and sport performance in a highly event-specific fashion, leading athletes to pursue extreme and occasionally dangerous techniques to alter anthropometrics to obtain an athletic advantage. These practices are most common for athletes competing in events with either a weight class or figure-sensitive component. Numerous dietary strategies are utilized for manipulation of body weight and composition such as dehydration, excessive energy restriction, and high protein diets in addition to other methods such as increased aerobic exercise or the use of saunas, diuretics, or excessive clothing. In addition to weight loss, some athletes seek weight gain for improved muscular strength and/or size. This chapter summarizes

TABLE 12.1
Summary of Various Sports and Athletic Events That Use Weight Classes or Weight Consciousness

Weight Class Athletics	Weight-Conscious Athletics
Wrestling	Gymnastics
Boxing	Figure skating
Mixed martial arts	Football
Body building	Basketball
Weightlifting	Soccer
Judo/tae kwon do	Swimming/diving
Kickboxing	Dance

many of the considerations as well as safety and efficacy of dietary strategies for weight maintenance and management for the weight conscious athlete.

12.1 INTRODUCTION

Body composition and body mass are important factors that directly influence athletic performance in a number of sporting events and physical competitions. Not surprisingly, numerous athletic competitions result in altered body composition and weight, usually in a seasonal or cyclic fashion. Despite the common practice of body mass manipulation among athletes, there are a few regulations governing the methods used to cause weight and fat loss. In general, athletes remain interested in reducing body mass to achieve eligibility within lower weight classes, reduce body fat for cosmetic purposes, or as a by-product of increased training intensity. Table 12.1 summarizes activities for which athletes commonly use weight reduction techniques, although this is not an exhaustive list.

12.2 BODY COMPOSITION AND WEIGHT MANAGEMENT

Body composition is an important indicator of health status and also an important variable for athletes and fitness enthusiasts. Body composition is typically categorized by either fat mass (FM) or lean body mass (LBM), which represents the mass of water, muscle, internal organs, ligaments, tendons, and bone. Of the FM stored within the body, roughly 3% is found within the bone marrow, heart, lungs, liver, spleen, kidneys, intestines, muscles, and other lipid-rich tissues and is therefore considered essential (Turocy et al. 2011). Body composition and distribution differs between genders because of sex-specific adipose storage (such as the breasts and hips of women). In addition to essential fat, fat is layered subcutaneously, which offers storage for future substrate liberation (Turocy et al. 2011). Minimal fat requirements (~5% for men and ~12% for women) are necessary for normal function and development (Turocy et al. 2011). While there are no maximum body fat requirements, healthy ranges are considered 10%–22%, and 20%–32% in physically mature adolescent males and females, respectively (Turocy et al. 2011). Excess body fat is associated with health consequences such as insulin resistance, cardiovascular disease, and premature death, as well as possible decrements in sports performance (Foster and Burton 1985). Owing to its importance with healthy weight control, manipulation, and management, the subject of body composition and energy expenditure has been dealt with in Chapter 2.

12.3 WEIGHT MANAGEMENT

12.3.1 COMMON UNSAFE WEIGHT MANAGEMENT PRACTICES

A multitude of methods are heavily advertised for athletes and active people to lose body fat and maximize performance, although many of these methods are underresearched for efficacy and safety, especially in adolescent and teenage populations. Many methods to enhance performance require manipulation of diet, weight, or body composition to achieve an ideal and sport-specific physique. Unfortunately, many of these methods of physique manipulation may be unsafe and lead to dehydration, self-starvation, and disordered eating potentially contributing to nutritional deficiency. The most common unsafe physique manipulations are combinations of dehydration, excessive exercise, and food restriction predominantly to reduce body fat.

12.3.2 Benefits of Exercise

The strong link between exercise and healthy blood pressure, blood triglycerides, HDL cholesterol, fasting blood glucose, abdominal adiposity, waist circumference, and body weight have been well established (Church 2011). Metabolic syndrome, characterized as a combination of poor clinical values in any three of the aforementioned health indicators, is tightly correlated with the development of heart disease. Epidemiological reports have demonstrated the powerful ability of regular exercise to reduce the development of insulin resistance (Church 2011; Sawada et al. 2003; Shaper et al. 1997; Weinstein et al. 2004). In those with type 2 diabetes, regular exercise and heightened physical fitness reduces risk of cardiovascular disease development in a nearly linear fashion leading to reduced mortality (Church 2011; Church et al. 2005, 2009; Wei et al. 2000). The diabetes prevention program (DPP) demonstrated that proper nutrition, exercise, and the combination thereof, can substantially reduce incidence of insulin resistance (Knowler et al. 2002; Tuomilehto et al. 2001). The DPP study included more than 3000 at-risk men and women who were assigned to a control group, metformin therapy group, or lifestyle modification group (lifestyle modification was designed to stimulate at least 7% weight loss through diet and exercise). After nearly 3 years of the lifestyle modification intervention, the incidence of type 2 diabetes was a fraction of both the control and the metformin therapy groups. A thorough review of the benefits of exercise (including resistance training) is discussed elsewhere (Church 2011).

12.3.3 Proper Exercise Prescription

Exercise represents a fun and meaningful way to stimulate the mind and body while reducing risk of disease. It is important to recognize that all people, especially competitive athletes, have a unique and ever-changing relationship with physical activity and exercise. Even so, there are some general recommendations of a typical exercise regimen or prescription. For the general population, the American College of Sports Medicine (ACSM) recommends at least 30 min of planned exercise at least 5 days per week to maintain general health. While 150 min per week represents a minimum recommendation to promote health, the ACSM also recognizes and promotes the dose-dependency of the benefits of exercise. In other words, if moderate amounts of exercise (150 min per week) promote several health benefits, high amounts of exercise (300 min per week) equates to more health benefits. Children and adolescents require 1 h or more of moderate-intensity to vigorous physical activity every day; however, approximately only 1 in 4 ages 12–15 meet these recommendations (Fakhouri et al. 2014). Additionally, muscle-strengthening activities should be performed at least 3 days a week as part of the 60-min activity.

Another important consideration is the intensity of exercise. Perhaps not surprisingly, the higher the intensity of exercise, the less it is required to reap health benefits. More recently, an increasing trend of high-intensity interval training (HITT) has become a popular exercise method, during which short and frequent bursts of maximal or near-maximal efforts are performed with limited rest between bouts. While HITT represents a viable training technique capable of stimulating even the most complex of muscular adaptations, it is important to recognize that maximal or near-maximal bouts can only be sustained for short durations. The limitation of HITT is that shorter durations of even the highest intensity exercise can only contribute subtly to energy expenditure. Therefore, athletes seeking weight loss will most likely also need to engage in regular cardiovascular exercises at lower intensities (50%–70% VO_{2max}). An adequate exercise prescription should promote cardiovascular and musculoskeletal fitness in addition to flexibility and a healthy body composition. It is important that athletes address these four components of fitness in a sport-specific way, while simultaneously perfecting techniques required for athletic competition.

12.3.4 Dehydration and Weight Management

Voluntary dehydration has been used since the late 1930s as a method of rapid weight loss to achieve a reduced body weight for competition. Athletes can actively withhold fluid intake, try to enhance sweat rate through exercise/or clothing manipulation, and use pharmacological methods. Active dehydration occurs when athletes increase exercise intensity to heighten heat production by skeletal muscle and sweat rate (Nadel 1985, 1984, 1983; Nadel et al. 1971). Fluid and heat loss through sweat evaporation during exercise are protective cooling methods, but are also effective at causing dehydration when the athlete abstains from fluid consumption. Additionally, sweat rate is often stimulated by saunas and excessive or nonbreathable clothing, reducing evaporative cooling effects of sweating, thereby promoting an elevated core temperature (Nadel 1985, 1984, 1983; Nadel et al. 1971). Dehydration was commonly used by wrestlers and boxers; however, recent data suggest that dehydration is a less common practice, probably as a result of changes in weigh-in procedures (Steen and Brownell 1990; Tipton and Tcheng 1970). In addition to dehydration, food restriction and food- and beverage-induced diuresis are often used in conjunction to promote weight reduction. Furthermore, pharmacological methods for stimulating dehydration are also routinely used. Diuretics, vomiting, and diet pills are common for rapid weight reduction for both weight-class athletic events as well as cosmetic purposes for sports such as bodybuilding.

12.3.5 Effects of Dehydration on Performance

Dehydration between 1% and 2% has been shown to diminish athletic performance in both children and adults, specifically through reduction of VO_{2max} and increased core temperature (Baror et al. 1992; Turocy et al. 2011). Additional dehydration up to 6% leads to more significant suppression of VO_{2max}, muscular strength, and endurance time. Additionally, temperature regulation is severely impaired as dehydration gets progressively worse. Interestingly, creatine phosphate metabolism is unaffected by dehydration, suggesting events exclusively requiring short bursts of high-intensity movements may not suffer huge decrements in performance (Turocy et al. 2011). Together, the effects of dehydration can reduce performance, increase blood pressure, and promote heat-related illness. Pharmacologically induced dehydration can also stimulate muscle cramps, more so than exercise- or sauna-induced dehydration (Tipton and Tcheng 1970; Turocy et al. 2011).

12.3.6 Excessive Caloric Restriction

Severe energy and nutrient restriction is another common method used to reduce or maintain body weight or manipulate body composition. Very low-calorie diets can damage the cardiovascular system, contribute to hypotension, bradycardia, ventricular arrhythmias, and sudden cardiac death (Ahmed et al. 2001; Stevens et al. 2002; Swenne and Larsson 1999). Low-calorie diets also suppress the endocrine system, reducing the effects of several important hormones in development (Douyon and Schteingart 2002; Turocy et al. 2011). Improved energy intake leads to growth catch-up, but may be insufficient and lead to stunted height and underdeveloped bone and muscle mass (Lanes and Soros 2004; Lantzouni et al. 2002). Thyroid function, specifically thyroxine (T4) and triiodothyronine (T3) are suppressed, leading to increased response of thyroid-stimulating hormone (TSH) and ultimately a lower metabolic rate (Douyon and Schteingart 2002; Turocy et al. 2011). The result is an increased adrenal production of free cortisol, without changes in adrenocorticotropic hormone, leading to increased adipose deposition (Douyon and Schteingart 2002; Turocy et al. 2011).

Lastly, sex hormones are suppressed, initiating with the suppression of gonadotropin-releasing hormone (GnRH) from the hypothalamus (Turocy et al. 2011). Subsequent luteinizing hormone (LH) and follicle-stimulating hormone (FSH) from the anterior pituitary cause reductions in circulating testosterone and estrogen, leading to delayed or slowed maturation, menstrual dysfunction, and possibly osteoporosis (Academy of Nutrition and Dietetics (AND) 2009b; Turocy et al. 2011).

Female athletes in weight-conscious sports are at further risk for development of the female athlete triad characterized by disordered eating, irregular menstrual function, and abnormal bone mineralization (Turocy et al. 2011). Amenorrhea, or loss of menstruation, occurs as a result of suppressed sex hormones following suppression of hypothalamic function (Hausenblas and Carron 1999). Additionally, deregulated hormones and suppressed estrogen contribute to increased risk of osteoporosis and higher incidence of stress fractures (Douyon and Schteingart 2002).

12.3.7 High Protein Intake

12.3.7.1 Benefits of High Protein Intake

High protein intake is a common, and often misunderstood nutritional strategy for athletes to enhance muscular size and density, improve body composition, and stimulate athletic performance. Protein is an essential macromolecule, important for a variety of biological functions ranging from hormones to contractile units of skeletal muscle. The major reason most athletes consume a high-protein diet is to increase muscle mass, particularly popular among athletes competing in sports where strength and muscular size are an advantage (Tipton 2011).

Officially, the recommended dietary allowance (RDA) for protein for nonathletes is 0.8 g/kg, which often corresponds with the acceptable macronutrient distribution range (AMDR) of 10%–35% of total energy intake (Berning and Horswill 2014; Phillips et al. 2007; Tipton and Witard 2007). For athletes, protein needs can range from 1.2 to 1.7 g/kg body weight/day (Berning and Horswill 2014; Phillips et al. 2007; Tipton and Witard 2007). Some athletes feel the need to exceed these recommended intakes, occasionally by more than 100%, because protein intake is vital for intramuscular protein synthesis. In fact, despite these well-established recommendations, some athletes commonly consume over 3 g of protein/kg/day (Phillips 2004, 2006). High-protein diets provide a benefit for muscle hypertrophy with concurrent training by providing amino acids to rebuild muscle proteins (Phillips 2004; Wilkinson et al. 2008). Additionally, resistance training leads to damaged muscle proteins and myofibers (Gibala et al. 2000; Stupka et al. 2001), leading to increased protein requirements (Academy of Nutrition and Dietetics (AND) and the American College of Sports Medicine (ACSM) 2009a; Campbell et al. 2007; Lemon 2000; Phillips 2004; Phillips et al. 2007). A study demonstrated that protein ingestion of 20–25 g improves protein synthesis following resistance exercise (Moore et al. 2009). As such, it is not surprising that recovery from intense exercise (especially resistance exercise) represents another situation in which high-protein diets may provide some additional benefits (Howatson and van Someren 2008).

In addition to promoting hypertrophy, weight loss with lean body mass preservation represents another situation when athletes may opt to increase protein intake. Calorie restriction through the reduction of carbohydrate content with a high percentage of total energy coming from protein seems to promote weight and fat loss in overweight and obese individuals (Tipton and Witard 2007). Additionally, lean body mass is more efficiently preserved with high-protein calorie restriction, further improving/maintaining energy expenditure (Layman 2004; Layman et al. 2003; Meckling and Sherfey 2007; Westerterp-Plantenga 2008). Table 12.2 summarizes several levels of protein needs based on various body weights, a topic that is covered in greater detail in Chapter 4.

12.3.7.2 Safety of High-Protein Diets

Chronic high-protein consumption is purported to lead to clinical problems, including declining kidney function and reduced bone mineralization (Lowery and Devia 2009; Metges and Barth 2000; Tipton 2011). Currently, there is no established upper limit on protein intake, particularly for younger athletes, because there is insufficient evidence to causally link high protein intake

TABLE 12.2
Summary of Estimated Protein Needs Based on Varying Body Weights for Specific Athletic Requirements

Athlete Weight		Protein Needs (g/day)		
Pounds	Kilogram	0.8 g/kg	1.2 g/kg	1.7 g/kg
80	36	29	44	62
90	41	33	49	70
100	45	36	55	77
110	50	40	60	85
120	55	44	65	93
130	59	47	71	100
140	64	51	76	108
150	68	55	82	116
160	73	58	87	124
170	77	62	93	131
180	82	65	98	139
190	86	69	104	147
200	91	73	109	155
210	95	76	115	162
220	100	80	120	170
230	105	84	125	178
240	109	87	131	185
250	114	91	136	193

with poor health outcomes and pathology due to the lack of clear cause and effect of high protein intake with health problems (Tipton 2011). The greatest concern of excess protein is the potential impact it could have on renal function (Tipton 2011). It has been hypothesized that the heightened need to eliminate nitrogenous waste constantly stimulates kidney function, possibly contributing to increased risk of renal disease, although this hypothesis has yet to be shown experimentally in healthy individuals (Brenner et al. 1982; Tipton 2011). It was also noted that the interactions between other lifestyle choices imposed by athletes (such as training routines) may further alter kidney function in an unknown fashion (Lowery and Devia 2009; Tipton 2011).

Currently available data have yet to show a substantial link between high protein intake and poor kidney function in athletes (Brandle et al. 1996; Poortmans et al. 2010). In addition to kidney disease, it has also been hypothesized that high protein intake will contribute to ongoing dehydration as a by-product of urea excretion (Lowery and Devia 2009; Tipton 2011). During exercise fluid losses increase, and because of the undeniable link between hydration status and heat-related-injury, athletes should always prioritize fluid replacement. The other major concern about regular high protein intake is the loss of bone mineralization. Increased calcium excretion (calciuria) is commonly used as an indicator of bone loss; however, loss of bone caused by high protein intake is not adequately supported by the available data (Tipton 2011). Additionally, many of those who consume a high-protein diet also participate in behaviors that improve bone mineralization such as resistance training and other weight-bearing exercises (Tipton 2011).

Although there is little evidence linking high-protein diets to pathology in healthy people, there is also lack of evidence supporting the efficacy of very high protein intakes. Athletes should consider achieving adequate protein intake of between 1.2 and 1.7 g/kg, predominantly from food sources rather than supplements. It must also be stressed that adequate carbohydrate consumption is necessary to promote muscle glycogen content, an important predictor of athletic performance.

Despite this widely accepted fact, many athletes regularly turn to and rely on supplements for their protein intake, usually as a result of convenience.

12.4 DISORDERED EATING AND WEIGHT MANAGEMENT

Disordered eating occurs in both male and female athletes, and is most common among athletes participating in weight class and figure-conscious activities (Sundgotborgen 1993; Turocy et al. 2011). Incidence of disordered eating appears to peak during adolescence and is more common in females than males (Martinsen et al. 2014). Moreover, disordered eating is more common in competitive adolescent athletes than similar "control" adolescents (Avdeev et al. 2014; Martinsen and Sundgot-Borgen 2013). Roughly 15% of boys who participate in weight-sensitive sports practice unhealthy weight loss behaviors, and more than 1 in 10 are estimated to have clinical eating disorders (Garner et al. 1998; Turocy et al. 2011). Approximately half of young wrestlers are estimated to be at risk of developing an eating disorder (Turocy et al. 2011), and 60% of average-weight female swimmers were reported to actively pursue weight loss (Dummer et al. 1987). Athletes are at a high risk for developing disordered eating when they believe their body is not ideal for their event which occurs in both genders (Turocy et al. 2011).

12.5 ASSESSING SUCCESSFUL WEIGHT CHANGE

Weight alterations are a necessary goal for many athletes and can be a challenging task. Weight loss and weight gain are common goals among athletes, especially those who have a well-defined weight class. Often, athletes attempt to gain as much lean mass during the off season as possible, and then lose much of their excess body fat prior to competition. Weight gain is a common goal for many athletes, especially among those competing in power and strength events. Initially, athletes should work to accurately predict or estimate energy needs required to maintain their current body weight (this estimate should include physical activity and current training routine). One method to accomplish this is to keep an accurate and detailed food log during a time of weight stability. Once the athlete has an estimate of the amount of food required to maintain their current body weight, the athlete can add a standard amount of an additional food. To promote the building of lean muscle mass, the athlete needs to consume an additional 500–1000 kcal/day. Athletes, as well as their coaches and parents, should regularly track changes in weight and body composition to determine the type of weight that the athlete is gaining. Weight gain greater than 2–3 lb/week is not all lean muscle mass, and should be slowed to avoid the deposition of excess body fat.

For weight loss, athletes should create an energy deficit of approximately 500–1000 kcal/day, while consuming a protein intake in the upper range of the AMDR to help preserve lean tissue. The energy deficit will most ideally come from a combination of increased aerobic exercise and dietary restriction. Initial estimates of energy needs can be determined through methods described for those attempting to gain weight; however, testing with indirect calorimetry may prove more accurate and useful for athletes who have a well-defined time line to make competition weight. The estimate of energy needs used to predict the necessary dietary restriction should include current physical activity levels, and be regularly reassessed based on amount of weight loss. As weight loss progresses, it will be necessary to restrict intake or increase aerobic exercise to levels beyond those initially required to facilitate weight loss. Most athletes have the best success subtly increasing aerobic training with subtle decreases in dietary intake. During prolonged dietary restrictions, it is important for these athletes to choose nutrient dense foods whenever possible and to consider a daily multivitamin and mineral supplement. In general, the initial weight loss plan should include goals of approximately 1–2 lb of weight loss per week. Weight loss in excess of this range tends to be a product of dehydration, overrestriction, or other unsafe behaviors that will negatively affect performance and health.

12.6 GENERAL NUTRITIONAL RECOMMENDATIONS FOR ATHLETES

12.6.1 DIETARY GUIDELINES

The Dietary Guidelines for Americans is a document released every 5 years to accurately summarize the vast field of nutritional recommendations, which will best help Americans meet nutritional needs and reduce chronic disease. In general, the Dietary Guidelines for Americans recommends that Americans consume more fruits, vegetables, whole grains, and fat-free or low-fat milk and milk products, as well as regularly include lean meats, poultry, fish, beans, eggs, and nuts for quality, low-fat protein. The Dietary Guidelines for Americans also encourages Americans to reduce the consumption of saturated fats, *trans* fats, cholesterol, salt (sodium), and added sugars. All of the recommendations are appropriate for athlete health, and helpful in their quest for improved athletic performance. Another primary focus of the Dietary Guidelines for Americans is to promote a prudent dietary lifestyle by discouraging overconsumption of total energy. Total energy requirements are of course estimated with consideration for physical activity, which is unique for each athlete. For a more detailed discussion, general dietary recommendations are provided in chapter 1 and the most recent version of the Dietary Guidelines for Americans can be found at the following website: http://health.gov/dietaryguidelines/2015/guidelines/ (U.S. Department of Health and Human Services 2015).

12.6.2 PREDICTED AND MEASURED ENERGY NEEDS

While covered in greater detail in Chapter 2, the estimation of energy requirements is a valuable tool that can assist athletes in appropriately predicting the amount of calories required for a stage of training, a key aspect of manipulating one's body mass. From the estimated energy requirement (EER), athletes can then estimate approximate quantities of macronutrients required to sustain athletic performance and possibly stimulate desired weight change, as visually represented in Figure 12.1. An EER can be estimated in a variety of ways. The most accurate approach is to first measure resting metabolic rate (RMR), most commonly through indirect calorimetry. Once the energy requirements for the athlete are determined for resting conditions, the athlete can then add a correction for activity level. For athletes who lack access to indirect calorimetry, population-specific predictive equations that estimate metabolic rate based on age, size, and sex can serve as another viable tool for estimating energy needs of athletes (Academy of Nutrition and Dietetics (AND) and the American College of Sports Medicine (ACSM) 2000; Manore 2002). Although these equations have been validated for many populations and are used by clinicians to estimate energy needs of compromised patients, there are limitations and inherent imperfections with predictive equations. To contest these limitations, athletes and clinicians alike can use the predicted energy requirement as a place to begin calorie consumption and then adjust based on athlete (or patient) weight change (or lack thereof). The athlete's caloric intake goals should always be based on the athletes desired body weight.

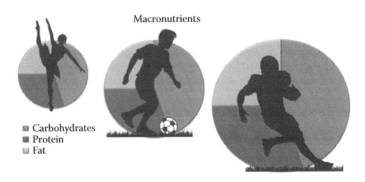

FIGURE 12.1 Representation of various macromolecule needs (shade) and total energy needs (size) for different athletes.

12.6.3 DIFFICULT NUTRIENTS FOR ATHLETES

Athletes often have needs beyond that of the general population, making some nutrient needs difficult for athletes to achieve. Moreover, choosing foods based on likes and dislikes, food tolerance, nutrient timing, and weight goals can further complicate matters. In general, athletes' diets are often low in vitamins such as B vitamins, and vitamins C, D, and E. Additionally, athletes may also consume inadequate amounts of minerals such as iron, zinc, magnesium, and selenium (Berning and Horswill 2014). They can increase intakes of these and other nutrients by choosing nutrient-dense foods, including fruits, vegetables, and complex grains.

Athletes may have difficulty meeting total energy requirements during times of intense training or attempts to add lean muscle mass. During these times, athletes may choose foods that are calorie and nutrient dense such as nut-butters, which provide protein in addition to polyunsaturated fats. In general, athletes can reduce risk of deficiencies and inadequacies by following the Dietary Guidelines for Americans with adjusted portions for increased physical activity. Athletes who practice food avoidance behaviors such as vegetarianism, veganism, and other restrictive diets may wish to seek further, more tailored nutritional advice from a registered dietitian or certified sports dietitian (CSSD). Although athletes can meet 100% of their dietary needs from a well-balanced intake, many athletes may choose to consume a multivitamin and mineral supplement to ensure adequate vitamin and mineral intake. It is imperative that the athlete only uses the supplement as an insurance policy so to speak, and does not rely on a supplement as a replacement for consistent and well-balanced food choices.

12.7 MAINTAINING BODY COMPOSITION AND WEIGHT WITH DIET AND EXERCISE

It is now widely accepted that a healthy lifestyle should include a combination of both proper nutrition and exercise. Evidence has repeatedly demonstrated that exercise alone or diet alone is less effective than the combination of both behaviors. Most ideally, an athlete's nutritional intake will meet needs as best described by the dietary guidelines while still allowing the athlete to compete in ideal weight classes and similar competition subdivisions. Athletes should seek recommendations from registered dietitians, especially board-CSSD, who are specially trained to encourage proper eating habits to meet a variety of nutritional goals while maintaining high standards of food-choice quality based on the latest guidelines. A limitation of this recommendation is that access to licensed healthcare professionals, including RDs and CSSDs, can be limited, and will usually be associated with an increased cost to athletes (especially for athletes not affiliated with professional or university associations).

12.8 GENERAL RECOMMENDATIONS FOR THE WEIGHT-CONSCIOUS ATHLETE

Recently, the ACSM issued a series of up-to-date recommendations that target the needs of athletes both in season and out of season while addressing the needs of those seeking to maintain weight or lose weight (Rodriguez et al. 2009). In general, most dietitians and healthcare providers believe that both athletes and nonathletes can meet 100% of their needs from a well-balanced dietary intake. As discussed above, some micronutrients can be difficult for some athletes to meet, depending on food likes/dislikes, food availability, religious practices, and many other reasons for which supplementation may be beneficial.

In general, the recommendations for athletes are similar to dietary guidelines for healthy Americans over 2 years of age. Specifically, athletes are encouraged to meet energy needs (depending on weight goals) by consuming between 50% and 70% of total energy from carbohydrates, and absolute quantity may vary greatly depending on the size of the athlete, along with training strategy and intensity (Berning and Horswill 2014). Consumption of adequate carbohydrates ensures

TABLE 12.3
Suggested Distribution of Caloric Intake of Each Macromolecule

Acceptable Macronutrient Distribution Range

Macronutrient	Percent Total Calories
Carbohydrates	45%–65%
Protein	10%–35%
Fat	25%–35%
Saturated fat	<10%
Trans fat	As little as possible

that athletes have ample glycogen storage, an independent predictor of exercise performance and onset of fatigue. Also similar to the general dietary guidelines, athletes are encouraged to consume 10%–35% of total energy intake from protein, corresponding with 1.2–1.7 g/kg body weight/day (Berning and Horswill 2014; Phillips et al. 2007; Tipton and Witard 2007). Fat intake should contribute between 25% and 35% of total calories, with saturated fats contributing less than 10% of total calories. *Trans* fats should be avoided whenever possible (Berning and Horswill 2014; Trumbo et al. 2002). Table 12.3 summarizes the AMDR from the dietary guidelines.

In addition to macronutrients, micronutrients (vitamins and minerals) should be consumed at quantities that approximate the RDA. Fluid needs are also important for athletes to consider, because dehydration can profoundly reduce athletic performance. Dehydration occurs following a loss of 2% or more of preexercise body weight. Due to hydration status having an essential role in dissipating body heat and preventing potentially catastrophic heat-related illnesses, it is especially important for athletes competing in high-intensity events, long-duration events, or events in hot and humid environments to maintain adequate hydration status (American College of Sports Medicine (ACSM) 2007; Berning and Horswill 2014). Athletes can meet both hydration and electrolyte needs using a variety of sources; however, many athletes prefer the convenience of performance beverages. In general, performance beverages will contribute approximately 6%–8% carbohydrate, with 110–165 mg of sodium per serving (Berning and Horswill 2014; Convertino et al. 1996). Performance beverages offer convenience along with appropriate concentrations of electrolytes and carbohydrate to facilitate maximum absorption and reduce gastrointestinal irritation. While performance beverages represent an ideal method for replacing electrolytes and fluid in athletes, it is most likely unnecessary for fitness enthusiasts engaging in moderately intense exercise for an hour or less.

12.8.1 Nutrition for Weight Modification

Weight modifications are both sport and season specific, and attempts to modify weight should ideally be performed in the off season (Berning and Horswill 2014; Turocy et al. 2011). The primary consideration should be the appropriateness of the athlete's desire to lose or gain weight. In order to determine the appropriateness, parents, coaches, athletes, and others who work with them should consider the athlete's physical maturity, their current body composition, and an honest assessment of current nutritional habits. The first and perhaps the most important consideration (physical maturity) should be assessed by an appropriate professional (for athletes under 18 years, a pediatrician is the most appropriate). The athlete should recognize that muscle maturity, body composition, and other factors are influenced to a great extent by developmental variables, and attempts to change these factors should not be rushed. Additionally, athletes who wish to reduce body weight should consider their stage of development because the continuous dietary restriction or excessive levels of physical activity required to maintain a lower than ideal body weight may have pronounced effects on bone density, body composition, and normal development as described above.

Once an athlete has determined the level of effort required to alter current body weight, the practitioner should begin by assessing current nutritional intake patterns and current training strategies. Most ideally, the athlete will keep detailed training and food-intake logs to provide information for ongoing assessment. Assessment of initial body weight and body composition should be performed and reassessed at regular intervals thereafter. For assessment of body weight and composition, it is important that the athlete is weighed or measured by a professional under similar conditions each time (i.e., first thing in the morning following bowl voiding, on an empty stomach, in standard clothes or nude).

12.8.1.1 Principles of Weight Gain

Weight gain is a common goal for many athletes, especially among males interested in competition in body building or power and strength events. Thermodynamically, when energy intake exceeds that of energy expenditure, the body is in a state of anabolism, or storage. Initially, athletes should work to accurately predict or estimate energy needs required to maintain their current body weight (this estimate should include physical activity and current training routine). An easy way to perform this is to keep an accurate and detailed food log (consisting of accurate food description, preparation method, and amount) during a time period when the athlete is weight stable. Once the athlete has gained an idea of the standard food required to maintain his or her body weight, the athlete can add a standard amount of an additional food (e.g., a twice daily peanut butter sandwich). It is important to ensure that the athlete is still consuming macronutrients within the AMDR; however, athletes seeking to gain lean muscle mass are encouraged to consume protein at the upper range of the AMDR. To facilitate the gain of lean muscle mass, the athlete should consume an additional 500–1000 kcal/day (in combination with an emphasis on a resistance training program). Despite numerous marketing advertisements from a variety of sources, weight gain in excess of 2–3 lb/week is not all lean muscle mass.

12.8.1.2 Principles of Weight Loss

Weight loss is also a common goal among athletes, especially those who have a well-defined weight class. Oftentimes, athletes attempt to gain as much lean mass during the off season as possible, and then lose much of their excess body fat prior to competition. The recommendations are not the complete inverse and opposite for athletes attempting to lose weight compared with those trying to gain weight. While it is accurate and appropriate for athletes trying to lose weight to create an energy deficit of approximately 500–1000 kcal/day, the athlete is still encouraged to maintain protein intake in the upper range of the AMDR to help preserve lean tissue. Initial estimation of calorie needs should include current physical activity levels, and should be based on an accurate nutrition log. And although athletes seeking weight loss should place a much larger emphasis on aerobic training, they should still incorporate regular resistance training, which will further promote the preservation of lean tissue.

Also similar to weight-gaining practices, athletes undergoing weight loss should assess their initial body weight and body composition, which should be reassessed at regular intervals thereafter under standard measurement conditions. As weight loss progresses, it will be necessary to restrict intake or increase aerobic exercise to levels beyond those initially required to facilitate weight loss. Most athletes have the best success subtly increasing aerobic training with subtle decreases in dietary intake. During extended periods of dietary restrictions, it is important for these athletes to choose nutrient-dense foods whenever possible and to consider a daily multivitamin and mineral supplement.

12.8.2 EXERCISE AND NUTRITIONAL TIMING

Preexercise is normally defined as the 4 h leading up to the bout of exercise. Adequate nutrition comprising sufficient fuels and fluid prior to exercise has been linked to improved performance (Berning and Horswill 2014; Moseley et al. 2003). Most ideally, a preexercise meal rich in complex carbohydrates and low in fiber should be consumed prior to exercise to maintain blood glucose during exercise. Athletes who consume sufficient carbohydrates prior to competition will more effectively maintain ideal blood glucose levels during exercise, which acts to spare muscle and liver glycogen. Muscle and liver glycogen are important predictors of athletic performance; therefore, it is also common for athletes to consume elevated amounts of carbohydrate days prior to competition.

The preexercise meal should be individualized, taking into consideration the optimal absorption and gastrointestinal emptying based on the athlete's past experiences. Athletes should experiment with a variety of preexercise meal and fluid combinations prior to competition and track which preexercise practices yield the best training results. The general recommendations for fluid and carbohydrate intake prior to competition is 4 h prior to exercise, drink 12–20 oz of fluid to optimize hydration, and allow sufficient time for excretion. Athletes should also consume approximately 3–4 g of carbohydrates per kilogram body weight 3–4 h prior to competition.

12.8.3 Nutrition during Exercise

Nutrition during exercise is most important for extended exercise because energy stores may become exhausted. In addition to depletion of muscle and liver glycogen, athletes also lose substantial amounts of fluids and should consider nutritional replacement of carbohydrates, fluids, and electrolytes during exercise. An individualized approach to during-exercise nutritional replacement is required to avoid excessive volume consumption leading to gastrointestinal upset and hyper-hydration. In general, fluid replacement should start early during the event as a preventative measure and be continuous throughout the activity. Athletes should also consume approximately 30–60 g of carbohydrate per hour to maintain blood glucose and extend performance (although the exact amount will depend on the athlete's size and preference, the intensity of the exercise, and the convenience of consumption during the event). Many sports performance beverages are specially formulated to provide sufficient fluid, electrolytes, and carbohydrates to provide convenience and adequate nutrition.

12.8.4 Nutrition for Postexercise Recovery

Following exercise, the body will likely be in a state of depletion (including glycogen, hydration, electrolytes, and musculoskeletal damage). Common postexercise dietary practices should include consumption of adequate carbohydrate, fluids, and electrolytes to replenish glycogen stores and promote rehydration. It is also important for athletes to prioritize protein consumption after exercise to promote protein synthesis within muscles that were contracted during exercise. Adequate protein and energy consumption will foster the building and repair of muscle tissue. The restoration of these deficiencies is especially important for athletes who are competing in multiple competitions in the same day. Ideally, athletes will begin replenishing losses immediately following exercise.

The general recommendations for postexercise consumption are 1.0–1.5 g of high-glycemic, low-fiber carbohydrates per kilogram of body weight, with approximately 10–30 g of protein. This combination will facilitate the resynthesis of glycogen and repair of muscle tissue (Berning and Horswill 2014; Moore et al. 2009). To further promote recovery, the athlete can repeat the immediate postexercise mixture of 1.0–1.5 g of high-glycemic low-fiber carbohydrates per kilogram of body weight with approximately 10–30 g of protein approximately 2 h postexercise. For fluid replacement, the volume consumed should be approximately 1.5 times that of fluids lost. One recommendation is to consume 16–24 oz of fluid for every pound lost during exercise; however, this requires an accurate preexercise weight, which is not always performed.

REFERENCES

Academy of Nutrition and Dietetics (AND). 2009b. Position of the American Dietetic Association: Weight management. *Journal of the American Dietetic Association* 109 (2):330–346. doi: 10.1016/j.jada.2008.11.041.

Academy of Nutrition and Dietetics (AND) and the American College of Sports Medicine (ACSM). 2000. Position of the American Dietetic Association, Dietitians of Canada, and the American College of Sports Medicine: Nutrition and athletic performance. *Journal of the American Dietetic Association* 100 (12):1543–1556.

Academy of Nutrition and Dietetics (AND) and the American College of Sports Medicine (ACSM). 2009a. Position of the American Dietetic Association, Dietitians of Canada, and the American College of Sports Medicine: Nutrition and athletic performance. *Journal of the American Dietetic Association* 109 (3):509–527. doi: 10.1016/j.jada.2009.01.005.

American College of Sports Medicine (ACSM). 2007. Selected issues in injury and illness prevention and the team physician: A consensus statement. *Medicine & Science in Sports & Exercise* 39 (11):2058–2068. doi: 10.1249/mss.0b013e31815a76ea.

Ahmed, W., M. A. Flynn, and M. A. Alpert. 2001. Cardiovascular complications of weight reduction diets. *American Journal of the Medical Sciences* 321 (4):280–284. doi: 10.1097/00000441-200104000-00007.

Avdeev, I., M. Martinsen, and A. Francis. 2014. Rate- and temperature-dependent material behavior of a multilayer polymer battery separator. *Journal of Materials Engineering and Performance* 23 (1):315–325. doi: 10.1007/s11665-013-0743-4.

Baror, O., C. J. R. Blimkie, J. A. Hay, J. D. Macdougall, D. S. Ward, and W. M. Wilson. 1992. Voluntary dehydration and heat intolerance in cystic-fibrosis. *Lancet* 339 (8795):696–699. doi: 10.1016/0140-6736(92)90597-V.

Berning, J. R. and C. A. Horswill. 2014. Active Voice: Guidance for Athletes Who Manipulate Body Weight. American College of Sports Medicine—Active Voice: Guidance for Athletes Who Manipulate Body Weight. Accessed April 24, 2014. http://www.multibriefs.com/briefs/acsm/active12-17.htm.

Brandle, E., H. G. Sieberth, and R. E. Hautmann. 1996. Effect of chronic dietary protein intake on the renal function in healthy subjects. *European Journal of Clinical Nutrition* 50 (11):734–740.

Brenner, B. M., T. W. Meyer, and T. H. Hostetter. 1982. Dietary-protein intake and the progressive nature of kidney-disease—The role of hemodynamically mediated glomerular injury in the pathogenesis of progressive glomerular sclerosis in aging, renal ablation, and intrinsic renal-disease. *New England Journal of Medicine* 307 (11):652–659.

Campbell, B., R. B. Kreider, T. Ziegenfuss, P. La Bounty, M. Roberts, D. Burke, J. Landis, H. Lopez, and J. Antonio. 2007. International Society of Sports Nutrition position stand: Protein and exercise. *Journal of the International Society of Sports Nutrition* 4 (8). doi: 10.1186/1550-2783-4-8.

Church, T. 2011. Exercise in obesity, metabolic syndrome, and diabetes. *Progress in Cardiovascular Diseases* 53 (6):412–418. doi: 10.1016/j.pcad.2011.03.013.

Church, T. S., M. J. LaMonte, C. E. Barlow, and S. N. Blair. 2005. Cardiorespiratory fitness and body mass index as predictors of cardiovascular disease mortality among men with diabetes. *Archives of Internal Medicine Journal* 165 (18):2114–2120. doi: 10.1001/archinte.165.18.2114.

Church, T. S., A. M. Thompson, P. T. Katzmarzyk, X. Sui, N. Johannsen, C. P. Earnest, and S. N. Blair. 2009. Metabolic syndrome and diabetes, alone and in combination, as predictors of cardiovascular disease mortality among men. *Diabetes Care* 32 (7):1289–1294. doi: 10.2337/dc08-1871.

Convertino, V. A., L. E. Armstrong, E. F. Coyle, G. W. Mack, M. N. Sawka, L. C. Senay, and W. M. Sherman. 1996. American College of Sports Medicine position stand—Exercise and fluid replacement. *Medicine & Science in Sports & Exercise* 28 (1):R1–R7. doi: 10.1097/00005768-199610000-00045.

Douyon, L. and D. E. Schteingart. 2002. Effect of obesity and starvation on thyroid hormone, growth hormone, and cortisol secretion. *Endocrinology and Metabolism Clinics of North America* 31 (1):173–189. doi: Pii S0889-8529(01)00023-8 doi 10.1016/S0889-8529(01)00023-8.

Dummer, G. M., L. W. Rosen, W. W. Heusner, P. J. Roberts, and J. E. Counsilman. 1987. Pathogenic weight-control behaviors of young competitive swimmers. *Physician and Sports Medicine* 15 (5):75–84.

Fakhouri, T. H., J. P. Hughes, V. L. Burt, M. Song, J. E. Fulton, and C. L. Ogden. 2014. Physical activity in U.S. youth aged 12–15 years, 2012. *NCHS Data Brief* 141:1–8.

Foster, W. R. and B. T. Burton. 1985. Health implications of obesity—National-Institutes-of-Health Consensus Development Conference—Introduction. *Annals of Internal Medicine* 103 (6):981–982.

Garner, D. M., L. W. Rosen, and D. Barry. 1998. Eating disorders among athletes—Research and recommendations. *Child and Adolescent Psychiatric Clinics of North America* 7 (4):839–857.

Gibala, M. J., S. A. Interisano, M. A. Tarnopolsky, B. D. Roy, J. R. MacDonald, K. E. Yarasheski, and J. D. MacDougall. 2000. Myofibrillar disruption following acute concentric and eccentric resistance exercise in strength-trained men. *Canadian Journal of Physiology and Pharmacology* 78 (8):656–661. doi: 10.1139/cjpp-78-8-656.

Hausenblas, H. A. and A. V. Carron. 1999. Eating disorder indices and athletes: An integration. *Journal of Sport & Exercise Psychology* 21 (3):230–258.

Howatson, G. and K. A. van Someren. 2008. The prevention and treatment of exercise-induced muscle damage. *Sports Medicine* 38 (6):483–503.

Knowler, W. C., E. Barrett-Connor, S. E. Fowler, R. F. Hamman, J. M. Lachin, E. A. Walker, D. M. Nathan, and Diabetes Prevention Program Res G. 2002. Reduction in the incidence of type 2 diabetes with lifestyle intervention or metformin. *New England Journal of Medicine* 346 (6):393–403.

Lanes, R. and A. Soros. 2004. Decreased final height of children with growth deceleration secondary to poor weight gain during late childhood. *Journal of Pediatrics* 145 (1):128–130. doi: 10.1016/j.jpeds.2004.03.053.

Lantzouni, E., G. R. Frank, N. H. Golden, and R. I. Shenker. 2002. Reversibility of growth stunting in early onset anorexia nervosa: A prospective study. *Journal of Adolescent Health* 31 (2):162–165. doi: Pii S1054-139x(02)00342-7 doi: 10.1016/S1054-139x(02)00342-7.

Layman, D. K. 2004. Protein quantity and quality at levels above the RDA improves adult weight loss. *Journal of the American College of Nutrition* 23 (6):631s–636s.

Layman, D. K., R. A. Boileau, D. J. Erickson, J. E. Painter, H. Shiue, C. Sather, and D. D. Christou. 2003. A reduced ratio of dietary carbohydrate to protein improves body composition and blood lipid profiles during weight loss in adult women. *Journal of Nutrition* 133 (2):411–417.

Lemon, P. W. R. 2000. Beyond the zone: Protein needs of active individuals. *Journal of the American College of Nutrition* 19 (5):513s–521s.

Lowery, L. M. and L. Devia. 2009. Dietary protein safety and resistance exercise: What do we really know? *Journal of the International Society of Sports Nutrition* 6 (3). doi: 10.1186/1550-2783-6-3.

Manore, M. M. 2002. Dietary recommendations and athletic menstrual dysfunction. *Sports Medicine* 32 (14):887–901.

Martinsen, M., R. Bahr, R. Borresen, I. Holme, A. M. Pensgaard, and J. Sundgot-Borgen. 2014. Preventing eating disorders among young elite athletes: A randomized controlled trial. *Medicine & Science in Sports & Exercise* 46 (3):435–447. doi: 10.1249/MSS.0b013e3182a702fc.

Martinsen, M. and J. Sundgot-Borgen. 2013. Higher prevalence of eating disorders among adolescent elite athletes than controls. *Medicine & Science in Sports & Exercise* 45 (6):1188–1197. doi: 10.1249/MSS.0b013e318281a939.

Meckling, K. A. and R. Sherfey. 2007. A randomized trial of a hypocaloric high-protein diet, with and without exercise, on weight loss, fitness, and markers of the metabolic syndrome in overweight and obese women. *Applied Physiology Nutrition and Metabolism—Physiologie Appliquee Nutrition Et Metabolisme* 32 (4):743–752. doi: 10.1139/H07-059.

Metges, C. C. and C. A. Barth. 2000. Metabolic consequences of a high dietary-protein intake in adulthood: Assessment of the available evidence. *Journal of Nutrition* 130 (4):886–889.

Moore, D. R., M. J. Robinson, J. L. Fry, J. E. Tang, E. I. Glover, S. B. Wilkinson, T. Prior, M. A. Tarnopolsky, and S. M. Phillips. 2009. Ingested protein dose response of muscle and albumin protein synthesis after resistance exercise in young men. *American Journal of Clinical Nutrition* 89 (1):161–168. doi: 10.3945/ajcn.2008.26401.

Moseley, L., G. I. Lancaster, and A. E. Jeukendrup. 2003. Effects of timing of pre-exercise ingestion of carbohydrate on subsequent metabolism and cycling performance. *European Journal of Applied Physiology* 88 (4–5):453–458. doi: 10.1007/s00421-002-0728-8.

Nadel, E. R. 1983. Factors affecting the regulation of body-temperature during exercise. *Journal of Thermal Biology* 8 (1–2):165–169. doi: 10.1016/0306-4565(83)90097-9.

Nadel, E. R. 1984. Temperature regulation and hyperthermia during exercise. *Clinics in Chest Medicine* 5 (1):13–20.

Nadel, E. R. 1985. Recent advances in temperature regulation during exercise in humans. *Federation Proceedings* 44 (7):2286–2292.

Nadel, E. R., R. W. Bullard, and J. A. Stolwijk. 1971. Importance of skin temperature in regulation of sweating. *Journal of Applied Physiology* 31 (1):80–87.

Phillips, S. M. 2004. Protein requirements and supplementation in strength sports. *Nutrition* 20 (7–8):689–695. doi: 10.1016/j.nut.2004.04.009.

Phillips, S. M. 2006. Dietary protein for athletes: From requirements to metabolic advantage. *Applied Physiology Nutrition and Metabolism—Physiologie Appliquee Nutrition Et Metabolisme* 31 (6):647–654. doi: 10.1139/H06-035.

Phillips, S. M., D. R. Moore, and J. E. Tang. 2007. A critical examination of dietary protein requirements, benefits, and excesses in athletes. *International Journal of Sport Nutrition and Exercise Metabolism* 17:S58–S76.

Poortmans, J. R., E. S. Rawson, L. M. Burke, S. J. Stear, and L. M. Castell. 2010. A–Z of nutritional supplements: Dietary supplements, sports nutrition foods and ergogenic aids for health and performance. Part 11. *British Journal of Sports Medicine* 44 (10):765–766. doi: 10.1136/bjsm.2010.076117.

Rodriguez, N. R., N. M. Di Marco, and S. Langley. 2009. American College of Sports Medicine position stand: Nutrition and athletic performance. *Med Sci Sports Exerc* 41:709–731.

Sawada, S. S., I. M. Lee, T. Muto, K. Matuszaki, and S. N. Blair. 2003. Cardiorespiratory fitness and the incidence of type 2 diabetes—Prospective study of Japanese men. *Diabetes Care* 26 (10):2918–2922. doi: 10.2337/diacare.26.10.2918.

Shaper, A. G., S. G. Wannamethee, and M. Walker. 1997. Body weight: Implications for the prevention of coronary heart disease, stroke, and diabetes mellitus in a cohort study of middle aged men. *British Medical Journal* 314 (7090):1311–1317.

Steen, S. N. and K. D. Brownell. 1990. Patterns of weight-loss and regain in wrestlers—Has the tradition changed. *Medicine & Science in Sports & Exercise* 22 (6):762–768.

Stevens, A., D. P. Robinson, J. Turpin, T. Groshong, and J. D. Tobias. 2002. Sudden cardiac death of an adolescent during dieting. *Southern Medical Journal* 95 (9):1047–1049.

Stupka, N., M. A. Tarnopolsky, N. J. Yardley, and S. M. Phillips. 2001. Cellular adaptation to repeated eccentric exercise-induced muscle damage. *Journal of Applied Physiology* 91 (4):1669–1678.

Sundgotborgen, J. 1993. Prevalence of eating disorders in elite female athletes. *International Journal of Sport Nutrition* 3 (1):29–40.

Swenne, I. and P. T. Larsson. 1999. Heart risk associated with weight loss in anorexia nervosa and eating disorders: Risk factors for QT(c) interval prolongation and dispersion. *Acta Paediatrica* 88 (3):304–309. doi: 10.1080/08035259950170079.

Tipton, C. M. and T. K. Tcheng. 1970. Iowa wrestling study—Weight loss in high school students. *Journal of the American Medical Association* 214 (7):1269–1274. doi: 10.1001/jama.214.7.1269.

Tipton, K. D. 2011. Symposium 2: Exercise and protein nutrition efficacy and consequences of very-high-protein diets for athletes and exercisers. *Proceedings of the Nutrition Society* 70:205–214. doi: 10.1017/S0029665111000024.

Tipton, K. D. and O. C. Witard. 2007. Protein requirements and recommendations for athletes: Relevance of ivory tower arguments for practical recommendations. *Clinical Journal of Sport Medicine* 26 (1):17–36. doi: 10.1016/j.csm.2006.11.003.

Trumbo, P., S. Schlicker, A. A. Yates, and M. Poos. 2002. Dietary reference intakes for energy, carbohydrate, fiber, fat, fatty acids, cholesterol, protein and amino acids. *Journal of the American Dietetic Association* 102 (11):1621–1630. doi: 10.1016/S0002-8223(02)90346-9.

Tuomilehto, J., J. Lindstrom, J. G. Eriksson, T. T. Valle, H. Hamalainen, P. Ilanne-Parikka, S. Keinanen-Kiukaanniemi et al. 2001. Prevention of type 2 diabetes mellitus by changes in lifestyle among subjects with impaired glucose tolerance. *New England Journal of Medicine* 344 (18):1343–1350. doi: 10.1056/Nejm200105033441801.

Turocy, P. S., B. F. DePalma, C. A. Horswill, K. M. Laquale, T. J. Martin, A. C. Perry, M. J. Somova, A. C. Utter, and Association National Athletic Trainers. 2011. National Athletic Trainers' Association position statement: Safe weight loss and maintenance practices in sport and exercise. *Journal of Athletic Training* 46 (3):322–336.

U.S. Department of Health and Human Services and U.S. Department of Agriculture. 2015–2020 Dietary Guidelines for Americans. 8th Edition. December 2015. Accessed on March 24, 2015. Available at http://health.gov/dietaryguidelines/2015/guidelines/.

Wei, M., L. W. Gibbons, J. B. Kampert, M. Z. Nichaman, and S. N. Blair. 2000. Low cardiorespiratory fitness and physical inactivity as predictors of mortality in men with type 2 diabetes. *Annals of Internal Medicine* 132 (8):605–611.

Weinstein, A. R., H. D. Sesso, I. M. Lee, N. R. Cook, J. E. Manson, J. E. Buring, and J. M. Gaziano. 2004. Relationship of physical activity vs body mass index with type 2 diabetes in women. *JAMA—Journal of the American Medical Association* 292 (10):1188–1194. doi: 10.1001/jama.292.10.1188.

Westerterp-Plantenga, M. S. 2008. Protein intake and energy balance. *Regulatory Peptides* 149 (1–3):67–69. doi: 10.1016/j.regpep.2007.08.026.

Wilkinson, S. B., S. M. Phillips, P. J. Atherton, R. Patel, K. E. Yarasheski, M. A. Tarnopolsky, and M. J. Rennie. 2008. Differential effects of resistance and endurance exercise in the fed state on signalling molecule phosphorylation and protein synthesis in human muscle. *Journal of Physiology—London* 586 (15):3701–3717. doi: 10.1113/jphysiol.2008.153916.

13 Dietary Supplement Considerations for the Young Athlete

Paul E. Luebbers

CONTENTS

Abstract 219
13.1 Introduction 219
13.2 Dietary Supplement Use among Young Athletes 221
13.3 Commonly Used Dietary Supplements by Youth and Adolescent Athletes 221
    13.3.1 Creatine 221
        13.3.1.1 Creatine Supplementation Research in Youth 223
        13.3.1.2 Potential Negative Effects of Creatine Supplementation 224
        13.3.1.3 Views of Creatine Supplementation in Youth by National Organizations 225
    13.3.2 Caffeine 225
        13.3.2.1 Caffeine Supplementation and Youth 226
        13.3.2.2 Potential Negative Effects of Caffeine 228
        13.3.2.3 Views on Caffeine Use and Energy Drink Consumption in Youth by National Organizations 228
    13.3.3 Protein 229
13.4 Considerations for Choosing a Dietary Supplement 230
    13.4.1 Good Manufacturing Practices and Third-Party Testing 231
13.5 Conclusions 233
References 233

ABSTRACT

Optimum athletic performance is a common goal for many of today's young athletes. While one can likely reach their full athletic potential through proper training and diet, it is not uncommon for athletes to consider dietary supplements in an effort to enhance performance. Although a "food-first" approach is encouraged, the fact that supplement use is common among youth, particularly those involved in athletics, should not be ignored. This chapter will focus on the most common nutritional supplements taken by youth, their mechanisms of action, potential ergogenic effects, their regulation by the government, safety concerns, and resources for making an informed decision regarding supplement use.

13.1 INTRODUCTION

Dietary supplement sales in the United States reached a record level of $36 billion in 2014. This represents a 60% increase from the $22.5 billion spent in 2006. This upward trend is expected to continue with an annual growth rate of approximately 7.1% through 2020 [1].

The dietary supplement industry encompasses a wide variety of consumer goods, which are often categorized into vitamins and minerals, meal replacements and weight-loss formulas, herbs and botanicals, and other specialty products. Dietary supplementation targeted toward sports nutrition comprise another category, and when combined with sales data on energy drinks, account for approximately $21 billion a year, well over half of all dietary supplement sales [1].

Dietary supplement use is widespread in the U.S. population and while it is difficult to determine exactly who is consuming which product and for what purpose, it is not unreasonable to assume that most sports supplements and likely many energy drinks are being purchased in hopes of enhancing athletic performance. While age demographics of those purchasing dietary supplements are not available, the use of dietary supplements among youth and especially adolescents is becoming increasingly popular.

A dietary supplement, as defined by the Dietary Supplement Health and Education Act of 1994 (DSHEA) [2], is

> a product (other than tobacco) intended to supplement the diet that bears or contains one or more of the following dietary ingredients: a vitamin, mineral, amino acid, herb or other botanical; or a dietary substance for use to supplement the diet by increasing the total dietary intake; or a concentrate, metabolite, constituent, extract, or combination of any ingredient described above; and intended for ingestion in the form of a capsule, powder, softgel, or gelcap, and not represented as a conventional food or as a sole item of a meal or the diet.
>
> **DSHEA**
> *Public Law 103-417, October 25, 1994*

Some of these ingredients—vitamins and minerals—are discussed in Chapter 6 of this book, and are not being examined in-depth in this chapter. A misperception among some consumers is that certain dietary supplements—those used for sports performance—are forms of anabolic steroids. There is a very clear distinction between dietary supplements and steroids. For further information regarding steroids and other illicit drugs, refer to Chapter 9.

The word "ergogenic" is derived from two words in the Greek language: "ergon," which means "work," and "genman," which means to "generate" or "create" [3]. Therefore, an ergogenic aid is anything that augments one's ability to do work. For an athlete, this means an improved ability to train and perform. While several classifications of ergogenic aids exist (see Table 13.1), this chapter will focus on nutritional ergogenic aids, particularly those classified as dietary supplements.

TABLE 13.1
Ergogenic Aid Classifications

Ergogenic Aid	Description	Examples
Mechanical	Any device or piece of equipment used to enhance performance during training or competition	Knee wraps, spikes/cleats, weighted vest
Nutritional	Any supplement, food product, or dietary intervention that enhances work capacity or athletic performance	Amino acids, caffeine, creatine
Pharmacological	Any substance or compound classified as a drug or hormonal agent that is used to improve work output or sports performance	Caffeine, erythropoietin, growth hormone
Physiological	Any practice or substance that enhances the body's various systems (e.g., cardiovascular, muscular) and thus improves athletic performance	Lactate threshold training, resistance training, warming-up
Psychological	Any practice or treatment that changes mental state and thereby enhances sport performance	Hypnosis, music, visualization

Source: Adapted from Fink, H.H., Mikesky, A.E., and Burgoon, L.A., *Practical Applications in Sports Nutrition*, 3 ed., Jones & Bartlett Learning, Burlington, MA, 2012.

13.2 DIETARY SUPPLEMENT USE AMONG YOUNG ATHLETES

As seen with other parts of the U.S. population, dietary supplement use by youth and adolescents has increased. In reviewing this literature, it is difficult to get a clear view of supplement use among young athletes as the published research does not have conformity among the types of data collection instruments used, the population examined, the level of competition played, ages of the youth, sample sizes, and the types and/or classifications of potential supplements being used. However, there does seem to be an indication that many youth, particularly athletic and/or active youth, are taking ergogenic nutritional supplements, and that the prevalence of this use does seem to increase with age. Outlined in Table 13.2 is a summary of several published studies and provides information such as the population studied, supplement usage statistics, sports involved, and other such related findings.

13.3 COMMONLY USED DIETARY SUPPLEMENTS BY YOUTH AND ADOLESCENT ATHLETES

What follows is an overview of the most commonly used dietary supplements by youth as ergogenics, as determined by the studies cited above: creatine, energy drinks, and protein. When possible, attention is given to research that has been conducted with those supplements in a young population.

13.3.1 CREATINE

Creatine is a naturally occurring nonessential compound derived from the amino acids arginine, glycine, and methionine. Two main sources of creatine exist, the first being exogenous or dietary sources. Dietary intake of creatine is centered largely upon the ingestion of various sources of meat whereby a typical 4 oz serving yields modest amounts of creatine: herring (0.74 g), pork (0.57 g), salmon (0.52 g), beef (0.52 g), tuna (0.45 g), and cod (0.34 g) [13]. The other source of creatine is endogenous production within the body, primarily in the liver, as well as the kidney and pancreas to a lesser extent. For a healthy individual with a body mass of 70 kg, the creatine requirement is approximately 2 g/day, which is typically met with 1 g coming from endogenous production and another gram from the diet. However, if one is following a vegetarian style of diet, the requirements of endogenous production will likely be higher. To this point, typical dietary intake of creatine has been linked to the classification of some individuals as "responders and nonresponders" to creatine supplementation. In this respect, presupplementation creatine levels are known to be a primary predictor of the responsiveness of creatine supplementation and those individuals who are vegetarian are likely to be more responsive to creatine supplementation and conversely for those people who consume high amounts of meat in their diet [14,15].

Skeletal muscle is the primary storage site for creatine (90%–95%), with smaller amounts found in the brain and heart. A healthy 70-kg individual will store an average of 120 g of total creatine in the skeletal muscles. Approximately 60%–65% of the intramuscular creatine is stored as phosphocreatine (PCr—a creatine molecule with a phosphate attached) and the remaining as free creatine. The body utilizes approximately 1%–2% (1.5–2.5 g) of this creatine pool daily, thus resulting in the approximate 2 g/day requirement. This turnover is measured via creatinine, the metabolic waste product of creatine utilization, which is excreted from the body via urine [16]. PCr operates as a foundational substrate to an energy system that the body relies upon for rapid energy production, particularly activities and exercise tasks of near-maximal intensity not exceeding 15 s. Depletion of creatine and phosphocreatine in muscle has been shown to severely limit the muscles' potential to perform high-intensity work [17]. Research indicates that the average capacity of creatine storage is around 160 g [17–19], thus increasing the muscular concentrations of creatine via supplementation has become a popular strategy to improve high-intensity exercise performance.

TABLE 13.2
Dietary Supplement Use in Youth and Adolescent Populations

Population	Key Findings	References
U.S.—high school	*Population*: 328 students (55% boys, 45% girls, 15.2 ± 1.3 years) *Usage statistics*: Creatine use of 8.2% (26 boys, 1 girl) *Sports*: Football (29%), soccer, and hockey *Perceived efficacy*: 79% felt it improved their performance *Frequency*: 35% daily, 35% weekly, 30% rate usage *Dosing*: 55% could not recall dosage, 23% (5 g/day), 23% (5–10 g/day) *Primary information source*: Friends	Smith and Dahm [4]
U.S.—middle and high school	*Population*: 1103 (55% boys, 45% girls, Grades 6–12) *Usage statistics*: Creatine use (8.8% boys, 1.8% girls). Creatine use was stable (3.4%) from grades 6–10, 12% use in 11th grade and 44% use in 12th grade *Sports*: Strength and power sports (football, wrestling, hockey) *Reasons to take*: Improve performance (72%), improve appearance (61%), and improve speed (40%) *Reasons not taking*: Safety concerns (46%), lack of perceived benefit (20%), expense (13%)	Metzl [5]
U.S.—high school	*Population*: 270 athletic high school boys (45%) and girls (55%), 13–18 years *Usage statistics*: Sports drinks were most common (59%), vitamin/minerals (46%), creatine (21% in boys, 3% in girls), amino acids (8% in boys, 1% girls) *Reasons to take*: Gain muscle, increase energy, prevent illness *Primary information source*: Coaches, doctors, and parents were primary sources of nutrition and dietary supplement information; parents have largest influence on use	Kayton [6]
Australia—middle and high school	*Population*: 78 students, grades 7–11, 11–18 years *Usage statistics*: Sports drink (56%), vitamin/minerals (49%), energy drinks (42%), creatine (5%), protein supplements (4%). Creatine was taken only by boys, all others were consumed by both gender *Reasons for taking*: Energy production or boost *Misc.*: Athletes had little to no knowledge of adverse events	O'Dea [7]
Canada—high school	*Population*: 333 high school boys (57%) and girls (42%), 15.4 ± 1.1 years *Usage statistics*: Vitamin/minerals (43%), protein (14%), creatine (5.3%). Boys reported similar use of vitamin/minerals as girls, greater protein and creatine use when compared to girls *Reasons for taking*: Students taking protein (43%) and creatine (42%) believed it would help their performance	Bell [8]
U.S.—high school	*Population*: 3248 students in grades 8–12 *Usage statistics*: Vitamin/minerals (59%), energy drinks (32%), protein (15%), and creatine (7%). Boys reported greater use of energy drinks, protein, and creatine with progressively higher levels of protein (40% of 12th grade boys) and creatine (22% of 12th grade boys) use occurring with age *Primary information source*: Teachers (36%) and parents (16%). As grade levels increased, parents, friends, coaches, athletic trainers, and Internet sites take on larger roles	Hoffman [9]
U.K.—young elite athletes	*Population*: 403 elite athletes (12–21 years, 17.7 ± 2.0 years) *Usage statistics*: Energy drinks (87%), vitamin/minerals (47%), whey protein (44%), and creatine (28%) *Sports*: Rugby, soccer, and swimming *Misc.*: Large majority (78%) did not believe nutritional supplementation was needed to achieve success in sports	Petroczi et al. [10]

(Continued)

TABLE 13.2 (*Continued*)
Dietary Supplement Use in Youth and Adolescent Populations

Population	Key Findings	References
Germany— young elite athletes	*Population*: 1138 Olympic-level competitors (14–18 years, 56% boys, 44% girls) *Usage statistics*: Vitamin/minerals (34%–69%), energy drinks (64%), protein (38%), creatine (12%)	Diehl et al. [11]
U.S.—youth	*Population*: 73.7 million U.S. children (10.8 ± 0.2 years, 57% older than age of 10) *Usage statistics*: 1.64% (1.2 million) used some form of supplement to enhance sport performance in last 30 days. 94.5% used vitamin/minerals, 44% used fish oils, 34% used creatine, 26% used fiber *Misc.*: Boys were twice as likely to use something. Independent of gender, usage increased with age (47% of 9–12 graders)	Evans [12]

Supplementation with creatine has been shown to increase intramuscular creatine levels by 20%. Common dosing protocols employ daily ingestion of 20 g (4 doses of 5 g spread throughout the day) for a minimum of 3 days and then are maintained with a daily 2 g dose [18,20]. Dosing relative to one's body mass has also been proposed as an attempt to provide a dose that matches an individual's lean tissue mass. Lehmkuhl et al. successfully utilized 0.3 g/kg/day for 1 week followed by 0.03 g/kg/day for 7 weeks. Regardless of which dosing method is used—absolute or relative—the initial, short-term high-dose of creatine supplementation is commonly referred to as the "loading" phase and the smaller, long-term follow-up dosage as the "maintenance" phase [21]. Cessation of the 2 g/day maintenance dose led to total creatine content returning to presupplementation values within 30 days [18,20].

The potential ergogenic effects of creatine supplementation have been thoroughly examined within the scientific community, with the majority of the research being conducted since creatine first became commercially available as a supplement in the early 1990s. Owing to the role creatine plays in energy production, particularly during short-term, high-intensity muscular work, the vast majority of research has focused on activities and exercise that are highly dependent on short-term, explosive movements. Several reviews and a meta-analysis [22–26] indicate that the primary potential ergogenic effects of creatine supplementation are

- *Increased body mass/muscle size*: This is possibly the most commonly experienced effect of creatine supplementation, and can be accounted for in two ways. First, increase in intracellular creatine has an osmotic effect, which pulls water into the cells. Second, the increased capacity to perform high-intensity work could lead to increased muscle protein content if an appropriate training stimulus is provided (e.g., resistance training).
- *Increased maximal force/strength*: This has been demonstrated in several studies utilizing 1-RM (one repetition maximum) protocols, usually with supine bench press and/or incline leg press.
- *Increased power output*: Creatine has been shown to improve power output in a number of modalities, including cycling, jumping, sprinting, and swimming.
- *Improved repeat performance during interval work*: Enhanced performance during repeated maximal or near-maximal work lasting less than 60 s, with short periods of intervening recovery. This has primarily been demonstrated with cycling and swimming protocols.

13.3.1.1 Creatine Supplementation Research in Youth

It is important to note that in the research cited above, the participants were all adults, ranging from young to middle age. Creatine supplementation in a youthful population has not been as extensively studied as it has in young and older adults, but a growing body of research does exist. Some of the earliest research in this age group focused on creatine's use with certain medical conditions. In 1996, Stockler and Hanefeld reported a case study that examined creatine supplementation in a 23-month-old infant born with a deficiency in guanidinoacetate methyltransferase (GAMT), which is a condition that causes depletion in brain and body creatine [27]. A 4–8 g/day dose was administered for 25 months. Muscle creatine, which accounts for 90% of total body creatine, was restored within the first few weeks, and the infant's extrapyramidal signs (inability to roll and hold its head) had resolved. The potential for improvements in strength and body composition in boys with Duchenne muscular dystrophy (DMD) was reported by Tarnopolsky et al. [28]. Thirty boys were administered creatine monohydrate at 0.10 g/kg/day for 4 months. In addition to the creatine administration being well tolerated, increases in fat-free mass (FFM), and dominant-hand grip strength as well as reductions in bone breakdown among the boys were also recorded [28]. A component in the chemotherapy treatment for acute lymphoblastic leukemia (ALL) is corticosteroid administration. This treatment is known to cause body weight gain by increasing body fat. A study utilizing 59 children afflicted with ALL was conducted examining various measures of body size and mass over a 38-week period. Only the children receiving creatine supplementation (0.1 g/kg/day for two 16-week periods [separated by a 6-week wash-out period]) demonstrated an attenuation of body fat percentage [29]. In 2008, Sakellaris et al. [30] examined a 6-month creatine dose of 0.4 g/kg/day in 39 children and adolescents with traumatic brain injury (TBI) between the ages of 1–18. They were investigating the potential neuroprotective effects of creatine supplementation on certain parameters of TBI. Significant improvements were seen in headaches, dizziness, and fatigue in all patients. No adverse side effects were observed.

In addition to research on clinical populations in youth, a small number of studies have also explored the impact of creatine supplementation on youth athletes and performance. Grindstaff et al. [31] demonstrated that short-term creatine monohydrate supplementation (9 days, 21 g/day) was effective in young competitive junior swimmers (15.3 ± 0.6 years) for improving performance in 50- and 100-m sprint times. Subjects did not report any adverse side effects from the supplementation. Dawson and colleagues [32] studied the effects of a 4-week creatine supplement regimen on 20 young (10 boys, 10 girls, 16.4 ± 1.8 years) competitive junior swimmers. Ten randomly assigned swimmers received creatine (loading for 5 days at 20 g/day, followed by 22 days of maintenance at 5 g/day) while the other ten received a placebo. Neither group experienced improvements in body mass or composition, nor in single sprint performance (50 and 100 m). However, the creatine group did see significant improvement in scores on a biokinetic swim bench test (2×30-s trials with 10-min passive recovery between). In 2004, Ostojic [33] examined creatine supplementation in 20 teenage boy soccer players (16.6 ± 1.9 years). Players were given either a placebo or creatine monohydrate (3×10 g doses) for 7 days. Before and after the one-week protocol, all players underwent a battery of skill tests including a dribble test, sprint-power test, vertical jump test, and a shuttle-run test. The experimental creatine group showed significant improvements in all tests with the exception of the shuttle run, while the control group did not improve on any measure. The experimental group also reported no untoward side effects from the supplementation. Juhasz et al. [34] administered 4.5 g/day of creatine monohydrate for 5 days to 16 boys who were highly trained competitive swimmers (15.9 ± 1.6 years). They observed an increase in power output, improved maximal 100 m swim times, and decreased lactate levels.

13.3.1.2 Potential Negative Effects of Creatine Supplementation

Creatine has been in wide use since the early- to mid-1990s. During this time, concerns have arisen about potential negative side effects of creatine supplementation, such as impaired kidney and liver function, muscle dehydration and cramping, and gastrointestinal distress. There have been numerous clinical investigations researching these concerns. To date, there is little scientific evidence that creatine supplementation by healthy individuals in recommended dosages (e.g., 5 g/day) leads to any of these adverse effects [35–45]. However, as yet, beyond what has been reported in the literature cited above, there have been no studies investigating these or other potential negative effects on children or adolescents supplementing with creatine.

As noted earlier, creatine supplementation has an osmotic effect that pulls water into the muscle cell, increasing intracellular fluid volume, effectively causing water retention. This shift in water from the extracellular space can be a cause for concern if proper hydration is not maintained. A decreased amount of extracellular fluid reduces how much is available for normal body functions, particularly during exercise and environmental conditions that may compromise thermoregulatory capability of the body. This effect has also been anecdotally linked to an increased incidence of muscle strains and cramping. A study completed by Powers et al. [46] reported that the normal distribution of water in the body does not appear to change. While creatine supplementation did increase water retention (as measured by total body water), the ratio of the increased measures of intracellular and extracellular fluid were consistent with what was normally seen in persons not supplementing with creatine. Therefore, as long as adequate amounts of fluid are consumed, creatine supplementation does not appear to alter overall body hydration status as the increased intracellular fluid is matched by increased extracellular fluid. Additionally, research by Kreider and Greenwood in collegiate football and baseball populations have reported those individuals who were supplementing with creatine were no more likely to experience muscle cramping and strains than those who were not supplementing [39,40].

13.3.1.3 Views of Creatine Supplementation in Youth by National Organizations

The use of creatine is not banned by any prominent athletic authority or organization. However, many organizations have spoken out against the use of ergogenic supplements in general by children and adolescents. The most notable may be the position statement published by the National Federation of State High School Associations (NFHS) in 2012 [47], and the 2005 policy statement by the American Academy of Pediatrics' (AAP) Committee on Sports Medicine and Fitness [48], both of which discourage the use of supplements, not only in high school and youth sports and activities, but also in general by any adolescent unless medically warranted.

Conversely, while acknowledging that there is not a large body of literature regarding creatine supplementation and youth, the International Society of Sports Nutrition also states that there does not appear to be any evidence that demonstrates that creatine supplementation is harmful to adolescents. Their official position stand published in 2007 is that "younger athletes should consider a creatine supplement only if the following conditions are met:

1. The athlete is past puberty and is involved in serious/competitive training that may benefit from creatine supplementation;
2. The athlete is eating a well-balanced, performance-enhancing diet;
3. The athlete and his/her parents understand the truth concerning the effects of creatine supplementation;
4. The athlete's parents approve that their child takes the supplemental creatine;
5. Creatine supplementation can be supervised by the athlete's parents, trainers, coaches and/or physician;
6. Quality supplements are used; and
7. The athlete does not exceed the recommended dosages."

13.3.2 Caffeine

Caffeine is a natural organic substance found in many types of plants, such as coffee, leaves (tea), and cocoa. Caffeine can also be produced synthetically and is added to many products, such as soft drinks, various snacks, and most recently, energy drinks. It has been approximated that 80%–90%

TABLE 13.3
Ergogenic and Nonergogenic Outcomes of Caffeine Use

Ergogenic Outcomes of Caffeine Use
- Increased aerobic capacity
- Increased work capacity
- Increased power output
- Increased muscular endurance
- Increased fat oxidation
- Improved mood
- Improved concentration and focus
- Decreased rate of fatigue
- Decreased rating of perceived exertion (RPE)

Nonergogenic Outcomes of Caffeine Use
- Increased resting heart rate
- Increased resting blood pressure
- Increased resting blood flow
- Sleeplessness

of Americans consume caffeine with the majority of this consumption being in beverage form (i.e., coffee, tea, soft drinks, etc.) [49]. Caffeine is easily absorbed by the intestine after ingestion with an uptake of approximately 95% in dosages of up to 10 mg/kg body mass. Depending upon the source (food, beverage, or tablet), caffeine can reach peak serum levels in approximately 30–60 min with half-life levels ranging from 2 to 10 h. When consumed, caffeine generally has a stimulatory effect, leading to feelings of increased alertness and energy. Caffeine acts through numerous mechanisms, and because caffeine can cross most cellular membranes in the body, including those in the CNS, all organs, and muscle, it is difficult to determine exactly how much of a role any one mechanism may be playing when caffeine's influence is being felt.

From an ergogenic perspective, early research supported caffeine's ability to increase fatty acid utilization [50,51], although not all research supports these findings [52] (Table 13.3). Consequently, increasing fat oxidation could theoretically reduce the reliance of glucose during prolonged exercise, thus sparing glycogen stores, leaving them on reserve until the end of an exercise session or race to effectively delay fatigue and increase performance [53,54], but these findings are not universal [55]. While the literature is not conclusive, most of the research that does support caffeine as an ergogenic supplement has largely been conducted with endurance types of exercise and/or activity [56,57], while a smaller body of literature supports its use in some short-term, high-intensity activity [58,59].

Finally, caffeine is known to possess a mild diuretic effect, and therefore it is often recommended that one be cautious with caffeine intake during situations where hydration is of upmost importance (e.g., long-duration exercise, exercise in a hot/humid environment). While monitoring hydration status is very important during these types of instances, there appears to be little evidence that caffeine use at "normal" levels, for example, less than 250 mg (3.57 mg/kg for a 70-kg athlete) exacerbates dehydration or negatively alters fluid balance, while doses larger than 300 mg may have an acute diuretic effect (4.29 mg/kg for a 70-kg athlete) [60]. Whether or not regular caffeine use in child or adolescent athletes who are exercising in a hot and humid environment would synergistically operate to further challenge fluid balance and thermoregulation remains to be seen.

13.3.2.1 Caffeine Supplementation and Youth

Caffeine and its effects on exercise performance have been thoroughly researched for the past several decades. But, as with creatine, research looking specifically at caffeine's potential to be an ergogenic with children and adolescents is limited [61]. Possibly the earliest known exercise study on caffeine and children was conducted in 1982 by Barta et al. [62], who reported differences in caffeine's effect (4 mg/kg) on free-fatty acid, glucose, and lactate levels in obese (n = 16) and nonobese (n = 6) children prior to and following a 4-min bout of aerobic stepping exercise. The nonobese group had a higher free-fatty acid level both at rest and after the exercise when compared to the placebo session, although no differences were noted for glucose or lactate levels. The obese group experienced no differences on any measure.

Research on caffeine, children, and exercise then remained relatively rare until just after the turn of the century. In 2006, Turley [63] investigated the effects of caffeine (5 mg/kg) on measures of cardiovascular, metabolic, and respiratory responses during aerobic exercise in 52 children (7–9 years old, 26 boys and 26 girls). Heart rate (HR) was significantly lower in the caffeine group compared to the placebo group at rest and during the two stages of the cycle ergometer trial (25 and 50 W). Blood pressure (BP) was higher in the caffeine group when measured prior to exercise and during exercise, with the exception of the girls during the 50 W stage. VO_2 and respiratory exchange ratio (RER) were not different between groups or genders during exercise.

It has been suggested that children may be more sensitive to caffeine than their adult counterparts [64]. Turley et al. [65] examined this in relation to exercise in 2007 when they studied the physiological responses to caffeine between 26 boys (8.8 ± 0.7 years) and 26 young men (22.6 ± 2.9 years). All participants randomly completed two-cycle ergometer tests (before and during which HR, BP, VO_2, and RER were monitored), with one trial being a control (no caffeine) and the other the treatment (5 mg caffeine per kg body mass). Neither the boys nor the men experienced any change in VO_2 or RER due to the treatment, and BP response was similar as well. However, the boys did see a significant decrease in pre-exercise HR during the caffeine treatment session, while the men did not experience the same effect.

Turley and colleagues [66] again turned to caffeine and children in 2008 as they examined various exercise responses to different dosages of caffeine in 40 boys and girls (8.1 ± 0.8 years). The children were randomly assigned to one of four groups and received (1) no, (2) 1 mg/kg, (3) 3 mg/kg, or (4) 5 mg/kg caffeine. The researchers examined BP, HR, and RER during a staged VO_{2peak} cycle ergometer test. In brief, they found that while caffeine did increase pre-exercise BP, the differences from the placebo disappeared during exercise. Moreover, pre-exercise HR was lower in the caffeine groups compared to the placebo, although during exercise, HR did increase more in the 3 and 5 mg/kg groups. Finally, RER measured indicated no differences in substrate utilization during exercise among any of the groups.

More recently, the effects of caffeine on anaerobic performance in young boys were examined [67]. Twenty-four boys (8–10 years) were randomly assigned to either a placebo group or a treatment group (5 g/kg). All participants completed a static hand-grip test and a 30-s Wingate cycle ergometer test, four separate times. There were no observed differences between the two groups in hand-grip strength or in peak power as measured by the Wingate. However, the caffeine group did have a higher peak HR (190 ± 10 vs. 185 ± 10 bpm) and a higher average power output (180 ± 36 vs. 173 ± 28 W).

While caffeine is generally the most common active ingredient in energy drinks, numerous other ingredients are usually present as well. Ingredients such as sugar, taurine, and B12 are common, but amounts and their inclusion can vary widely between brands. This inconsistent nature of the exact ingredients and their amounts make it difficult to compare the ergogenic effect of one drink to another as there are simply too many variables to consider. However, research on the ergogenic effect of energy drinks is emerging. But as with most supplements, research on energy drinks, exercise, and adolescents remains limited, as most of the research on energy drinks and youth is focused on behavior or overall health [68–70].

Gwacham et al. [71] examined the effect of a low-calorie caffeine–taurine drink on repeated sprint performance in NCAA DI football players. Twenty participants (19.7 ± 1.8 years) completed two separate trials of the test (six, 35-m sprints with a 10-s rest between each). In one of the randomized trials, participants drank a placebo; in the other trial, they consumed a serving of the energy drink (11 g carbohydrate, 200 mg of taurine, 120 mg of caffeine plus numerous other ingredients). Analysis determined that there was no difference between the sprint time performances of the placebo or energy drink. However, the authors note that there was a significant interaction effect between regular caffeine use and the treatment, indicating that those who were not as habituated with caffeine were more likely to have an improved performance.

A similar study was conducted in 2012 by Astorino and colleagues [72], in which repeated sprint performance was evaluated in young female collegiate soccer players (19.5 ± 1.1 years). Fifteen participants completed two randomized trials of three sets of eight bouts of a modified t-test, which included forward, backward, and lateral running. The control session consisted of a placebo drink, while the treatment session consisted of 255 mL (1.3 mg/kg caffeine and 1 g of taurine) of an energy drink. No differences were evident between sessions in any measure, including sprint performance, rating of perceived exertion, or HR.

Overall, the limited research on energy drinks (irrespective of study participant's age) has demonstrated mixed results, with some studies showing slight improvement in endurance-related tests [73–77], while others have shown no effect in either aerobic- or anaerobic-related performance [73,78–80]. The limited research on caffeine and youth is mixed as well, and energy drinks and exercise performance research exclusively conducted with children and/or adolescents is still lacking.

13.3.2.2 Potential Negative Effects of Caffeine

Caffeine is no longer a substance banned by the World Anti-Doping Agency (WADA) or the International Olympic Committee (IOC) as it was removed from their lists in 2004. However, the National Collegiate Athletic Association (NCAA) still has a limit on its use (at levels above 15 μg/mL of urine), although the amount of caffeine needing to be consumed to reach this level is considerably high (e.g., 70-kg athlete drinking 6–7 cups of coffee [~9 mg/kg] 1 h prior to testing could potentially approach the limit). This allows for "normal" consumption of caffeinated beverages without risk of exceeding the limit.

While moderate doses of caffeine have been shown to be safe (e.g., 2.5 mg/kg body mass) in healthy adults, there does not appear to be a clear consensus regarding acceptable adolescent or pediatric dosages. Additionally, the safety of the consumption of energy drinks has yet to be determined [81]. This is likely due to the potential interactions of the numerous ingredients in addition to caffeine found in energy drinks, as well as the apparent proclivity for these types of drinks to be consumed in excess by youth. Some of the potential negative side effects of excessive caffeine use include, but are not limited to, light headedness, agitation, tremors, bloating, diarrhea, dehydration, impaired sleep, impaired motor control, and heart arrhythmias.

13.3.2.3 Views on Caffeine Use and Energy Drink Consumption in Youth by National Organizations

In recent years, there has been growing concern about the increase in energy drink consumption by youth. This is likely due to the potential for numerous health consequences when energy drinks are consumed in excess or in other inappropriate manners. While evidence is needed to link energy drink performance to any of these potential side effects, the impact of consuming caffeine and sugar in high amounts are linked to side effects such as restlessness, arrhythmias, and dental caries. More pointedly, the overall nutritional quality of such drinks is quite poor with many calories coming from sugar and little other nutritional contributions. From that fact alone, young athletes are encouraged to minimize their consumption of caffeine and other caffeine-containing drinks in favor of other food items that will better facilitate their adaptations to exercise training and biological growth and development.

Several organizations have spoken publicly about the need for further education about the potential risks of energy drink consumption by children and adolescents and strongly caution their use.

The most prominent again being the NFHS and ISSN, which both have position statements regarding energy drinks [82,83], and the AAP, which has published a clinical report on the topic [84].

13.3.3 PROTEIN

Other topics related to protein are discussed in greater detail in Chapter 4. This section will focus on the common dietary proteins used as dietary supplements: whey, casein, and soy. By using a food-first approach and consuming a well-balanced diet that offers adequate energy and macronutrients, athletes will likely achieve a dietary protein intake that will be adequate for maintenance of health, muscle building, tissue repair, and recovery. However, it should be accepted that instances will arise when protein supplements may be warranted (e.g., travel, lengthy events, busy schedules, need for convenience, etc.).

The two milk proteins, whey and casein, are the most popular protein supplements used in the United States. Approximately 20% of protein in bovine milk protein is whey while 80% is casein. Both proteins provide all of the nine essential amino acids, and are particularly high in the three branched-chain amino acids (BCAA), a group of specialized amino acids that comprise 33% of skeletal muscle protein, and may play an important role in muscle protein synthesis and maintenance [85,86].

In comparison to other forms of protein, whey protein is known to be a "fast" digesting protein. Faster digestion and absorption rates translate into sharper and faster increases in serum amino acid levels, which some research has translated into greater accretion of muscle protein when compared to casein [87–89]. In addition, whey protein has higher leucine content, an essential amino acid that evokes strong signals inside the muscle cell to stimulate protein synthesis [90,91]. Finally, compared to casein, whey contains several bioactive protein subfractions that may be important to overall health [92,93].

Whey is available in a variety of forms, the differences coming primarily from how they are processed. While the processing method does make some slight changes to the amino acid profile and macronutrient content, the differences are minor with more research being needed to determine if one protein type is superior to another. Whey protein concentrate (WPC) from a reputable company is generally 70%–85% protein (70–85 g of protein per 100 g of the final product). Concentrate forms of whey protein are very popular and the least expensive. Whey protein isolates are commonly greater than 90% protein. To yield an isolated product, concentrate forms are passed through either cross-flow microfiltration or ion exchange and fats and lactose are further removed. Ion exchange methods are known to reduce some of the healthy subfraction peptides from the protein. Hydrolyzed protein supplements will usually have a protein content similar to isolates (90%–95%), but the protein is "pre-digested" using a chemical or enzymatic process to break apart (hydrolyze) the original protein product. Hydrolyzed proteins are generally absorbed faster relative to other forms of whey. Whether this increased absorption rate is of any additional benefit to an athlete has not yet been determined.

In contrast, casein is often referred to as a "slow" protein due largely to the clotting or clumping that occurs to the protein upon mixing with acids in the stomach. This clumping slows the digestion and absorption speed and promotes a slower rise in serum amino acid levels as compared with whey. Casein is often marketed as a "sustained-release" protein, meaning that the amino acids do not rise and fall rapidly in the system, but rather are released at a slow, steady pace over a period of several hours, providing the muscles with a continual supply of amino acids. Owing to its slightly lower leucine content and slower release time, casein may have a more "anticatabolic" effect than whey, which is more likely to have an "anabolic" effect on skeletal muscle [87]. Casein is also available in a variety of forms: micellar, caseinates, and hydrolysate. Micellar casein is typically found in the best-selling casein powders and typically contains 80% protein by weight. Caseinates are another form of casein and are usually in the forms of calcium, potassium, or sodium caseinates. They too are approximately 80% protein, but unlike micellar casein, caseinates are produced via a high-temperature ultrafiltration process that alters the protein structure and makes them more soluble. As a result, caseinates are easier to mix in fluids and for this reason are commonly used in protein powders, bars, shakes, etc. These differences are important as micellar casein retains the slow rate of assimilation inside the body and may better operate as a slow-digestion and anticatabolic protein.

Soy protein is derived from the soybean plant and like whey and casein provides all of the essential amino acids. Research using soy has indicated it can be as effective as whey in promoting lean muscle tissue and strength gains when used in conjunction with resistance training [94,95], although not all research is in agreement [96,97]. Soy is also considered a "fast" protein with digestion and absorption rates typically faster than casein [98]. Since soy is a plant-based protein, it is often a primary choice for athletes who follow a vegan diet or have allergies to milk-based proteins. The isoflavones found in soy appear to have the potential to provide certain health benefits. Genistein and daidzein have both been associated with reduced risk of some cancers [99], and daidzein alone is thought to promote bone health [100]. In addition, research has indicated that the isoflavones may also improve cardiovascular health profiles [101,102]. The isoflavones are also phytoestrogens, which has led to some concern about potential negative health outcomes, particularly in males. However, when soy consumption does not exceed recommended amounts, there does not appear to be any deleterious effects on blood concentrations of sex hormones [103,104]. Soy is available in various forms, much like whey and casein, with concentrates and isolates being among the most commonly used. Concentrates are typically 70%–80% protein by weight, low in fat and relatively high in fiber; however, the processing steps to produce a concentrate often removes most health-promoting isoflavones. Soy isolates are typically 80%–90% protein by weight and due to processing are void of sugars and fibers making them fast-digesting. The isoflavone content is largely retained in isolates giving them higher isoflavone levels than concentrates, but less than soybeans.

13.4 CONSIDERATIONS FOR CHOOSING A DIETARY SUPPLEMENT

A primary concern with taking dietary supplements is the safety of the product. Several instances can be referenced in which consumers have inadvertently put themselves at risk by consuming products that were tainted with potential harmful ingredients that were not listed on the label. Possibly one of the best-known examples of this occurred in 2009, when the online supplement retailer Bodybuilding.com, working in conjunction with the FDA, conducted a voluntary recall of 65 supplements that were believed to be tainted with illegal steroids [105].

In other instances, athletes have taken supplements under the presumption that all of the listed ingredients were allowable by their sporting organization, only to discover they had used a product that contained a banned ingredient. In 2011, a Grand Valley State football player was suspended for five games after a drug test revealed he had taken the stimulant methylhexaneamine (1,3-dimethylamylamine), a substance banned by the NCAA. This stimulant was an ingredient in a pre-workout supplement that the player had been taking, unaware that it was a banned substance [106]. Since the time of this occurrence, the FDA has removed this stimulant from the market due to safety concerns [107]. A year later, in 2012, 10 Menomonie, Wisconsin high school football players were suspended for three games for consuming a pre-workout product that contained synephrine, a stimulant banned for use by many sport governing bodies, including the Wisconsin Interscholastic Athletic Association [108]. In both of these instances, the ingredients in question were included on the product's label. The issue, it appears, was that because the supplements were available to purchase over-the-counter, the athletes assumed that they were acceptable to use.

In the United States, dietary supplements are regulated by the Food and Drug Administration (FDA) under the Dietary Supplement and Health Education Act of 1994 (DSHEA) [2]. Oversight of supplement advertising is conducted by the Federal Trade Commission (FTC). Under DSHEA, manufacturers do not need FDA approval prior to the production and or marketing of the dietary supplements. Although DSHEA does stipulate that companies must ensure the labeling of products is accurate, manufacturers are allowed to make claims about their product that go beyond the limited structure/function claims allowed on food products, as long as the label includes a disclaimer that the statements have not been evaluated by the FDA and that the product is not intended to "diagnose, treat, cure, or prevent any disease" [109].

The primary role and responsibilities of the FDA and FTC lies in the post-marketing of the product: the monitoring of the labeling, claims, and advertising accompanying the supplements. In addition, they respond to any health concerns associated with a product. This is essentially a passive and reactive process as the FDA relies on reports from the public regarding adverse effects of a product [110]. Consumers are encouraged to report product concerns to the FDA either by talking to their health professional, who can help fill out and submit the adverse event form, or by contacting the FDA directly and submitting the report themselves, via phone, mail, or online submission. The adverse event reporting form and instructions for completion and submission are available to the public on the FDA website [109].

Once multiple reports indicating possible health issues have been received, the FDA will begin a review process examining the reported concerns and the potential of the product to cause harm to consumers. The review can lead to a wide range of regulatory actions, from requiring that warning labels be added to the product in question up to the removal of the product from the market. The recall of supplements containing ephedra and the subsequent banning of the sale of ephedra and/or ephedra alkaloids is perhaps the best-known example of this regulatory process. Ephedra alkaloids had been a very popular ingredient in supplements sold primarily to enhance weight loss, increase energy, and/or enhance athletic performance. The FDA received numerous adverse event reports about these products, ranging from mild to serious, including some instances of death. An extensive review process was completed and it ultimately led to ephedra alkaloids being banned from use in the United States in 2004 [111].

13.4.1 Good Manufacturing Practices and Third-Party Testing

To address concerns about the quality of dietary supplements, the FDA announced in 2007 a ruling that established current good manufacturing practices (cGMPs) requirements for dietary supplements. In brief, the ruling requires that manufacturers "evaluate the identity, purity, quality, strength, and composition of dietary supplements" [112]. The intent is to establish high levels of quality control within the industry in order to protect consumers from substandard products that could potentially be harmful. By 2010, all manufacturers of dietary supplements were required to be in compliance with the regulations. It should be noted that GMPs are intended only to try to ensure that a product actually is what it claims to be, that it is free of contaminants, and that it is safe when used as directed. In other words, GMPs do not address the efficacy of a product. GMPs effectively provide a level of government oversight in the production of dietary supplements. It still remains that the manufacturers themselves are responsible for ensuring that their facilities and production processes meet GMP standards. In order to address this concern, the FDA and the U.S. Anti-Doping Agency (USADA) both encourage consumers to consider products that have been certified or verified via third-party testing [113,114].

Third-party testing is a voluntary process in which manufacturers of dietary supplements submit a product or products to an independent organization for testing and verification. While the level of verification processes vary, these organizations generally test products to make sure that the supplement contains the ingredients listed on the label and in the reported amounts, that the product is free of ingredients not listed on the label, and that there are no contaminants present. Some third-party organizations also inspect the manufacturing plants themselves to make sure that they meet GMP standards as well as review the companies who supply the supplement manufacturer with ingredients. Once a product has passed the given tests, it will be verified or certified by the third-party organization. This will generally be indicated on the product itself by means of a verification symbol or label.

While there are several third-party testing companies that examine all varieties of dietary supplements, some have developed certification programs specifically for sports-oriented supplements. The primary goal of these programs is to ensure that a supplement is not contaminated with an ingredient or substance that is banned by an athletic authority (e.g., WADA, USADA, IOC, NCAA). To date, the most prominent of these organizations are NSF's Certified for Sport, Informed Choice, and Banned Substance Control Group. Information about each of these organizations, their testing procedures, and which products meet their certification standards can be found at their respective websites, the addresses of which can be found below.

Finally, certain resources are available for parents, coaches, athletes, trainers, and any other individuals seeking information about dietary supplements. While the majority of these resources were developed for the collegiate athlete, approximately two-thirds of college athletes who use dietary supplements began using supplements while in high school or middle school [115]. Consequently, the resources found in Sidebar 13.1 may be of benefit to younger athletes, their parents, and coaches, who are interested in competing beyond high school or who may simply wish to further their own education about the topic.

SIDEBAR 13.1   SELECTED DIETARY SUPPLEMENT RESOURCES

ACSM's and USADA's Professionals Against Doping in Sports (PADS)

http://www.nodope.org/
A joint effort by these two associations with an aim to establish ethical principles regarding drug and supplement use in sports.

ATLAS and ATHENA

http://www.atlasathena.org
Athletes Training and Learning to Avoid Steroids (ATLAS)
Athletes Targeting Healthy Exercise and Nutrition Alternatives (ATHENA)
Developed by Oregon Health & Science University, these are gender-specific, health promotion, and substance abuse programs for high school athletic teams. Athletes are taught about sports nutrition and strength training, as well as educated about the effects of steroids, alcohol, supplements, and illicit drugs on athletic performance.

Banned Substances Control Group

http://www.bscg.org
A third-party, quality assurance program for sports supplements.

Drug Free Sport's Resource Exchange Center

http://www.drugfreesport.com/rec/rec-home.asp
This is an online service developed to provide athletes, coaches, and sport organizations information and educational resources regarding dietary supplements and banned substances.

FDA's MedWatch

http://www.fda.gov/Safety/MedWatch/
The online safety information and adverse event reporting program for dietary supplements and medical products.

Informed Choice

http://www.informed-choice.org/
A third-party, quality assurance program for sports supplements.

NSF Certified for Sport
http://www.nsfsport.com/
A third-party, quality assurance program for sports supplements.

USADA's Supplement 411
http://www.usada.org/supplement411
This site provides athletes, parents, and coaches information regarding supplement use, how to reduce the risk of taking a harmful supplement, and how to make an informed decision in choosing a dietary supplement.

13.5 CONCLUSIONS

Dietary supplement sales continue to be on an upward trend in the United States with no signs of this trend changing in coming years. Supplements specifically taken for their potential ergogenic effect comprise a substantial portion of these sales. While generally well-researched in the adult population, the literature on the efficacy of ergogenic supplements with young athletes is limited at this time. Although optimum performance can likely be achieved with a "food-first" approach, and despite the paucity of research, surveys indicate that these types of supplements are being used by many young athletes, with creatine, energy drinks, and protein supplements being among the most commonly consumed.

The oversight of the production of dietary supplements by the FDA is limited and action concerning potential adverse health effects is largely reactive. Several prominent associations have either discouraged the complete use of some of these supplements or have at least cautioned in their use, largely due to safety concerns. To address some of these concerns, the USADA and other organizations have developed resources for parents, coaches, and athletes, to further educate them about potential benefits and risks of using dietary supplements.

REFERENCES

1. Nutrition Business Journal. NBJ's supplement business report 2015. *Nutr Bus J*, Penton Media, Inc., 2015.
2. Federal Drug Administration. Dietary Supplement Health and Education Act of 1994.
3. Fink, H.H., A.E. Mikesky, and L.A. Burgoon, *Practical Applications in Sports Nutrition*. 3rd ed., 2012, Burlington, MA: Jones & Bartlett Learning.
4. Smith, J. and D.L. Dahm, Creatine use among a select population of high school athletes. *Mayo Clin Proc*, 2000. 75(12): p. 1257–63.
5. Metzl, J.D. et al., Creatine use among young athletes. *Pediatrics*, 2001. 108(2): p. 421–5.
6. Kayton, S. et al., Supplement and ergogenic aid use by competitive male and female high school athletes. *Med Sci Sports Exerc*, 2002. 34(5): p. S193.
7. O'Dea, J., Consumption of nutritional supplements among adolescents: Usage and perceived benefits. *Health Educ Res*, 2003. 18: p. 98–107.
8. Bell, A. et al., A look at nutritional supplement use in adolescents. *J Adolesc Health*, 2004. 34(6): p. 508–16.
9. Hoffman, J. et al., Nutritional supplementation and anabolic steroid use in adolescents. *Med Sci Sports Exerc*, 2008. 40: p. 15–24.
10. Petroczi, A. et al., Nutritional supplement use by elite young UK athletes: Fallacies of advice regarding efficacy. *J Int Soc Sports Nutr*, 2008. 5(1): p. 22.
11. Diehl, K. et al., Elite adolescent athletes' use of dietary supplements: Characteristics, opinions, and sources of supply and information. *Int J Sport Nutr Exerc Metab*, 2012. 22(3): p. 165–74.
12. Evans, M.W., Jr. et al., Dietary supplement use by children and adolescents in the United States to enhance sport performance: Results of the National Health Interview Survey. *J Prim Prev*, 2012. 33(1): p. 3–12.
13. Balsom, P.D., K. Soderlund, and B. Ekblom, Creatine in humans with special reference to creatine supplementation. *Sports Med*, 1994. 18(4): p. 268–80.

14. Lukaszuk, J.M. et al., Effect of a defined lacto-ovo-vegetarian diet and oral creatine monohydrate supplementation on plasma creatine concentration. *J Strength Cond Res*, 2005. 19(4): p. 735–40.
15. Syrotuik, D.G. and G.J. Bell, Acute creatine monohydrate supplementation: A descriptive physiological profile of responders vs. nonresponders. *J Strength Cond Res*, 2004. 18(3): p. 610–7.
16. Wyss, M. and R. Kaddurah-Daouk, Creatine and creatinine metabolism. *Physiol Rev*, 2000. 80(3): p. 1107–213.
17. Hultman, E. et al., Energy metabolism and fatigue during intense muscle contraction. *Biochem Soc Trans*, 1991. 19(2): p. 347–53.
18. Harris, R.C., K. Soderlund, and E. Hultman, Elevation of creatine in resting and exercised muscle of normal subjects by creatine supplementation. *Clin Sci (Lond)*, 1992. 83(3): p. 367–74.
19. Greenhaff, P.L., Creatine supplementation: Recent developments. *Br J Sports Med*, 1996. 30(4): p. 276–7.
20. Hultman, E. et al., Muscle creatine loading in men. *J Appl Physiol*, 1996. 81(1): p. 232–7.
21. Lehmkuhl, M. et al., The effects of 8 weeks of creatine monohydrate and glutamine supplementation on body composition and performance measures. *J Strength Cond Res*, 2003. 17(3): p. 425–38.
22. Branch, J.D., Effect of creatine supplementation on body composition and performance: A meta-analysis. *Int J Sport Nutr Exerc Metab*, 2003. 13(2): p. 198–226.
23. Bemben, M.G. and H.S. Lamont, Creatine supplementation and exercise performance: Recent findings. *Sports Med*, 2005. 35(2): p. 107–25.
24. Cooper, R. et al., Creatine supplementation with specific view to exercise/sports performance: An update. *J Int Soc Sports Nutr*, 2012. 9(1): p. 33.
25. Haussinger, D. et al., Cellular hydration state: An important determinant of protein catabolism in health and disease. *Lancet*, 1993. 341(8856): p. 1330–2.
26. Berneis, K. et al., Effects of hyper- and hypoosmolality on whole body protein and glucose kinetics in humans. *Am J Physiol*, 1999. 276(1 Pt 1): p. E188–95.
27. Stockler, S., F. Hanefeld, and J. Frahm, Creatine replacement therapy in guanidinoacetate methyltransferase deficiency, a novel inborn error of metabolism. *Lancet*, 1996. 348(9030): p. 789–90.
28. Tarnopolsky, M.A. et al., Creatine monohydrate enhances strength and body composition in Duchenne muscular dystrophy. *Neurology*, 2004. 62(10): p. 1771–7.
29. Bourgeois, J.M. et al., Creatine monohydrate attenuates body fat accumulation in children with acute lymphoblastic leukemia during maintenance chemotherapy. *Pediatr Blood Cancer*, 2008. 51(2): p. 183–7.
30. Sakellaris, G. et al., Prevention of traumatic headache, dizziness and fatigue with creatine administration. A pilot study. *Acta Paediatr*, 2008. 97(1): p. 31–4.
31. Grindstaff, P.D. et al., Effects of creatine supplementation on repetitive sprint performance and body composition in competitive swimmers. *Int J Sport Nutr*, 1997. 7(4): p. 330–46.
32. Dawson, B., T. Vladich, and B.A. Blanksby, Effects of 4 weeks of creatine supplementation in junior swimmers on freestyle sprint and swim bench performance. *J Strength Cond Res*, 2002. 16(4): p. 485–90.
33. Ostojic, S.M., Creatine supplementation in young soccer players. *Int J Sport Nutr Exerc Metab*, 2004. 14(1): p. 95–103.
34. Juhasz, I. et al., Creatine supplementation improves the anaerobic performance of elite junior fin swimmers. *Acta Physiol Hung*, 2009. 96(3): p. 325–36.
35. Kreider, R.B. et al., Long-term creatine supplementation does not significantly affect clinical markers of health in athletes. *Mol Cell Biochem*, 2003. 244(1–2): p. 95–104.
36. Gualano, B. et al., Effects of creatine supplementation on renal function: A randomized, double-blind, placebo-controlled clinical trial. *Eur J Appl Physiol*, 2008. 103(1): p. 33–40.
37. Kim, H.J. et al., Studies on the safety of creatine supplementation. *Amino Acids*, 2011. 40(5): p. 1409–18.
38. Lugaresi, R. et al., Does long-term creatine supplementation impair kidney function in resistance-trained individuals consuming a high-protein diet? *J Int Soc Sports Nutr*, 2013. 10(1): p. 26.
39. Greenwood, M. et al., Cramping and injury incidence in collegiate football players are reduced by creatine supplementation. *J Athl Train*, 2003. 38(3): p. 216–9.
40. Greenwood, M. et al., Creatine supplementation during college football training does not increase the incidence of cramping or injury. *Mol Cell Biochem*, 2003. 244(1–2): p. 83–8.
41. Gualano, B. et al., Creatine supplementation does not impair kidney function in type 2 diabetic patients: A randomized, double-blind, placebo-controlled, clinical trial. *Eur J Appl Physiol*, 2011. 111(5): p. 749–56.
42. Gualano, B. et al., Effect of short-term high-dose creatine supplementation on measured GFR in a young man with a single kidney. *Am J Kidney Dis*, 2010. 55(3): p. e7–9.

43. Mayhew, D.L., J.L. Mayhew, and J.S. Ware, Effects of long-term creatine supplementation on liver and kidney functions in American college football players. *Int J Sport Nutr Exerc Metab*, 2002. 12(4): p. 453–60.
44. Neves, M., Jr. et al., Effect of creatine supplementation on measured glomerular filtration rate in postmenopausal women. *Appl Physiol Nutr Metab*, 2011. 36(3): p. 419–22.
45. Taes, Y.E. et al., Creatine supplementation does not affect kidney function in an animal model with pre-existing renal failure. *Nephrol Dial Transplant*, 2003. 18(2): p. 258–64.
46. Powers, M. E. et al., Creatine supplementation increases total body water without altering fluid distribution. *J Athl Train*, 2003. 38(1): p. 44–50.
47. Supplements Position Statement, 2012, National Federation of State High School Associations Sports Medicine Advisory Committee.
48. Committee on Sports Medicine and Fitness, Use of performance-enhancing substances. *Pediatrics*, 2005. 115(4): p. 1103–6.
49. Somogyi, L. P., Caffeine Intake by the U.S. Population. 2012. Available from: http://www.fda.gov/downloads/AboutFDA/CentersOffices/OfficeofFoods/CFSAN/CFSANFOIAElectronicReadingRoom/UCM333191.pdf.
50. Costill, D.L., G.P. Dalsky, and W.J. Fink, Effects of caffeine ingestion on metabolism and exercise performance. *Med Sci Sports*, 1978. 10(3): p. 155–8.
51. Ivy, J.L. et al., Influence of caffeine and carbohydrate feedings on endurance performance. *Med Sci Sports*, 1979. 11(1): p. 6–11.
52. Graham, T.E. et al., Does caffeine alter muscle carbohydrate and fat metabolism during exercise? *Appl Physiol Nutr Metab*, 2008. 33(6): p. 1311–8.
53. Erickson, M.A., R.J. Schwarzkopf, and R.D. McKenzie, Effects of caffeine, fructose, and glucose ingestion on muscle glycogen utilization during exercise. *Med Sci Sports Exerc*, 1987. 19(6): p. 579–83.
54. Spriet, L.L. et al., Caffeine ingestion and muscle metabolism during prolonged exercise in humans. *Am J Physiol*, 1992. 262(6 Pt 1): p. E891–8.
55. Laurent, D. et al., Effects of caffeine on muscle glycogen utilization and the neuroendocrine axis during exercise. *J Clin Endocrinol Metab*, 2000. 85(6): p. 2170–5.
56. Ganio, M.S. et al., Effect of caffeine on sport-specific endurance performance: A systematic review. *J Strength Cond Res*, 2009. 23(1): p. 315–24.
57. Warren, G.L. et al., Effect of caffeine ingestion on muscular strength and endurance: A meta-analysis. *Med Sci Sports Exerc*, 2010. 42(7): p. 1375–87.
58. Woolf, K., W.K. Bidwell, and A.G. Carlson, The effect of caffeine as an ergogenic aid in anaerobic exercise. *Int J Sport Nutr Exerc Metab*, 2008. 18(4): p. 412–29.
59. Astorino, T.A. et al., Minimal effect of acute caffeine ingestion on intense resistance training performance. *J Strength Cond Res*, 2011. 25(6): p. 1752–8.
60. Maughan, R.J. and J. Griffin, Caffeine ingestion and fluid balance: A review. *J Hum Nutr Diet*, 2003. 16(6): p. 411–20.
61. Temple, J.L., Caffeine use in children: What we know, what we have left to learn, and why we should worry. *Neurosci Biobehav Rev*, 2009. 33(6): p. 793–806.
62. Barta, L. et al., The effect of caffeine and physical exercise on blood lactate levels of obese children. *Acta Paediatr Acad Sci Hung*, 1982. 23(3): p. 343–7.
63. Turley, K.R. and J.W. Gerst, Effects of caffeine on physiological responses to exercise in young boys and girls. *Med Sci Sports Exerc*, 2006. 38(3): p. 520–6.
64. Nehlig, A., J.L. Daval, and G. Debry, Caffeine and the central nervous system: Mechanisms of action, biochemical, metabolic and psychostimulant effects. *Brain Res Brain Res Rev*, 1992. 17(2): p. 139–70.
65. Turley, K.R., T. Desisso, and J.W. Gerst, Effects of caffeine on physiological responses to exercise: Boys versus men. *Pediatr Exerc Sci*, 2007. 19(4): p. 481–92.
66. Turley, K.R., J.R. Bland, and W.J. Evans, Effects of different doses of caffeine on exercise responses in young children. *Med Sci Sports Exerc*, 2008. 40(5): p. 871–8.
67. Turley, K.R. et al., Effects of caffeine on anaerobic exercise in boys. *Pediatr Exerc Sci*, 2012. 24(2): p. 210–9.
68. Kaminer, Y., Problematic use of energy drinks by adolescents. *Child Adolesc Psychiatr Clin N Am*, 2010. 19(3): p. 643–50.
69. Seifert, S.M. et al., Health effects of energy drinks on children, adolescents, and young adults. *Pediatrics*, 2011. 127(3): p. 511–28.
70. Blankson, K.L. et al., Energy drinks: What teenagers (and their doctors) should know. *Pediatr Rev*, 2013. 34(2): p. 55–62.

71. Gwacham, N. and D.R. Wagner, Acute effects of a caffeine–taurine energy drink on repeated sprint performance of American college football players. *Int J Sport Nutr Exerc Metab*, 2012. 22(2): p. 109–16.
72. Astorino, T.A. et al., Effects of Red Bull energy drink on repeated sprint performance in women athletes. *Amino Acids*, 2012. 42(5): p. 1803–8.
73. Forbes, S.C. et al., Effect of Red Bull energy drink on repeated Wingate cycle performance and bench-press muscle endurance. *Int J Sport Nutr Exerc Metab*, 2007. 17(5): p. 433–44.
74. Ivy, J.L. et al. Improved cycling time-trial performance after ingestion of a caffeine energy drink. *Int J Sport Nutr Exerc Metab*, 2009. 19(1): p. 61–78.
75. Rahnama, N., A.A. Gaeini, and F. Kazemi, The effectiveness of two energy drinks on selected indices of maximal cardiorespiratory fitness and blood lactate levels in male athletes. *J Res Med Sci*, 2010. 15(3): p. 127–32.
76. Del Coso, J. et al., Effects of a caffeine-containing energy drink on simulated soccer performance. *PLoS One*, 2012. 7(2): p. e31380.
77. Duncan, M.J. et al., The acute effect of a caffeine-containing energy drink on mood state, readiness to invest effort, and resistance exercise to failure. *J Strength Cond Res*, 2012. 26(10): p. 2858–65.
78. Candow, D.G. et al., Effect of sugar-free Red Bull energy drink on high-intensity run time-to-exhaustion in young adults. *J Strength Cond Res*, 2009. 23(4): p. 1271–5.
79. Eckerson, J.M. et al., Acute ingestion of sugar-free Red Bull energy drink has no effect on upper body strength and muscular endurance in resistance trained men. *J Strength Cond Res*, 2013. 27(8): p. 2248–54.
80. Pettitt, R.W. et al., Do the noncaffeine ingredients of energy drinks affect metabolic responses to heavy exercise? *J Strength Cond Res*, 2013. 27(7): p. 1994–9.
81. Higgins, J.P., T.D. Tuttle, and C.L. Higgins, Energy beverages: Content and safety. *Mayo Clin Proc*, 2010. 85(11): p. 1033–41.
82. National Federation of State High School Associations Sports Medicine Advisory Committee, 2012. Position Statement and Recommendations for the Use of Energy Drinks by Young Athletes.
83. Campbell, B. et al., International Society of Sports Nutrition position stand: Energy drinks. *J Int Soc Sports Nutr*, 2013. 10(1): p. 1.
84. Committee on Nutrition and the Council on Sports Medicine and Fitness, Sports drinks and energy drinks for children and adolescents: Are they appropriate? *Pediatrics*, 2011. 127(6): p. 1182–9.
85. Louard, R.J., E.J. Barrett, and R.A. Gelfand, Effect of infused branched-chain amino acids on muscle and whole-body amino acid metabolism in man. *Clin Sci (Lond)*, 1990. 79(5): p. 457–66.
86. Blomstrand, E. and E.A. Newsholme, Effect of branched-chain amino acid supplementation on the exercise-induced change in aromatic amino acid concentration in human muscle. *Acta Physiol Scand*, 1992. 146(3): p. 293–8.
87. Boirie, Y. et al., Slow and fast dietary proteins differently modulate postprandial protein accretion. *Proc Natl Acad Sci U S A*, 1997. 94(26): p. 14930–5.
88. Dangin, M. et al., The digestion rate of protein is an independent regulating factor of postprandial protein retention. *Am J Physiol Endocrinol Metab*, 2001. 280(2): p. E340–8.
89. Pennings, B. et al., Whey protein stimulates postprandial muscle protein accretion more effectively than do casein and casein hydrolysate in older men. *Am J Clin Nutr*, 2011. 93(5): p. 997–1005.
90. Kimball, S.R. and L.S. Jefferson, Signaling pathways and molecular mechanisms through which branched-chain amino acids mediate translational control of protein synthesis. *J Nutr*, 2006. 136(1 Suppl): p. 227S–31S.
91. Burd, N.A. et al., Greater stimulation of myofibrillar protein synthesis with ingestion of whey protein isolate v. *micellar casein at rest and after resistance exercise in elderly men*. *Br J Nutr*, 2012. 108(6): p. 958–62.
92. Walzem, R.L., C.J. Dillard, and J.B. German, Whey components: Millennia of evolution create functionalities for mammalian nutrition: What we know and what we may be overlooking. *Crit Rev Food Sci Nutr*, 2002. 42(4): p. 353–75.
93. Krissansen, G.W., Emerging health properties of whey proteins and their clinical implications. *J Am Coll Nutr*, 2007. 26(6): p. 713S–23S.
94. Brown, E. et al., Soy versus whey protein bars: Effects on exercise training impact on lean body mass and antioxidant status. *Nutr J*, 2004. 3(1): p. 22.
95. Candow, D.G. et al., Effect of whey and soy protein supplementation combined with resistance training in young adults. *Int J Sport Nutr Exerc Metab*, 2006. 16(3): p. 233–44.
96. Wilkinson, S.B. et al., Consumption of fluid skim milk promotes greater muscle protein accretion after resistance exercise than does consumption of an isonitrogenous and isoenergetic soy-protein beverage. *Am J Clin Nutr*, 2007. 85(4): p. 1031–40.

97. Tang, J.E. et al., Ingestion of whey hydrolysate, casein, or soy protein isolate: Effects on mixed muscle protein synthesis at rest and following resistance exercise in young men. *J Appl Physiol*, 2009. 107(3): p. 987–92.
98. Bos, C. et al., Postprandial kinetics of dietary amino acids are the main determinant of their metabolism after soy or milk protein ingestion in humans. *J Nutr*, 2003. 133(5): p. 1308–15.
99. Xu, X. et al., Effects of soy isoflavones on estrogen and phytoestrogen metabolism in premenopausal women. *Cancer Epidemiol Biomarkers Prev*, 1998. 7(12): p. 1101–8.
100. Uehara, M., Isoflavone metabolism and bone-sparing effects of daidzein-metabolites. *J Clin Biochem Nutr*, 2013. 52(3): p. 193–201.
101. Zhan, S. and S.C. Ho, Meta-analysis of the effects of soy protein containing isoflavones on the lipid profile. *Am J Clin Nutr*, 2005. 81(2): p. 397–408.
102. Reynolds, K. et al., A meta-analysis of the effect of soy protein supplementation on serum lipids. *Am J Cardiol*, 2006. 98(5): p. 633–40.
103. Kurzer, M.S., Hormonal effects of soy in premenopausal women and men. *J Nutr*, 2002. 132(3): p. 570S–3S.
104. Munro, I.C. et al., Soy isoflavones: A safety review. *Nutr Rev*, 2003. 61(1): p. 1–33.
105. FDA, Bodybuilding.com Is Conducting a Voluntary Nationwide and International Recall of 65 Dietary Supplements That May Contain Steroids. 2009; Available from: http://www.fda.gov/safety/recalls/ucm188929.htm. Retrieved on February 16, 2016.
106. Zuidema, M., *Tough to Swallow: Banned Supplement has Grand Valley State Football Standout Sidelined*, The Grand Rapids Press, Grand Rapids, Michigan, 2011.
107. FDA, DMAA in Dietary Supplements. 2013; Available from: http://www.fda.gov/Food/DietarySupplements/ProductsIngredients/ucm346576.htm. Retrieved on February 16, 2016.
108. Hart, B. 10 MHS athletes suspended for consuming energy drink. The Dunn County News. 2012. Available from: http://chippewa.com/dunnconnect/news/local/mhs-athletes-suspended-for-consuming-energy-drink/article_bf21683e-cb79-11e1-bd1a-0019bb2963f4.html. Retrieved on March 12, 2016.
109. FDA, Structure/Function Claims, 1997, United States Food and Drug Administration.
110. FDA, How Consumers Can Report an Adverse Event or Serious Problem to FDA. 1993; Available from: http://www.fda.gov/Safety/MedWatch/HowToReport/ucm053074.htm. Retrieved on February 16, 2016.
111. FDA, FDA Acts to Remove Ephedra-Containing Dietary Supplements from Market. 2004; Available from: http://www.fda.gov/NewsEvents/Newsroom/PressAnnouncements/2004/ucm108379.htm. Retrieved on February 16, 2016.
112. FDA, Current Good Manufacturing Practices (CGMPs) for Dietary Supplements. 2007; Available from: http://www.fda.gov/Drugs/DevelopmentApprovalProcess/Manufacturing/ucm090016.htm. Retrieved on February 16, 2016.
113. FDA, Voluntary Third-Party Certification Programs for Foods and Feeds. 2009; Available from: http://www.fda.gov/RegulatoryInformation/Guidances/ucm125431.htm. Retrieved on February 16, 2016.
114. USADA, Third Party Testing. 2012.
115. NCAA, R.S., NCAA Study of Substance Use Habits of College Student-Athletes. 2006.

14 Exercise Prescription and Strength and Conditioning Considerations

Adriana Coletta, Kyle Levers, Elfego Galvan, and Richard B. Kreider

CONTENTS

Abstract 240
14.1 Introduction 240
14.2 Cardiovascular Exercise 240
    14.2.1 General Benefits 240
    14.2.2 Guidelines to Promote General Fitness 241
        14.2.2.1 Type of Activity 241
        14.2.2.2 Intensity 241
        14.2.2.3 Frequency and Duration 242
        14.2.2.4 Progression of Activities 242
    14.2.3 Advanced Training Guidelines for Performance 243
        14.2.3.1 Aerobic Conditioning and Power 243
        14.2.3.2 Type of Activity 244
        14.2.3.3 Intensity 244
        14.2.3.4 Frequency and Duration 245
        14.2.3.5 Progression of Activities 245
14.3 Muscular Strength and Endurance 246
    14.3.1 General Benefits 247
        14.3.1.1 Special Considerations 248
    14.3.2 Guidelines to Promote General Fitness 248
        14.3.2.1 Type of Activity 248
        14.3.2.2 Intensity and Volume 249
        14.3.2.3 Duration and Frequency 251
        14.3.2.4 Progression of Activities 251
    14.3.3 Advanced Training Guidelines 252
        14.3.3.1 Intensity and Volume 252
        14.3.3.2 Duration and Frequency 253
        14.3.3.3 Progression of Activities 253
14.4 Stretching and Flexibility 253
    14.4.1 General Benefits 253
    14.4.2 General Recommendations 254
    14.4.3 Special Considerations 255
14.5 Healthy Training for Performance 255
    14.5.1 Consequences of an Unhealthy Training Regimen 256
    14.5.2 Benefits of a Healthy Training Regimen 257
    14.5.3 Considerations for a Healthy Training Regimen 258
References 258

ABSTRACT

The popularity and number of young children and adolescents who are participating in formalized exercise training programs throughout the year continue to rise. While a multitude of physical, psychological, and emotional benefits can be derived, the need for a program to be properly developed is important. This chapter summarizes the recommended exercise training principles that should be followed by young athletes and those individuals who are coordinating and supervising the workouts. Guidelines for aerobic exercise are first introduced followed by resistance exercise and then stretching and flexibility. With proper prescription and progression of exercise, young athletes can safely train to further enhance a number of physical goals, which will aid in their development as well as their athletic performance.

14.1 INTRODUCTION

Initial recommendations for physical activity in school-aged children and adolescents were basic. Recommendations consisted primarily of encouraging children to participate in unstructured, spontaneous activity (Health 2001; Nettle and Sprogis 2011). Given the increased incidence of childhood obesity (Nettle and Sprogis 2011), more specific physical activity guidelines have been established to promote overall health/wellness and prevent early onset of disease secondary to obesity (i.e., type 2 diabetes, chronic heart failure, obstructive sleep apnea, and hypertension). Current guidelines for physical activity in school-aged children and adolescents are as follows: at least 60 minutes per day of cardiovascular activity, most days per week, at moderate to vigorous intensity, with muscle- and bone-strengthening activities 3 days per week within the 60-minute sessions of cardiovascular activity (Committee 2008).

While the increased incidence of childhood obesity is likely related to decrease in lifestyle and physical activity for the majority of the population, preadolescent and adolescent participation in organized sport has increased over time (Nettle and Sprogis 2011). This has prompted a growing pool of evidence for specific exercise guidelines to promote optimal sport performance, while still ensuring adequate growth and development. Specific exercise guidelines are now available for the youth athlete within the following areas: cardiovascular exercise, muscular strength and endurance, flexibility, body composition, and promotion of a healthy training regimen. The purpose of this chapter is to present a thorough review of exercise guidelines to promote general health and wellness, and athletic performance in school-aged children and adolescents. General nutritional guidelines to promote performance, growth, and development will also be discussed, as the topics of exercise and nutrition for optimal health and performance are often hand in hand. Table 14.1 explains general considerations for developing exercise prescription in youth and adolescents.

14.2 CARDIOVASCULAR EXERCISE

14.2.1 GENERAL BENEFITS

Developing healthy habits, including lifestyle and physical activity, as early as childhood improves the chance for the behavior to translate into adulthood, when significant chronic conditions may manifest themselves (Epstein et al. 2001). Engaging in cardiovascular exercise on a consistent basis reduces the risk of obesity, diabetes, hypertension, cardiovascular disease, and certain cancers, and improves biomarkers associated with adverse health events, such as the blood lipid profile (Candeias et al. 2010). Activity promoting cardiovascular health generally consists of modes of exercise easily accessible to the general public. The following section will review general guidelines and advanced training guidelines for cardiovascular exercise, including type of activity, frequency, duration, and recommended progression of activity.

TABLE 14.1
Considerations for Exercise Prescription in Youth and Adolescents

Area for Consideration	Rationale
Initial knowledge	Understanding aspects of aerobic and resistance training as it relates to overall fitness and athletic performance enhancement will enable appropriate selection of exercises.
Psychological maturity	Stage of maturity will enable appropriate selection of intensity, volume, and frequency of exercises within the individual or team training regimen. This will also allow one to select the best exercises given the team dynamic.
Physiological maturity	A direct relationship exists between developmental stage and athletic performance. Age should not be used as a primary indicator of athletic ability. The four developmental stages are as follows: 1. Early childhood: 0–7 years old 2. Prepubertal: 7–11 years for females and 7–12 years for males 3. Circumpubertal: 11–15 years for female, 12–15 years old for males 4. Late adolescence: 15+ and 16+ years of age for female and males, respectively (Stages 1 and 2 may also be referred to as prepubescent, while 3 and 4 are referred to as pubescent/postpubescent [Baquet et al. 2003])
Type of activity	Types of activities required by the sport will assist with selection of appropriate exercises to include in both the aerobic and resistance training regimens.
Movement analysis	Assist in identifying any biomechanical or structural deficiencies that may result in injury or obstruction of growth/development. Identification of deficiencies will also assist with appropriate selection of both aerobic and resistance training exercises.
Nutrition/diet	Analysis of diet is helpful to ensure adequate energy intake to promote training, performance, and adequate growth/development.

14.2.2 Guidelines to Promote General Fitness

14.2.2.1 Type of Activity

Assuming the exercise intensity, duration, and frequency among different types of cardiovascular exercises are consistent, when comparing the exercises, one type is not necessarily more advantageous than the other. The main objective of prescribing cardiovascular exercise in youth should be to promote enjoyment, while also gaining health and fitness/endurance benefits from appropriate physical challenge to the body. Development of positive attitudes about physical activity in children and adolescents can help establish a lifetime commitment to an active lifestyle. Conversely, negative attitudes about physical activity can develop in children and adolescents who participate in excessive training, competition, and/or if exercise is used as a form of punishment or discipline. It is also imperative to consider safety, effectiveness, and efficiency within the exercise selection. Examples of types of exercise that promote improvements in cardiovascular function include running, brisk walking, hiking, bicycling, jumping rope, swimming, rowing, and soccer.

14.2.2.2 Intensity

Most health benefits seem to be associated with exercise conducted at moderate-to-vigorous intensity levels (Ruiz et al. 2006). While it is known that exercise can improve various risk factors associated with the development of chronic disease, such as weight status, cardiovascular health, and insulin resistance (Rubin et al. 2008), if the exercise intensity is too low, the health and fitness benefits may be nonexistent.

Within the adult population, intensity is typically prescribed as a function of absolute heart rate (HR) or a percentage of maximal heart rate (HRmax). Within the pediatric population, absolute HR and HRmax measures can be highly variable between individuals (Baquet et al. 2003). Thus, measures of endurance exercise intensity via HR should not be used in prepubescent youth. However, HR measures have been validated for use in pubescent and postpubescent youth. Additionally, HR measures are typically used to measure intensity within more advanced cardiovascular/endurance training regimens.

When considering intensity levels for a general endurance/cardiovascular exercise regimen in youth, the Borg rating of perceived exertion scale (RPE) is a useful and more appropriate tool to use. RPE is defined as the reported degree of effort performed for a certain activity. For example, consider using a scale that ranges from zero to ten; zero will equal no exertion and ten will equal maximal exertion. Moderate-intensity physical activity will fall within the range of five or six, while vigorous-intensity physical activity will be classified as seven or eight (Nader et al. 2009).

Along with RPE, the pedometer is another tool that can be used to determine exercise intensity. Within investigations assessing a correlation between steps per day and exercise intensity in children and adolescents, it was determined that the lower range of moderate-intensity exercise for children is approximately 122 steps per minute (Tudor-Locke et al. 2011). Thus, the lower-range of moderate-intensity exercise is approximately 3600 steps in 30 minutes or about 7300 steps in 60 minutes. Along with this, vigorous-intensity exercise was calculated at approximately 150 steps per minute, which equates to approximately 4500 steps in 30 minutes and 9000 steps in 60 minutes (Tudor-Locke et al. 2011).

14.2.2.3 Frequency and Duration

In addition to exercise type and intensity, frequency (how often) and duration (length of time) should also be considered. Frequency of exercise is commonly expressed as the number of sessions or bouts per week, whereas duration is typically expressed in minutes per session. Once more, the current recommendation is to engage in exercise on most, preferably all days per week for an accumulation of 60 minutes or more per exercise bout (Organization 2010; Services 2008). Total time of exercise can be broken down into multiple exercise bouts throughout the day, with each bout lasting at least 20 minutes in length in order to gain endurance/cardiovascular benefits (Kreider et al. 2009b).

While the general recommendation encourages daily physical activity, some investigations suggest physical activity for at least 3 days per week to achieve general fitness and health benefits (Landry and Driscoll 2012; Nassis et al. 2005). Nassis and colleagues (2005) demonstrate significantly improved cardiorespiratory fitness, insulin sensitivity, and increased lower-limb fat-free mass after 12 weeks of cardiovascular exercise for only 3 days per week at 40 minutes per exercise bout in school-aged and adolescent females.

Along with this, Kimm and colleagues (2005) demonstrated increased prevalence of weight gain in adolescent girls participating in less than 30 minutes per day of exercise in comparison to those engaging in 60 minutes per day. Thus, the minimum requirements to achieve general health benefits and fitness appear to be no less than 40 total minutes per day, for at least 3 days per week. Furthermore, in order to improve endurance/fitness, each exercise bout should be held for at least 20 minutes.

14.2.2.4 Progression of Activities

When initiating the cardiovascular component of an exercise program in a relatively sedentary child or adolescent, it is important to introduce exercise gradually, in a stepwise fashion, with the eventual goal of meeting the general recommendation. It is imperative to remember that some physical activity, even if it does not initially meet the recommended guidelines, is better than no physical activity at all. Thus, if a child's current physical activity level is zero, then it would be appropriate to start off with 15–20 minutes of low-intensity exercise, 1–2 days per week. Duration, intensity, and frequency should increase gradually as the child's fitness levels and exercise tolerance improve. Table 14.2 provides an example of how to progress a cardiovascular/endurance exercise program in children and adolescents.

TABLE 14.2
Example of Progression of General Endurance/Cardiovascular Exercise Program in Children and Adolescents

Exercise Type	Intensity	Frequency (days per week)	Duration (min)
Preferred type per child preference and/or sport requirement	RPE of 5–6 (on Borg 10-point scale)	2–3	20
	RPE of 5–6 (on Borg 10-point scale)	3	20–30
	RPE of 5–6 (on Borg 10-point scale)	3–5	30–40
	RPE of 7–8 (on Borg 10-point scale)	3–5	30–40
	RPE of 7–8 (on Borg 10-point scale)	3–5	40–60
	RPE of 7–8 (on Borg 10-point scale)	5+	60+

14.2.3 Advanced Training Guidelines for Performance

Along with general guidelines for cardiovascular exercise to promote health and general fitness benefits, a specific set of guidelines has been created due to the increased prevalence in child and adolescent training and specialization in sport. Establishing a training regimen built upon the previously mentioned guidelines is necessary to provide health and fitness benefits while also improving athletic performance.

14.2.3.1 Aerobic Conditioning and Power

Obtaining a general understanding of the aerobic energy system, aerobic conditioning, and power may be helpful when developing the cardiovascular/endurance component of a training program. Briefly, aerobic activity is fueled by energy produced within the oxidative metabolic pathway (Stricker 2002). Primary energy sources metabolized within the oxidative pathway include carbohydrates and fats (Stricker 2002). Aerobic training increases the athlete's capacity to participate in endurance exercise and utilize fat as the primary fuel source as opposed to carbohydrate. Per gram, fat provides more energy in comparison to carbohydrates (9 kcal/g vs. 4 kcal/g).

Measuring cardiorespiratory fitness via maximal oxygen consumption, VO_2max, is the primary indicator of the effectiveness of an aerobic training regimen (Geithner et al. 2004; Stricker 2002). VO_2max measures the functionality and effectiveness of oxygen transport during aerobic exercise (Baquet et al. 2003). The ultimate goal of aerobic conditioning for performance is to increase VO_2max in a method applicable for the particular sport and athlete (Baquet et al. 2003).

VO_2max is also referred to as aerobic power and is measured as either an absolute value, in liters per minute (L/min), or relative value, milliliters per kilogram per minute (mL/kg/min). Several investigations have demonstrated a relationship between certain physiological parameters, such as cholesterol, fat mass, body fat percentage, peak growth velocity, and peak weight velocity, in relation to VO_2max during adolescence (Andersen and Haraldsdóttir 1994; Baquet et al. 2003; Geithner et al. 2004; Malina et al. 1995; Stricker 2002).

In healthy youth, absolute values of VO_2max increase with age, with no significant differences demonstrated between genders during the prepubescent period (Binkhorst et al. 1984; Krahenbuhl et al. 1985; Rutenfranz et al. 1981; Stricker 2002). Moreover, males exhibit higher absolute values of VO_2 in comparison to females at every age as depicted in Figure 14.1 (Geithner et al. 2004). Differences in VO_2 by gender has been further explained in multiple investigations such that relative VO_2max in males aged 8–16 years demonstrate a stable increase in oxygen consumption, while females experience a plateau and/or even slight decline in relative oxygen consumption after age 13 secondary to increases in fat mass from puberty (Armstrong and Welsman 1994; Geithner et al. 2004; Gumming et al. 1978; Krahenbuhl et al. 1985).

Additionally, in a longitudinal study conducted by Geithner and colleagues (2004), children and adolescents aged 10–18 years of both genders demonstrated increases in VO_2 correlated with increases

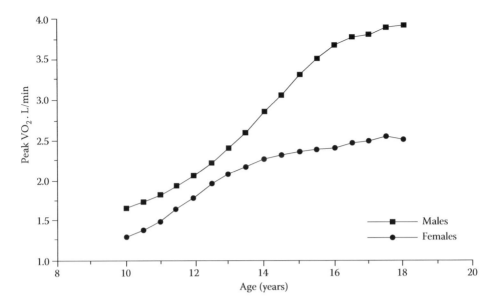

FIGURE 14.1 Changes in absolute VO$_2$max over time males and females. (From Geithner, C.A. et al. *Med Sci Sports Exerc*, 36, 1616–1624, 2004.)

in height. Maximal height does not, however, determine VO$_2$max since aerobic power capacity generally increases for several years after peak height velocity has been achieved. Trends in aerobic power between genders coincide with normative maturation patterns since the increase in VO$_2$max typically occurs earlier in females, but to a greater magnitude in males (Armstrong and Welsman 1994; Geithner et al. 2004; Krahenbuhl et al. 1985). Overall, while cardiovascular development for performance applications is highly variable and specific across age, developmental stages, and gender, a clear positive relationship is exhibited between age, aerobic power, and capacity; along with this, it is also clear that aerobic power and capacity is generally higher in males when compared to females at any age.

14.2.3.2 Type of Activity

There are two general methods of training to improve endurance performance: intensive training and traditional continuous submaximal training. Intensive training can be broken down into three subcategories: high-intensity interval training (Valovich McLeod et al. 2011), fast distance training, or pace training. Distance or submaximal training consists of two workout types: long, slow distance training (LSD), and medium-distance training (Rusko 1992). Table 14.3 provides examples of different types of exercises within each method of endurance training.

It has been suggested that intensive training may be best for younger athletes such that the short, intermittent nature of the activities grasp the attention of younger athletes, thus increasing enjoyment and compliance (Baquet et al. 2001). However, in order to gain greatest performance benefits, endurance training should be catered toward the needs of the athlete and energy system requirements of the particular sport and position. For example, a training program designed with only a submaximal distance component would not be applicable for a soccer player, since soccer is a dynamic sport requiring a combination of sprint intervals and continuous submaximal movement over the course of a 60–90-minute match. A mix of high-intensity interval training and fast distance training may be better suited for the youth athlete training for soccer.

14.2.3.3 Intensity

After types of exercises for the training regimen have been selected, intensity is the next major component to consider. As mentioned previously, within the pediatric population, absolute HR and

TABLE 14.3
Examples of Exercises within Each Method of Endurance Training

Method of Endurance Training	Exercise Examples
Intensive Training	
High-intensity interval training	Fartleks; repeated sprints with little rest (i.e., 5 × 100 m with 30-second rest)
Fast distance training	Tempo runs; 800 m repeats
Pace training	Run at a percentage of race pace for a given distance (i.e., 60% race pace × 7 miles)
Distance/Submaximal Training	
Long, slow distance	10+ mile run at a pace significantly less than race pace (i.e., 50% race pace)
Medium-distance training	4–9 mile run at a pace significantly less than race pace

HRmax measures can be highly variable (Baquet et al. 2003), and so HR measures are generally used with pubescent and postpubescent youth athletes only. Within advanced endurance training programs, exercise intensity among prepubescent youth is most often expressed as a percentage of an individual's fastest pace or time to complete a specific interval or total distance. Among pubescent and postpubescent youth, a commonly used method to calculate HRmax is as follows: 220 – age. An example of how to use HR to determine cardiovascular exercise intensity is provided in Table 14.4.

14.2.3.4 Frequency and Duration

Finally, when determining frequency and duration within an advanced cardiovascular training regimen, prepubescent children who engage in free play as an aside from their cardiovascular training regimen for sport should not have any limitations on play frequency and duration. However, cardiovascular training sessions in prepubescence and early puberty should not occur more than 2–3 days per week to allow for proper recovery and time for free play. Additionally, child athletes in prepubescence or early puberty should be limited to 30–45 minutes of cardiovascular training, including proper warm-up and cooldown, to prevent overuse injuries.

Regarding pubescent and postpubescent youth athletes, cardiovascular training for 5–6 days per week for at least 45 minutes has demonstrated improvements in aerobic power (Rusko 1992). Additionally, nonsport specific activity is encouraged *ad libitum* on nontraining days and during the off-season.

14.2.3.5 Progression of Activities

Prepubescent and early pubescent cardiovascular training should progress as tolerated by the child athlete. Activities focused on improving cardiovascular performance must include elements of fun

TABLE 14.4
Example of Cardiovascular/Endurance Training Intensities Based on HRmax Percentages for Pubescent and Postpubescent Youth Athletes

Training Method	Training Intensity
Intensive training: interval training, fast distance training, pace training	HR 0–25 bpm below maximum HR
Long, slow distance	HR 50–80 bpm below maximum HR
Medium-distance training	HR 20–50 bpm below maximum HR

Source: Adapted from Rusko, H.K., *Med Sci Sports Exerc*, 24, 1040, 1992.
Note: HR = heart rate, bpm = beats per minute.

TABLE 14.5
Example of Progression of Advanced Cardiovascular/Endurance Exercise Program in Children and Adolescents

Training Method	Intensity	Frequency	Duration (min)
Dependent on sport. May consist of intensive training or distance/ submaximal training	Prepubescent		
	60% fastest pace/race pace	1–2 days/wk × weeks 1–4	30
	70% fastest pace/race pace	2–3 days/wk × weeks 5–8	30–40
	80% fastest pace/race pace	2–3 days/wk × weeks 8–12	30–45
	Pubescent and postpubescent		
	HR 20–25 bpm < HRmax	4–5 days/wk × weeks 1–4	30
	HR 15–20 bpm < HRmax	5–6 days/wk × weeks 5–8	35–40
	HR 10–15 bpm < HRmax	5–6 days/wk × weeks 8–12	≥45

Note: HR = heart rate, bpm = beats per minute, HRmax = maximum heart rate, days/wk = days per week.

TABLE 14.6
Example of Progression of an Advanced Endurance Training Program in Pubescent/Postpubescent Youth

	HRmax Range (%)	Minutes	Days per Week
Week 1	70–80	20	2–3
Week 2	70–80	20	2–3
Week 3	70–80	20	2–3
Week 4	70–80	20	2–3
Week 5	70–80	30	2–3
Week 6	70–80	30	2–3
Week 7	70–80	30	3–4
Week 8	70–80	30	3–4
Week 9	70–80	40	3–4
Week 10	70–80	40	3–4
Week 11	70–80	40	3–4
Week 12	70–80	40	3–4

Source: Adapted from Kreider, R.B. et al. *Exercise & Sport Nutrition: Principles, Promises, Science and Recommendations*, Fitness Technologies Press, Santa Barbara, CA, 2009a.

and enjoyment to maximize adherence (Fraser-Thomas et al. 2008; Janssen 2007; Molinero et al. 2006; Salguero et al. 2003). As the child athlete progresses through puberty, exercise complexity, intensity, frequency, and duration should increase in a stepwise fashion based on performance goals for the season. The progression in these programs may closely resemble those prescribed for adult athletes (Janssen 2007). Table 14.5 provides an example of the progression of an advanced cardiovascular/endurance exercise program in children and adolescents. Additionally, Table 14.6 provides another example of progression of an advanced endurance training program in pubescent youth.

14.3 MUSCULAR STRENGTH AND ENDURANCE

While it is well known that cardiovascular exercise provides benefits to both pediatric and adult populations, resistance training, traditionally thought only to apply to adults, has also demonstrated benefits within the pediatric population. Increases in muscular strength are attributed to increases in muscle cross-sectional area, structural (muscle size and moment arm length), and neural adaptations (Bouchant et al. 2011; Lloyd et al. 2013). The mechanisms behind these training adaptations vary in youth depending on the stage of development and the type of tissue (connective vs. muscle) utilized. Multiple investigations conclude that muscular strength and endurance will increase in response to a resistance training program in prepubescent/early pubescent boys (<13 years) and girls (<12 years) with only a minor difference between genders on both absolute and relative strength gains. Once in the pubescent period, maturation is accompanied by increases in strength, power, and muscular endurance with differences demonstrated between genders (Faigenbaum et al. 1996, 2009; Falk and Eliakim 2003; Falk and Tenenbaum 1996; Lillegard et al. 1997; Pierce et al. 2008; Stratton et al. 2004).

There are multiple myths and misconceptions associated with risk of injury and growth impairment when considering a resistance training program in children and adolescent athletes. Acute resistance training injuries among youth athletes generally occur when the athletes are unsupervised or supervised by unqualified strength training professionals (Dahab and McCambridge 2009; Faigenbaum and Myer 2010b; Lloyd et al. 2013). Furthermore, the rate of accidental injuries (77%) associated with both youth and adult resistance training has been attributed to a lack of proper supervision, technical competency, and a safe training environment, all of which are avoidable (Lloyd et al. 2013; Myer et al. 2009).

Along with risk of bone or muscular injury, a common reservation among parents and coaches is risk of injury to the developing growth plates, which are generally considered 3–5 times weaker than the surrounding connective tissues (Faigenbaum and Myer 2010b; Micheli 2006). On the contrary, evidence supports resultant mechanical stress placed on the young musculoskeletal system as a result of resistance training to bone growth and formation (Faigenbaum and Myer 2010b; Lloyd et al. 2013). While there are some retrospective clinical case reports associating injuries of growth plates with resistance training, these cases have been attributed to equipment misuse, inappropriate weight lifted, improper technique, or lack of qualified supervision (Caine et al. 2006; Dahab and McCambridge 2009; Faigenbaum and Myer 2010b).

Overall, recent research has continually supported the notion that benefits from resistance training obtained in young athletes are similar to benefits obtained by adults (Behm et al. 2008; Faigenbaum et al. 2009). Since over 30 million children participate in sports every year in the United States, with most children participating in multiple sports and seasons, youth strength and conditioning programs are necessary (National Institute of Arthritis 2006). The following section will discuss the general benefits, special considerations, and general and advanced guidelines for resistance training in children and adolescents.

14.3.1 General Benefits

A primary goal of any strength and conditioning program is to minimize the risk of injury during sport activities. Current research indicates that properly supervised and designed resistance training programs for youth athletes will reduce the incidence of overuse injuries in children and adolescent athletes by approximately 50% (Lloyd et al. 2013; Valovich McLeod et al. 2011). More specifically, these multifaceted youth athlete resistance training programs help to increase muscular strength, enhance motor skills and movement mechanics, and improve functional capacities to aid in reducing the risk or severity of sports-related injuries (Dahab and McCambridge 2009; Lloyd et al. 2013; MacKay et al. 2004; Nóbrega et al. 2005). Increases in both muscular strength and endurance have been achieved beyond normal growth and maturation in youth (Behm et al. 2008; Faigenbaum et al. 2009). In fact, average strength gains of 30%–40%, even up to 80%, have been observed after only 8–20 weeks of structured resistance training in youth (Faigenbaum et al. 1993; Payne et al. 1997). The majority of increases in strength are attributed to improvements in neuromuscular function, since large increases in muscle size and hypertrophy are not typically seen (Blimkie 1992; Ramsay et al. 1990).

Additionally, there are a tremendous amount of neural benefits associated with proper resistance training progression in children and adolescents. Neural benefits of youth strength training allow stronger young athletes to more readily grasp proper techniques and make larger strides in their overall athletic development regardless of chronological age or maturation (Pierce et al. 2008). Neural benefits derived from strength training in youth sport are directly related to improvements in proprioception and balance, which will lead to a reduction in injury risk during maturation and growth.

Other general benefits of participation in youth resistance training programs include improvements in body composition, bone health, and insulin sensitivity (Annesi et al. 2005; Schwingshandl and Borkenstein 1995; Schwingshandl et al. 1999; Shabi et al. 2006; Sung et al. 2002). The aforementioned benefits are also associated with reduced risk of adverse health events, such as obesity, osteoporosis, fractures, and development of type 2 diabetes. Thus in addition to injury prevention and performance enhancement, resistance training may be related to disease prevention and promotion of overall health and wellness.

14.3.1.1 Special Considerations

To achieve the benefits from resistance training within the pediatric population, the following factors should be considered to mitigate risk of injury: technique and proper form of exercises, training load in relation to maturation stage of the athlete, and overall training regimen, including recovery time for the athlete (Faigenbaum et al. 2009; Faigenbaum and Myer 2010a,b). Emphasis should be placed on proper technique, form, and body position in order to prevent injury on account of incorrect movement patterns (Faigenbaum and Myer 2010a,b). To achieve proper body position for certain exercises, body size and weight must be considered.

Along with proper form, maturation stage may impact tolerance of training load such that two players on the same team may not be able to complete the same resistance training regimen. Maturation stage will vary regardless of age; thus it is imperative for the strength and conditioning coach to pay close attention to the athlete's cues related to tolerance of the training task and rate of progression within each training task (Faigenbaum and Myer 2010b). Large or rapid increases in training load and/or volume should be avoided in order to promote gradual improvements in performance and avoid injury (Faigenbaum and Myer 2010b).

Furthermore, with the increase in participation in team sports among adolescents (Nettle and Sprogis 2011); it is possible that the youth athlete is participating in multiple sports during one season or has been training across seasons without appropriate recovery. Thus in order to reduce the risk of overtraining or overuse injuries, it is important to understand the athlete's training and recovery schedule and appropriately plan time for resistance training within this schedule.

Overall, while technique, maturation stage, and training regimens are important factors to consider when designing a resistance training program, it is important to remember to keep the program fun for the child athlete. The more fun and enjoyable the workouts are, the more likely the young athlete will stick with the program. A detailed list of considerations for a resistance training program in youth is listed in Table 14.7.

14.3.2 GUIDELINES TO PROMOTE GENERAL FITNESS

When developing a resistance training program in youth, it is important to include the following principles: type of activity, intensity and volume, duration, and frequency. Table 14.8 provides an example of resistance training guidelines for youth.

14.3.2.1 Type of Activity

A variety of resistance training techniques within exercise programs have demonstrated improved fitness, muscular strength, and muscular endurance (Annesi et al. 2005; Behm et al. 2008; Faigenbaum et al. 1999, 2009; Faigenbaum and Micheli 2000; Faigenbaum and Myer 2010b; Lloyd et al. 2013). A specific type of resistance training, or gold standard, does not exist within the young athlete

TABLE 14.7
General Resistance Training Considerations for Youth

- A qualified individual should supervise and be present at all training sessions.
- Focus on proper exercise form and technique.
- Complete a 5–10-minute dynamic warm-up prior to training.
- Focus on full-body compound movements.
- Provide individualized workouts and monitor progress.
- Provide gradual increases in resistance (5%–10%).
- Ensure a fun and safe environment.
- Complete a 5–10-minute cooldown.

Source: Adapted from Faigenbaum, A.D. and Myer, G.D., *Br J Sports Med*, 44, 56–63, 2010b.

TABLE 14.8
Principles of Resistance Training for Youth

Principle	Recommendation
Frequency	2–3 days per week
Duration	30–60 minutes
Intensity	40%–60% 1RM
Volume:	
Repetitions	8–15
Sets	1–2
Number of exercises	8–12

Source: Adapted from Behm, D.G. et al. *Appl Physiol Nutr Metab*, 33, 547–61, 2008; Faigenbaum, A.D. et al. *J Strength Cond Res*, 23, S60–79, 2009.

population. Body weight exercises, traditional weightlifting, calisthenics, and plyometric training have all been deemed safe and effective strategies to improve muscular strength and endurance with minimal risk of injury when executed properly (Faigenbaum and Myer 2010a, 2012; Faigenbaum 2000; Faigenbaum et al. 2009). Activity type within resistant training is dependent upon specificity of sport, resistance training experience of the athlete, performance goals, and availability of equipment. Table 14.9 provides examples of different types of resistance exercise.

14.3.2.2 Intensity and Volume

In resistance training, exercise intensity is often expressed as a percentage of an individual's one repetition maximum (1RM). Training volume is often expressed as the total number of repetitions and sets of repetitions completed at a specific intensity (Behm et al. 2008). When standardized protocols and equipment are implemented under the supervision of qualified professionals, it is safe to perform strength and power testing for 1RM in youth (Baechle and Earle 2008; Faigenbaum et al. 2003; Lloyd et al. 2013). However, most youth coaches do not have access to facilities or equipment for 1RM testing, have limited time, or are likely not qualified to perform 1RM testing with child or adolescent athletes. Thus, alternative methods such as using submaximal loads and prediction equations to calculate 1RM may be more appropriate (Castro-Piñero et al. 2010a,b; Lloyd et al. 2013).

TABLE 14.9
Examples of Resistance Exercises

Chest	Bench press
	Incline bench press
	Chest flies (pec deck)
	Decline bench press
	Dips
	Lat pulls
	Seated rows
	Push-ups
Shoulders	Shoulder press
	Incline bench press
	Shoulder flies (front flexion, side abduction, extension)
	Shoulder front raises
	T-bar rows/upright rows
Lats/back/traps	Lat pulls
	Seated rows (two arm and single arm)
	Wide grip pull-ups
	Shoulder shrugs
	Back extension
Arms	Single and two arm biceps curls
	Lat pulls
	Seated rows
	Triceps extension (standing, supine)
	Bench press
	Closed grip bench press
	Dips
Forearms	Wrist curls and extension
Gluteals/upper Hamstrings	Leg press
	Squats
	Lunges
	Dead lifts
	Box squats
	Hip and back (hip extension)
Lower hamstrings	Leg curls
Quadriceps	Hip/leg press/sled
	Front/back/safety squats
	Leg extension
Hip adductors (groin)	Hip adduction/abduction machine
	Hip flexion
	Leg press/squats
	Lunges
Hip abductors	Hip abduction (multihip machine)
	Hip abduction/adduction machine
Calves	Leg press/squats
	Heel raises
Abdominals	Crunches
	Abdominal machine
	Reverse crunches
	Hanging hip flexion

Source: Adapted from Kreider, R.B. et al. *Exercise & Sport Nutrition: Principles, Promises, Science and Recommendations*, Fitness Technologies Press, Santa Barbara, CA, 2009a.

A variety of resistance training protocols have been shown to be effective in terms of improving muscular strength and endurance in youth (Behm et al. 2008; Faigenbaum et al. 1993, 1999, 2001, 2002; Faigenbaum and Myer 2012). The general consensus is such that youth should begin using low to moderate intensities, which are equivalent to 50%–70% of their 1RM (Faigenbaum et al. 2009). Proper form and technique should be the first priority before higher loads and volumes are used.

14.3.2.3 Duration and Frequency

Duration refers to the length of time to complete a training session. While a gold standard for duration of resistance training in children and adolescent athletes does not exist, a recent study has demonstrated improvements in muscular strength and endurance following 45 minutes of resistance exercise, 3 days per week (Annesi et al. 2005). Similarly, training sessions lasting 30–40 minutes have also been shown to improve muscular strength 11%–30% when completed 2 days per week (Faigenbaum et al. 2002).

Along with duration, frequency of resistance training consists of the number of times the exercise bout should be performed per week. Frequency is governed by the total training volume (number of repetitions and sets) and dictates the number of times a particular resistance training workout will appear in the training cycle or how often resistance training will occur throughout a training week (Lloyd et al. 2013). As little as 1 day per week of strength training has been shown to increase lower body muscular strength by 14% in children, and greater strength gains (25%), were observed when the frequency was increased to 2 days per week (Faigenbaum et al. 2002). Therefore, it is recommended that youth engage in resistance training 2–3 days per week (Behm et al. 2008). Resistance training should also be conducted on nonconsecutive days during the week to allow for adequate recovery in between workouts.

14.3.2.4 Progression of Activities

Once the child or adolescent athlete has demonstrated proper technique and improvements, progression strategies may be implemented. Progress in the resistance training program may be achieved by adjusting different components, or training variables, such as increasing the number of sets, increasing the intensity, adjusting rest periods, or incorporating more complex movements and exercises.

Progression should be conducted in a gradual, stepwise fashion to ensure safety. For example, if the individual is currently performing two sets of 12 repetitions at 50% of his/her 1RM, the load may be increased to 60% of his/her 1RM as long as proper technique can be maintained. Additionally, the number of sets or repetitions can be increased in increments of either five repetitions or one set, depending on the desired training goal. It has been suggested that varying the resistance training program every 8–12 weeks can help to avoid plateaus in training adaptations and facilitate improvements (Behm et al. 2008). Table 14.10 provides an example of resistance training

TABLE 14.10
Example of Progression Guidelines for Resistance Training in Youth

Training Principle	Level		
	Novice	Intermediate	Advanced
Exercise	Single or multiple joint	Single or multiple joint	Single or multiple joint
Intensity	50%–70% 1RM	60%–80% 1RM	70%–85% 1RM
Volume	1–2 sets × 10–15 reps	2–3 sets × 8–12 reps	≥ 3 sets × 6–10 reps
Rest intervals (minutes)	1	1–2	2–3
Frequency (days per week)	2–3	2–3	3–4

Source: Adapted from Faigenbaum, A.D. et al. *J Strength Cond Res*, 23, S60–79, 2009.

TABLE 14.11
Health-Related Fitness Program for Beginners

Program Component	Exercises	Time (min)	Goal
Warm-up	Walk Light stretching	5	Prepare for exercise
Endurance training	Walk, cycle, or row @ 60%–70% of HRmax (pubescent and postpubescent) or RPE 5–6 (prepubescent)	20	Promote improvements in cardiovascular fitness and positive adaptations in body composition
Resistance training	Perform 2–3 sets of the following lifts at 65%–70% of 1RM (10–15 repetitions) with 1–2 minutes rest recovery between sets Bench press Lat pulls Shoulder press Abdominal curls/crunches Back extension Bicep curl Elbow extension Leg press Leg extension Leg curl	30–40	Promote improvements in muscular strength and endurance and positive adaptations in body composition
Cooldown	Walk Light stretching	5	Promote proper recovery from exercise

Source: Adapted from Kreider, R.B. et al. *Exercise & Sport Nutrition: Principles, Promises, Science and Recommendations.* Fitness Technologies Press, Santa Barbara, CA, 2009a.

Note: Perform three times per week.

progression for youth athletes. Additionally, Table 14.11 provides an example of a fitness program, including resistance and cardiovascular exercise, for a beginner.

14.3.3 ADVANCED TRAINING GUIDELINES

Strength training among children and adolescents participating in sport varies from basic to more advanced youth resistance training programs. Within youth athletes, the type of activity is specific for the sport the athlete is training for. Once the type of activity is selected, intensity and volume, duration and frequency, and progression of activities can be prescribed.

14.3.3.1 Intensity and Volume

Training intensity should be based on the goals and phase of the resistance training program. For example, an endurance athlete may be prescribed 80%–90% of his/her 1RM to promote muscular endurance, whereas a wrestler or gymnast may lift 95%–100% of his/her 1RM to focus on muscular strength. For the youth athlete competing at a high/elite level, volume and intensity of a resistance training program should be altered each session or within a particular phase of the training program corresponding to the specific training goals of the individual athlete or team (Lloyd et al. 2013). Additionally, not all exercises prescribed in a youth resistance training program must be performed for the same number of sets and repetitions (Faigenbaum et al. 2009; Lloyd et al. 2013).

Intensity of a particular resistance training session or over an entire training cycle can also be dictated by the rest intervals between exercises or sets. In comparison to adults, children physiologically possess increased muscle tissue elasticity, which affords the ability to recover more rapidly from intense bouts of resistance training (Faigenbaum et al. 2008; Lloyd et al. 2013; Zafeiridis et al. 2005). Work-to-rest ratios should be increased for children and adolescents newly introduced to resistance exercise allowing for approximately one minute of recovery between sets. As the youth athlete gains more resistance training experience, more complicated exercises may require increased force and power production, thus leading to recovery time closer to 2–3 minutes between sets (Lloyd et al. 2013).

14.3.3.2 Duration and Frequency

Resistance training guidelines for duration and frequency in youth athletes are similar to general guidelines. Training should last for 30–60 minutes per session, and one should engage in resistance training initially 2–3 days per week with gradual progression to 3–5 days.

14.3.3.3 Progression of Activities

Among youth athletes competing at higher/elite levels, the resistance training program should progress from simplistic exercises, including single joint movements (i.e., bicep curls, leg extension, leg curls), to advanced multijoint movements (i.e., squats, deadlifts, leg press). Emphasis should be placed on proper technique and control through the full range of motion (Faigenbaum et al. 2009). Additionally, exercise intensity, volume, frequency, and intervals for rest should increase as tolerated as the young athlete becomes more fit, and time participating in a resistance training program has increased. See Table 14.10 for an example of resistance training progression for youth athletes.

14.4 STRETCHING AND FLEXIBILITY

Along with cardiovascular, and muscular strength and endurance exercises, stretching and flexibility are also important components of exercise prescription. Stretching exercises to improve flexibility may serve as a benefit to both general physical fitness and fitness for sport-specific activities. Recommendations for stretching from the American College of Sports Medicine were originally created for adults; however, these recommendations can be translated to the pediatric population due to limited research regarding stretching and flexibility in pediatrics (Landry and Driscoll 2012). Along with general recommendations, recent literature has developed sport-specific recommendations for stretching. The following section will explore potential benefits of stretching and flexibility, general guidelines, and special considerations.

14.4.1 General Benefits

Traditionally, stretching occurs both during the warm-up and cooldown phases of physical activity. Stretching is encouraged after exercise as part of the cooldown phase in order to prevent muscle stiffness and injury. In addition, stretching may also be beneficial during the warm-up. Stretching to improve flexibility of muscle-tendon units (MTU) is generally accepted as a method to prevent injury and, in some cases, improve performance (Witurouw et al. 2004). Theoretically, stretching and flexibility increases muscle compliance by decreasing stiffness, which should prevent injuries such as muscle tears and strains (McHugh and Cosgrave 2010). Safran and colleagues (1988) found a reduction in the risk of injury after following a stretching protocol when the MTU was warm, such that a warm MTU required greater length and force in comparison to a cold MTU in order to produce a muscle tear. As demonstrated in the work of McHugh and Cosgrave (McHugh and Cosgrave 2010), some studies have shown a significant reduction in risk of muscle strain when appropriate stretching protocols were followed prior to exercise.

Additionally, a goal of stretching prior to exercise is to increase range of motion, decrease resistance to stretch, and enable freer movement (McHugh and Cosgrave 2010). This is most applicable in sports and activities requiring wide joint range of motion, such as ballet (McHugh and Cosgrave 2010). Gymnastics, diving, and dance are other examples of activities requiring greater joint range of motion (Knudson 1999). Thus, one may infer that stretching prior to activity aimed at improving flexibility may result in improved athletic performance in sports requiring greater range of joint motion. While this relationship is not demonstrated for all types of sport, a review of the literature by Shrier (2004) has found a relationship between regular stretching within an exercise/training routine (either before or after exercise) and overall performance benefits, such that regular stretching increases velocity contraction and isometric force production. Overall, incorporation of stretching within an exercise/training regimen may improve flexibility of the MTUs resulting in improved performance and prevention of muscle strains and tears.

14.4.2 General Recommendations

Along with the general benefits of stretching/improving flexibility, there are general recommendations for each type of stretching exercise. The three different types of stretching exercises are as follows: ballistic stretching; proprioceptive neuromuscular facilitation (PNF); and static stretching, including both active and passive stretch exercises. Table 14.12 provides a description of each type of stretching exercise.

According to the American College of Sports Medicine Position Stand (Garber et al. 2011), within static or ballistic stretching, it is recommended to hold stretches for 10–30 seconds. Additionally, PNF stretching exercises should be held for 3–6 seconds at 20%–75% maximum contraction followed by 10–30 seconds of assisted stretching. Each PNF stretching exercise should be repeated two to four times (Garber et al. 2011). Furthermore, all stretching exercises should be conducted when the muscles and MTUs are warm (Garber et al. 2011; Knudson 1999; Safran et al. 1988). This is when stretching and flexibility exercises are most effective. Finally, the American College of Sports Medicine Position Stand (Garber et al. 2011) encourages engaging in flexibility exercises at least 2–3 days per week, or daily, to achieve larger gains in joint range of

TABLE 14.12
Types of Stretching Exercises

Stretching Exercise	Description
Ballistic stretching	Swinging a body segment in order to create a fast, momentum-assisted stretch (Knudson 1999)
	For example, leg-swings from hip joint, circular arm swings
Proprioceptive neuromuscular facilitation (PNF)	A series of stretches conducted in a cyclical fashion such that an isometric contraction is followed by static stretching of the same muscle group (Garber et al. 2011)
	For example, vinyasa yoga flow—plank to upward dog to downward dog to standing hamstring stretch
Static stretching	Holding a muscle or tendon group in a desired stretched position for a period of time, usually 10–30 seconds (Garber et al. 2011)
• Active static	Holding a stretch with strength from an agonist muscle (Garber et al. 2011)
	For example, arm overhead to stretch tricep while flexing bicep, stretching quadricep by flexing hamstring
• Passive static	Holding a stretch without any outside influences (i.e., partner, elastic band, or barre) (Garber et al. 2011)
	For example, hamstring stretch, quadricep stretch, tricep stretch, lunge

Source: Adapted from Garber, C.E. et al. *Med Sci Sports Exerc*, 43, 133401359, 2011; Knudson, D. *JOPERD*, 70, (7), 24–29, 1999.

motion. Regardless of the child's or adolescent's level of fitness (i.e., beginner, intermediate, or advanced/trained athlete), recommendations for stretching remain the same.

14.4.3 SPECIAL CONSIDERATIONS

Timing of stretching to prevent injury or improve performance is dependent upon the type of activity performed (Knudson 1999; McHugh and Cosgrave 2010; Witurouw et al. 2004). As mentioned previously, athletes engaging in sports that require greater range of motion in the joints benefit from stretching prior to activity during warm-up (Knudson 1999; McHugh and Cosgrave 2010). According to Witurouw and colleagues (2004), different types of sports require different levels of flexibility or "levels of musculo-tendinous compliance." For example, activities/sports requiring quick force through muscle contractions (isometric or concentric), such as swimming or cycling, may benefit from a stiffer MTU, such that stiffer MTUs lead to faster force transferred to bones and consequently faster movement of the joint (Witurouw et al. 2004). Therefore, when engaging in these endurance-like activities, also considered activities with low use of stretch-shortening cycles (SSCs), one may exhibit the most benefit from stretching after exercise during the cooldown phase as opposed to before exercise during the warm-up.

In opposition to activities requiring low SSCs, examples of activities requiring high use of SSCs include "explosive type skills" (Witurouw et al. 2004), such as football and soccer. A more flexible MTU is needed in these activities because MTUs can use the elastic energy from the stretched muscle during eccentric contractions to produce more power (Witurouw et al. 2004). Additionally, to prevent injury, stretching should be conducted during the warm-up in sports requiring high SSCs, and during the cooldown in sports requiring low SSCs (Witurouw et al. 2004). Thus, some sports may require stretching prior to exercise in order to achieve improved performance and subsequently prevention of injury, whereas others may favor stretching after exercise.

Along with timing of stretching, type of stretching should also be considered. When comparing the different types of stretching, ballistic and static stretching are comparable in terms of ability to improve flexibility, whereas PNF and static stretching are comparable in improving range of motion in joints (Garber et al. 2011). Additionally, PNF stretching activities may reportedly produce the largest gains in flexibility and joint range of motion (Garber et al. 2011). When stretching multiple people at once, such as team stretching, either type of static stretching, active or passive, is best to allow for greater efficiency with time (Knudson 1998).

While static and ballistic stretching are considered comparable, it is important to note that ballistic stretching has been associated with greater risk of injury (Knudson 1998; Weerapong et al. 2004). Thus ballistic stretching should be conducted under close supervision in order to ensure exercises are conducted safely and appropriately. Otherwise, it may be best to use static stretching techniques to achieve the same flexibility goals with a safer method.

Overall, when determining which stretching method is the best, static or ballistic stretching may be ideal for low-SSC sports/activities (endurance-like activities), since these stretches are suitable for improving flexibility. A combination of PNF and static stretching is ideal for high-SSC sports, explosive-like sports, and sports requiring high joint range of motion. Table 14.13 provides a summary of stretching/flexibility guidelines.

14.5 HEALTHY TRAINING FOR PERFORMANCE

A healthy training regimen in youth consists of a balance among mode of training, and attention and time devoted to training/competition. When implemented incorrectly, adverse psychological and physiological effects may occur, such as excessive cognitive stress and anxiety leading to athletes' burnout (Lewthwaite and Scanlan 1989; Sagar and Stoeber 2009; Stoeber and Becker 2008) and overuse injury (Smith et al. 1993). On the contrary, when a training regimen is implemented appropriately, the following positive benefits may result: improvement in academic performance (So 2012;

TABLE 14.13
Stretching Guidelines

Type of Activity	Timing	Type of Stretching Exercise
Wider range of motion i.e., gymnastics, diving, dance and/or Explosive skills i.e., football, soccer, basketball	Before exercise	PNF Either type of static stretching
Endurance-like activity i.e., swimming, cycling, running	After exercise	Ballistic stretching Either type of static stretching

Strong et al. 2005); reduction in anxiety, depression, and physiological response to psychological stress (Roemmich et al. 2009; Strong et al. 2005); and improvement in overall health, fitness, and athletic performance (Janssen and LeBlanc 2010; Nettle and Sprogis 2011).

14.5.1 Consequences of an Unhealthy Training Regimen

To prevent unnecessary psychological stress and anxiety, it is advised to avoid extra pressure from parents and coaches (Smith et al. 1993). Examples of pressure from parents and coaches include heavy emphasis on winning and sometimes negative consequences, such as extra practice and negative reinforcement, when winning is not achieved. This type of training environment (referred to as the performance climate) stresses winning, interpersonal comparisons between athletes, and unhealthy normative standards (Tsai and Chen 2009). A typical product of the performance climate consists of an unhealthy preoccupation with perfectionism, commonly referred to as maladaptive or negative perfectionism. Maladaptive perfectionism is when one obsesses over mistakes, doubts actions, feels dissonance between high expectations and actual achievements, experiences self-criticism, and fears failure to live up to expectations of other's or one's own standards (Stoeber and Otto 2006). Among youth athletes, a positive correlation between character traits of maladaptive perfectionism, notably fear of failure, and cognitive anxiety has been established (Lewthwaite and Scanlan 1989; Sagar and Stoeber 2009; Tsai and Chen 2009).

The combination of maladaptive perfectionism and resultant stress and anxiety is the perfect formula for athletes' burnout. Athletes' burnout can be defined as the emotional and physical disengagement from a sport one previously enjoyed on account of stress (Smith 1986). Research conducted in both youth and young adults has demonstrated a relationship between maladaptive perfectionism and incidence of burnout (Appleton et al. 2009). Examples of the psychological manifestations included in athletes' burnout are lack of enthusiasm regarding sport, feeling of fatigue, and challenges with completing daily tasks and routines (Brenner 2007). Thus, if a child or adolescent athlete trains and competes in an unhealthy environment, this will likely result in the following domino effect: onset of psychological stress and anxiety, development of athletes' burnout, negative interference with sport performance and likely other activities of daily living.

Additionally, the physical adaptations associated with emotional burnout include overtraining, resultant decline in athletic performance, and eventual overuse injury. According to Small (2002), when too much training occurs with inadequate time for recovery, psychological, hormonal, and physiological changes result, which causes decreased athletic performance. The physiological signs/symptoms of overtraining include chronic joint and muscle pain, and fatigue. As mentioned previously, overtraining will likely result in overuse injury. Overuse injury is defined as repeated stress, usually submaximum, to previously normal tissue or bone (Martin and Martin 2002). It is known that overuse injury can end a season for an athlete, and so it is important to implement the appropriate balance between mental and physical training to avoid this.

14.5.2 Benefits of a Healthy Training Regimen

The benefits of a healthy training regimen in school-aged children and adolescents are twofold, encompassing both mental and physical health. Demonstrated mental health benefits include improvement in academic performance, reduction in symptoms of anxiety and depression, and improved physiological response to psychological stress. According to a recent meta-analysis conducted by Fedewa and Ahn (2011), a relationship was found among academic performance, engagement in regular physical activity, and physical fitness, such that academic performance was positively associated with engagement in regular physical activity and levels of physical fitness. Adequate evidence was found in an additional systematic review to support the relationship of regular physical activity and improved academic performance (Strong et al. 2005).

When assessing the relationship between regular exercise and academic performance/cognitive function, frequency and mode of exercise have also been explored. So and colleagues demonstrated a positive relationship between exercise and academic performance when adolescent boys and girls participated in no more than 4 days per week of moderate cardiovascular exercise (So 2012). The general physical activity recommendation of 60 minutes per day at moderate to vigorous intensity also supports the relationship between regular activity and academic performance (Strong et al. 2005). Moreover, regular physical activity has been associated with reduced symptoms of anxiety and depression. Strong evidence supports reduction in symptoms of anxiety and depression when youth meet the general guidelines for physical activity (Strong et al. 2005).

In addition to improvements in academic performance and reduction in anxiety and depression, a more recent study conducted by Roemmich and colleagues (2009) assessed the relationship between physical activity and the physiological response to psychological stress. Two separate experiments were included in the study. In their first experiment, children were assigned to one of two conditions, either 25 minutes of exercise (exercise condition) or 25 minutes of TV watching (sedentary condition), followed by a 25-minute reading recovery period and subsequent cognitively stressful event, delivering an interpersonal speech. A significant difference was found in diastolic blood pressure (DBP), such that DBP was reactively lower in the exercise condition versus the sedentary condition. In the second experiment, each participant engaged in a sedentary condition and an exercise condition on separate days, with each condition followed by a recovery period and a stressful event (speech stressor). Within this experiment, significant differences were found such that systolic blood pressure (SBP), DBP, and HR were lower during the exercise condition. It was concluded that exercise was positively associated with reduction in physiological response to outside stressors. Overall, one may conclude that a healthy training regimen, consisting of an appropriate amount of physical activity, will promote academic performance, reduce anxiety and depression, and mitigate physiological stress response to outside stressors (Roemmich et al. 2009).

Along with the mental health benefits associated with a healthy training regimen, physical health benefits will also result. Evidence supporting physical health benefits and regular physical activity is growing among the pediatric population. Regular physical activity, along with a calorically appropriate and healthful diet, is recommended in part to prevent the onset of obesity. Increased prevalence of obesity among school-aged children and adolescents is associated with early onset of multiple health disparities such as type 2 diabetes, hypertension, orthopedic issues, and cardiovascular disease (Nettle and Sprogis 2011). According to recent systematic reviews, strong evidence has been found supporting an inverse relationship between regular physical activity and blood pressure/hypertension, cardiovascular health, musculoskeletal health, adiposity, and blood lipid profiles (Janssen and LeBlanc 2010; Strong et al. 2005). All in all, an appropriate amount of physical activity included in a healthy training regimen will reduce a child or adolescent's risk of experiencing adverse health events.

14.5.3 Considerations for a Healthy Training Regimen

When developing a training regimen for youth, the child's training/exercise regimen should promote overall wellness, mentally and physically. In terms of mental health, a positive training environment is encouraged. Smith and colleagues (1993) suggested, in opposition to parents selecting their child's sport/activity, to allow the child to select his/her sport based on her own desires and emotional needs. As mentioned previously, focus and pressure around winning should be avoided. Contrasting the performance climate, a mastery climate is encouraged. Mastery climate encourages intrapersonal standards, efforts, teamwork, and focuses on mastering skills and personal improvement (Tsai and Chen 2009).

To optimize health and performance, the training regimen should include all components of a general fitness program. Thus, strength, endurance, and flexibility exercises should be included (Smith et al. 1993). Additionally, in comparison to young and middle-aged adults, children and adolescents are at greater risk for developing injury during physical activity. The risk of injury in this population is related to coordination, skeletal maturity, flexibility, size, and stage of growth, specifically puberty (Demorest 2003). According to the American Academy of Pediatrics Council on Sports Medicine and Fitness, the following guidelines should be considered to prevent overtraining and burnout: include age-appropriate, interesting, and fun workouts; limit to one sport/mode of training no more than 5 days per week; allow at least 1 day per week for rest; and grant at least 2–3 months off per year from a specific sport/mode of training (OK for cross-training during this time) (Brenner 2007). The aforementioned guidelines will also help prevent overuse injury.

In terms of exercise intensity during training and competition, it is recommended to allow the child athlete some control over intensity of training and competition as opposed to parents and coaches (Smith et al. 1993). This technique will help prevent both acute and chronic injuries. Furthermore, a general rule for progressing training safely is to increase intensity, frequency, and/or duration, no more than 10% at one time (DiFiori 1999).

In summary, a healthy training regimen is imperative within the pediatric population in order to prevent adverse mental and physical health events while optimizing sport performance. When developing a healthy training regimen, the child athlete should have autonomy regarding selection of sport/activity and intensity of training/competition. It is also important to ensure a balance between daily living activities and free play, and time spent in training and competition both mentally and physically.

REFERENCES

Andersen, L.B. and J. Haraldsdóttir. 1994. Changes in CHD risk factors with age: A comparison of Danish adolescents and adults. *Med Sci Sports Exerc* 26 (8):967.

Annesi, J.J., W.L. Westcott, A.D. Faigenbaum, and J.L. Unruh. 2005. Effects of a 12-week physical activity protocol delivered by YMCA after-school counselors (Youth Fit for Life) on fitness and self-efficacy changes in 5–12-year-old boys and girls. *Res Q Exerc Sport* 76 (4):468–476.

Appleton, P.R., H.K. Hall, and A.P. Hill. 2009. Relations between multidimensional perfectionism and burnout in junior-elite male athletes. *Psychol Sport Exerc* 10:457–465.

Armstrong, N. and J.R. Welsman. 1994. Assessment arid interpretation of aerobic fitness in children and adolescents. *Exerc Sport Sci Rev* 22 (1):435–476.

Baechle, T.R. and R.W. Earle. 2008. *Essentials of Strength Training and Conditioning*. Champaign, IL: Human Kinetics.

Baquet, G., S. Berthoin, M. Gerbeaux, and E. Van Praagh. 2001. High-intensity aerobic training during a 10 week one-hour physical education cycle: Effects on physical fitness of adolescents aged 11–16. *Int J Sports Med* 22 (04):295–300.

Baquet, G., E. Van Praagh, and S. Berthoin. 2003. Endurance training and aerobic fitness in young people. *Sports Med* 33 (15):1127–1143.

Behm, D.G., A.D. Faigenbaum, B. Falk, and P. Klentrou. 2008. Canadian society for exercise physiology position paper: Resistance training in children and adolescents. *Appl Physiol Nutr Metab* 33 (3):547–561. doi: 10.1139/H08-020.

Binkhorst, R.A., M.C. De Jong-Van De Kar, and A.C.A. Vissers. 1984. Growth and aerobic power of boys aged 11–19 years. In J. Ilmarinen and I. Valimaki (eds), *Children and Sport*, 99–105. Berlin Heidelberg: Springer.

Blimkie, C.J. 1992. Resistance training during pre- and early puberty: Efficacy, trainability, mechanisms, and persistence. *Can J Sport Sci* 17 (4):264–279.

Bouchant, A., V. Martin, N.A. Maffiuletti, and S. Ratel. 2011. Can muscle size fully account for strength differences between children and adults? *J Appl Physiol* 110 (6):1748–1749.

Brenner, J.S. 2007. Overuse injuries, overtraining, and burnout, in child and adolescent athletes. *Pediatrics* 119:1242–1245. doi: 10.1542/peds.2007-0887.

Caine, D., J. DiFiori, and N. Maffulli. 2006. Physical injuries in children's and youth sports: Reasons for concern? *Br J Sports Med* 40 (9):749–760.

Candeias, V., T.P. Armstrong, and G.C. Xuereb. 2010. Diet and physical activity in schools: Perspectives from the implementation of the WHO global strategy on diet, physical activity and health. *Can J Public Health* 101:S28–S30.

Castro-Piñero, J., E.G. Artero, V. España-Romero, F.B. Ortega, M. Sjöström, J. Suni, and J.R. Ruiz. 2010a. Criterion-related validity of field-based fitness tests in youth: A systematic review. *Br J Sports Med* 44 (13):934–943.

Castro-Piñero, J., F.B. Ortega, E.G. Artero, M.J. Girela-Rejón, J. Mora, M. Sjöström, and J.R. Ruiz. 2010b. Assessing muscular strength in youth: Usefulness of standing long jump as a general index of muscular fitness. *J Strength Cond Res* 24 (7):1810–1817.

Committee, Physical Activity Guidelines Advisory. 2008. *Physical Activity Guidelines Advisory Committee Report*. Washington, D.C.: US Department of Health and Human Services.

Dahab, K.S. and T.M. McCambridge. 2009. Strength training in children and adolescents: Raising the bar for young athletes? *Sports Health* 1 (3):223–226.

Demorest, R. 2003. Prevention of pediatric sports injuries. *Curr Sports Med Rep* 2 (6):337–343.

DiFiori, J.P. 1999. Overuse injuries in children and adolescents. *Phys Sportsmed* 27 (1):75–89.

Epstein, L.H., R.A. Paluch, L.E. Kalakanis, G.S. Goldfield, F.J. Cerny, and J.N. Roemmich. 2001. How much activity do youth get? A quantitative review of heart-rate measured activity. *Pediatrics* 108 (3):E44. doi: 10.1542/peds.108.3.e44.

Faigenbaum, A., L. Zaichkowksy, W. Westcott, L. Micheli, and A. Fehlandt. 1993. The effects of twice per week strength training program on children. *Pediatr Exerc Sci* 5:339–346.

Faigenbaum, A.D. 2000. Strength training for children and adolescents. *Clin Sports Med* 19 (4):593–619.

Faigenbaum, A.D., W.J. Kraemer, C.J. Blimkie, I. Jeffreys, L.J. Micheli, M. Nitka, and T.W. Rowland. 2009. Youth resistance training: Updated position statement paper from the national strength and conditioning association. *J Strength Cond Res* 23 (5 Suppl):S60–S79. doi: 10.1519/JSC.0b013e31819df407.

Faigenbaum, A.D., R.L. Loud, J. O'Connell, S. Glover, J. O'Connell, and W.L. Westcott. 2001. Effects of different resistance training protocols on upper-body strength and endurance development in children. *J Strength Cond Res* 15 (4):459–465.

Faigenbaum, A.D. and L.J. Micheli. 2000. Preseason conditioning for the preadolescent athlete. *Pediatr Ann* 29 (3):156–161.

Faigenbaum, A.D., L.A. Milliken, R.L. Loud, B.T. Burak, C.L. Doherty, and W.L. Westcott. 2002. Comparison of 1 and 2 days per week of strength training in children. *Res Q Exerc Sport* 73 (4):416–424.

Faigenbaum, A.D., L.A. Milliken, and W.L. Westcott. 2003. Maximal strength testing in healthy children. *J Strength Cond Res* 17 (1):162–166.

Faigenbaum, A.D. and G. Myer. 2012. Effective strategies for developing young athletes. *ACSMs Health Fit J* 16 (5):9–16.

Faigenbaum, A.D. and G.D. Myer. 2010a. Pediatric resistance training: Benefits, concerns, and program design considerations. *Curr Sports Med Rep* 9 (3):161–168. doi: 10.1249/JSR.0b013e3181de1214.

Faigenbaum, A.D. and G.D. Myer. 2010b. Resistance training among young athletes: Safety, efficacy and injury prevention effects. *Br J Sports Med* 44 (1):56–63. doi: 10.1136/bjsm.2009.068098.

Faigenbaum, A.D., N.A. Ratamess, J. McFarland, J. Kaczmarek, M.J. Coraggio, J. Kang, and J.R. Hoffman. 2008. Effect of rest interval length on bench press performance in boys, teens, and men. *Pediatr Exer Sci* 20 (4):457–69.

Faigenbaum, A.D., W.L. Westcott, R.L. Loud, and C. Long. 1999. The effects of different resistance training protocols on muscular strength and endurance development in children. *Pediatrics* 104 (1):e5.

Faigenbaum, A.D., W.L. Westcott, L.J. Micheli, A.R. Outerbridge, C.J. Long, R. LaRosa-Loud, and L.D. Zaichkowsky. 1996. The effects of strength training and detraining on children. *J Strength Cond Res* 10 (2):109–114.

Falk, B. and A. Eliakim. 2003. Resistance training, skeletal muscle and growth. *Pediatr Endorinol Rev* 1 (2):120.

Falk, B. and G. Tenenbaum. 1996. The effectiveness of resistance training in children. *Sports Med* 22 (3):176–186.

Fedewa, A.L. and S. Ahn. 2011. The effects of physical activity and physical fitness on children's achievement and cognitive outcomes: A meta-analysis. *Res Q Exerc Sport* 82 (3):521–535.

Fraser-Thomas, J., J. Côté, and J. Deakin. 2008. Understanding dropout and prolonged engagement in adolescent competitive sport. *Psychol Sport Exerc* 9 (5):645–662.

Garber, C.E., B. Blissmer, M.R. Deschenes, B.A. Franklin, M.J. Lamonte, I.-M. Lee, D.C. Nieman, and D.P. Swain. 2011. The American College of Sports Medicine position stand, Cardiorespiratory, musculoskeletal, and neuromotor fitness in apparently healthy adults: Guidance for prescribing exercise. *Med Sci Sports Exerc* 43 (7):1334–1359.

Geithner, C.A., M.A. Thomis, B.V. Eynde, H.H.M. Maes, R.J.F. Loos, M. Peeters, A.L.M. Claessens, R. Vlietinck, R.M. Malina, and G.P. Beunen. 2004. Growth in peak aerobic power during adolescence. *Med Sci Sports Exerc* 36 (9):1616–1624.

Gumming, G.R., D. Everatt, and L. Hastman. 1978. Bruce treadmill test in children: Normal values in a clinic population. *Am J Cardiol* 41 (1):69–75.

Health, American Academy of Pediatrics Committee on Sports Medicine and Fitness and Committee in School. 2001. Organized sports for children and preadolescents. *Pediatrics* 107 (6):1459–1462.

Janssen, I. 2007. Physical activity guidelines for children and youth. *Can J Public Health* 98 (S2):S109–S121.

Janssen, I. and A.G. LeBlanc. 2010. Systematic review of the health benefits of physical activity and fitness in school-aged children and youth. *Int J Behav Nutr Phys Act* 7 (40):1–16. doi: 10.1186/1479-5868-7-40.

Kimm, S.Y.S., N.W. Glynn, E. Obarzanek, A.M. Kriska, S.R. Daniels, B.A. Barton, and K. Liu. 2005. Relation between the changes in physical activity and body-mass index during adolescence: A multicentre longitudinal study. *Lancet* 366 (9482):301–307. doi: 10.1016/s0140-6736(05)66837.

Knudson, D. 1998. Stretching: From science to practice. *JOPERD* 3 (69):38–42.

Knudson, D. 1999. Stretching during warm-up: Do we have enough evidence? *JOPERD* 70 (7):24–29.

Krahenbuhl, G.S., J.S. Skinner, and W.M. Kohrt. 1985. Developmental aspects of maximal aerobic power in children. *Exerc Sport Sci Rev* 13 (1):503–538.

Kreider, R.B., B. Leutholtz, F.I. Katch, and V.L. Katch. 2009a. *Exercise & Sport Nutrition: Principles, Promises, Science and Recommendations*. Santa Barbara, CA: Fitness Technologies Press.

Kreider, R.B., B.C. Leutholtz, F.I. Katch, and V. Katch. 2009b. *Exercise & Sport Nutrition: Principles, Promises, Science, Recommendations*. Santa Barbara, CA: Fitness Technologies Press.

Landry, B.W. and S.W. Driscoll. 2012. Physical activity in children and adolescents. *PM&R* 4 (11):826–32.

Lewthwaite, R. and T.K. Scanlan. 1989. Predictors of competitive trait anxiety in male youth sport participants. *Med Sci Sports Exerc* 21 (2):221–229.

Lillegard, W.A., E.W. Brown, D.J. Wilson, R. Henderson, and E. Lewis. 1997. Efficacy of strength training in prepubescent to early postpubescent males and females: Effects of gender and maturity. *Pediatr Rehabil* 1 (3):147–157.

Lloyd, R.S., A.D. Faigenbaum, M.H. Stone, J.L. Oliver, I. Jeffreys, J.A. Moody, C. Brewer, K.C. Pierce, T.M. McCambridge, and R. Howard. 2013. Position statement on youth resistance training: The 2014 International Consensus. *Br J Sports Med* 48 (7):498–505.

MacKay, M., A. Scanlan, L. Olsen, D. Reid, M. Clark, K. McKim, and P. Raina. 2004. Looking for the evidence: A systematic review of prevention strategies addressing sport and recreational injury among children and youth. *J Sci Med Sport* 7 (1):58–73.

Malina, R.M., G.P. Beunen, A.L. Claessens, J. Lefevre, B.V. Eynde, R. Renson, B. Vanreusel, and J. Simons. 1995. Fatness and physical fitness of girls 7 to 17 years. *Obes Res* 3 (3):221–231.

Martin, T.J. and J.S. Martin. 2002. Special issues and concerns for the high-school and college-aged athlete. *Pediatr Clin North Am* 49:533–552.

McHugh, M.P. and C.H. Cosgrave. 2010. To stretch or not to stretch: The role of stretching in injury prevention and performance. *Scand J Med Sci Sports* 20:169–181.

Micheli, L. 2006. Preventing injuries in sports: What the team physician needs to know. In *FIMS Team Physician Manual* (2nd ed.). Chan, K., Micheli, L., Smith, A., Rolf, C., Bachl, N., Frontera, W., and Alenabi, T., eds. Hong Kong: CD Concept, 555–572.

Molinero, O., A. Salguero, C. Tuero, E. Alvarez, and S. Márquez. 2006. Dropout reasons in young Spanish athletes: Relationship to gender, type of sport and level of competition. *J Sport Behav* 29 (3):255–69.

Myer, G.D., C.E. Quatman, J. Khoury, E.J. Wall, and T.E. Hewett. 2009. Youth versus adult "weightlifting" injuries presenting to United States emergency rooms: Accidental versus nonaccidental injury mechanisms. *J Strength Cond Res* 23 (7):2054–2060.

Nader, P.R., R.H. Bradley, R.M. Houts, S.L. McRitchie, and M. O'Brien. 2009. Moderate-to-vigorous physical activity from ages 9 to 15 years (vol 300, pg 295, 2008). *JAMA* 301 (20):2095–2098.

Nassis, G.P., K. Papantakou, K. Skenderi, M. Triandafillopoulou, S.A. Kavouras, M. Yannakoulia, G.P. Chrousos, and L.S. Sidossis. 2005. Aerobic exercise training improves insulin sensitivity without changes in body weight, body fat, adiponectin, and inflammatory markers in overweight and obese girls. *Metabolism* 54 (11):1472–1479. doi: 10.1016/j.metabol.2005.05.013.

National Institute of Arthritis, Musculoskeletal and Skin Diseases. 2006. *Childhood Sports Injuries and Their Prevention: A Guide for Parents with Ideas for Kids.* edited by NIH Pub.: NIH.

Nettle, H. and E. Sprogis. 2011. Pediatric exercise: Truth and/or consequences. *Sports Med Arthrosc* 19 (1):75–80.

Nóbrega, A.C.L., K.C. Paula, and A.C.G. Carvalho. 2005. Interaction between resistance training and flexibility training in healthy young adults. *J Strength Cond Res* 19 (4):842–846.

Organization, World Health. 2010. *Global Recommendations on Physical Activity for Health.*

Payne, V.G., J.R. Morrow Jr, L. Johnson, and S.N. Dalton. 1997. Resistance training in children and youth: A meta-analysis. *Res Q Exerc Sport* 68 (1):80–88.

Pierce, K., C. Brewer, M. Ramsey, R. Byrd, W.A. Sands, M.E. Stone, and M.H. Stone. 2008. Youth resistance training. *Profess Strength Cond* 10:9–23.

Ramsay, J.A., C.J. Blimkie, K. Smith, S. Garner, J.D. MacDougall, and D.G. Sale. 1990. Strength training effects in prepubescent boys. *Med Sci Sports Exerc* 22 (5):605–614.

Roemmich, J.N., M. Lambiase, S.J. Salvy, and P.J. Horvath. 2009. Protective effect of interval exercise on psychophysiological stress reactivity in children. *Psychophysiology* 46:852–861.

Rubin, D.A., R.G. McMurray, J.S. Harrell, A.C. Hackney, D.E. Thorpe, and A.M. Haqq. 2008. The association between insulin resistance and cytokines in adolescents: The role of weight status and exercise. *Metabolism* 57 (5):683–690. doi: 10.1016/j.metabol.2008.01.005.

Ruiz, J.R., N.S. Rizzo, A. Hurtig-Wennloef, F.B. Ortega, J. Warnberg, and M. Sjoestroem. 2006. Relations of total physical activity and intensity to fitness and fatness in children: The European Youth Heart Study (vol 84, pg 299, 2006). *Am J Clin Nutr* 89 (2):656–656. doi: 10.3945/ajcn.2008.27261.

Rusko, H.K. 1992. Development of aerobic power in relation to age and training in cross-country skiers. *Med Sci Sports Exerc* 24 (9):1040.

Rutenfranz, J., K. Lange Andersen, V. Seliger, F. Klimmer, I. Berndt, and M. Ruppel. 1981. Maximum aerobic power and body composition during the puberty growth period: Similarities and differences between children of two European countries. *Eur J Pediatr* 136 (2):123–133.

Safran, M.R., W.E. Garrett, A.V. Seaber, R.R. Glisson, and B.M. Ribbeck. 1988. The role of warmup in muscular injury prevention. *Am J Sports Med* 16 (2):123–129.

Sagar, S.S. and J. Stoeber. 2009. Perfectionism, fear of failure, and affective responses to success and failure: The central role of fear of experiencing shame and embarrassment. *J Sport Exerc Psychol* 31:602–627.

Salguero, A., R. Gonzalez-Boto, C. Tuero, and S. Marquez. 2003. Identification of dropout reasons in young competitive swimmers. *J Sports Med Phys Fitness* 43 (4):530–534.

Schwingshandl, J. and M. Borkenstein. 1995. Changes in lean body mass in obese children during a weight reduction program: Effect on short term and long term outcome. *Int J Obes Relat Metab Disord* 19 (10):752–755.

Schwingshandl, J. K. Sudi, B. Eibl, S. Wallner, and M. Borkenstein. 1999. Effect of an individualised training programme during weight reduction on body composition: A randomised trial. *Arch Dis Child* 81 (5):426–428.

Services, US Department of Health and Human. 2008. *2008 Physical Activity Guidelines for Americans.*

Shabi, G., M. Cruz, G. Ball, M. Weigensberg, G. Salem, N. Crespo, and M. Goran. 2006. Effects of resistance training on insulin sensitivity in overweight Latino adolescent males. *Med Sci Sports Exerc* 38:1208–1215.

Shrier, I. 2004. Does stretching improve performance? A systematic and critical review of the literature. *Clin J Sport Med* 14 (5):267–274.

Small, E. 2002. Chronic musculoskeletal pain in young athletes. *Pediatr Clin N Am* 49:655–662.

Smith, A.D., J.T. Andrish, and L.J. Micheli. 1993. Current comment from the American College of Sports Medicine. August 1993—"The prevention of sport injuries of children and adolescents". *Med Sci Sports Exerc* 25 (8 Suppl):1–7.

Smith, R.E. 1986. Toward a cognitive-affective model of athlete burnout. *J Sport Psychol* 8:36–50.

So, W.Y. 2012. Association between physical activity and academic performance in Korean adolescent students. *BMC Public Health* 12:258–265. doi: 10.1186/147-2458-12-258.

Stoeber, J. and C. Becker. 2008. Perfectionism, achievement motives, and attribution of success and failure in female soccer players. *Int J Psychol* 43 (6):980–987. doi: 10.1080/00207590701403850.

Stoeber, J. and K. Otto. 2006. Positive conceptions of perfectionism: Approaches, evidence, challenges. *Pers Soc Psychol Rev* 10 (4):295–319.

Stratton, G., M. Jones, K.R. Fox, K. Tolfrey, J. Harris, N. Maffulli, M. Lee, and S.P. Frostick. 2004. BASES position statement on guidelines for resistance exercise in young people. *J Sport Sci* 22 (4):383–390.

Stricker, P.R. 2002. Sports training issues for the pediatric athlete. *Pediatr Clin N Am* 49 (4):793–802.

Strong, W.B., R.M. Malina, C.J. Blimke, S.R. Daniels, R.K. Dishman, B. Gutin, A.C. Hergenroeder, A. Must, P.A. Nixon, J.M. Pivarnik, T. Rowland, S. Trost, and F. Trudeau. 2005. Evidence based physical activity for school-age youth. *J Pediatr* 146 (6):732–737.

Sung, R.Y., C.W. Yu, S.K. Chang, S.W. Mo, K.S. Woo, and C.W. Lam. 2002. Effects of dietary intervention and strength training on blood lipid level in obese children. *Arch Dis Child* 86 (6):407–410.

Tsai, Y.M. and L.H. Chen. 2009. Relation of motivational climate and fear of failure in Taiwanese adolescent athletes. *Psychol Rep* 104:627–632.

Tudor-Locke, C., C.L. Craig, M.W. Beets, S. Belton, G.M. Cardon, S. Duncan, Y. Hatano, D.R. Lubans, T.S. Olds, A. Raustorp, D.A. Rowe, J.C. Spence, S. Tanaka, and S.N. Blair. 2011. How many steps/day are enough? For children and adolescents. *Int J Behav Nutr Phys Act* 8:1–14. doi: 10.1186/1479-5868-8-78.

Valovich McLeod, T.C., L.C. Decoster, K.J. Loud, L.J. Micheli, J.T. Parker, M.A. Sandrey, and C. White. 2011. National Athletic Trainers' Association position statement: Prevention of pediatric overuse injuries. *J Athl Train* 46 (2):206.

Weerapong, P., P.A. Hume, and G.S. Kolt. 2004. Stretching: Mechanisms and benefits for sport performance and injury prevention. *Phys Ther Rev* 9 (4):189–206.

Witurouw, E., N. Mahieu, L. Danneels, and P. McNair. 2004. Stretching and injury prevention, an obscure relationship. *Sports Med* 34 (7):443–449.

Zafeiridis, A., A. Dalamitros, K. Dipla, V. Manou, N. Galanis, and S. Kellis. 2005. Recovery during high-intensity intermittent anaerobic exercise in boys, teens, and men. *Med Sci Sports Exerc* 37 (3):505–512.

Section III

A Hands-on, Practical Approach

15 How to Fuel Your Day

Jennifer McDaniel and Elizabeth Fox

CONTENTS

Abstract 266
15.1 Introduction 266
15.2 Planning Breakfast, Lunch, Dinner, and Snacks 266
    15.2.1 Basic Components of a Balanced Plate at Meals 266
    15.2.2 Breakfast, Lunch, and Dinner of "Champions" 266
        15.2.2.1 Breakfast 266
    15.2.3 Fluid Needs and Choices 268
        15.2.3.1 Helpful Tips to Meet Fluid Needs 269
    15.2.4 Snack Attack: What to Pack and Why 269
        15.2.4.1 Three W's of Snacking 269
        15.2.4.2 Example Snack Duo Power 270
        15.2.4.3 Five Favorite Dips 270
15.3 Healthy Eating on the Road 270
    15.3.1 Planning Fueling Opportunities before Travel 270
        15.3.1.1 Eating on the Road Checklist 270
    15.3.2 Choosing the Healthiest Options When Eating Out 270
    15.3.3 Questions Parents/Coaches Should Ask Regarding Individual Orders 271
        15.3.3.1 When Ordering Out, Keep in Mind 271
    15.3.4 Favorite Meal Ideas 271
        15.3.4.1 Our Five Favorite Fast Food Picks 272
    15.3.5 Air Travel 272
15.4 End of the Day Eating: How to Eat Healthy at Night 272
    15.4.1 Evening Eats to Avoid 273
    15.4.2 Ten Grocery/Gas Station Snacks 274
    15.4.3 Eating at Night Myths 274
15.5 Tackling the Grocery Store 274
    15.5.1 Before You Shop 274
    15.5.2 Navigating the Store Aisle by Aisle 275
        15.5.2.1 Aisle by Aisle 275
    15.5.3 Getting Kids Involved 276
    15.5.4 Label Reading 276
        15.5.4.1 Beware of Health Halo Labeling 276
15.6 Navigating the Cafeteria 277
    15.6.1 Building a "Champions" Plate 278
    15.6.2 Brown Bag Lunches 278
    15.6.3 Other Meal Suggestions for a Healthy Brown Bag 279
15.7 Helpful Resources for Parents/Coaches 279
References 280

ABSTRACT

This chapter provides an introduction to food and fluid recommendations for young athletes, including fueling strategies for parents, coaches, nurses, and other healthcare practitioners. Timing of food and fluid intake before and after exercise as well as ideal food and fluid choices for child and adolescent athletes are reviewed. Breakfast, lunch, dinner, and snack ideas are discussed in detail, as well as planning ahead for fueling opportunities while traveling. Developing a fueling schedule and including children and adolescents in meal and snack preparation is essential. Further concepts outlined in this chapter include navigation of the grocery store and cafeteria, packing optimal brown bag lunches, and tips for ordering when eating on the road.

15.1 INTRODUCTION

Life runs more smoothly when we plan ahead. Feeding a family can be a daunting task with the juggling of multiple lives and schedules. However, carving out time to plan meals can save precious time and energy. Healthy meals do not just happen; they require time management. In order to function effectively and efficiently on a daily basis, we have to plan ahead. For example, scheduling a doctor's appointment without interfering with work, school, or practice can be challenging. But if done in advance, as crazy as things may be, everything works out. It is important to apply these same time management skills in developing a plan for adequately fueling your child athlete for performance. This chapter provides simplified recommendations and fueling strategies for busy parents, coaches, nurses, and other health practitioners working with youth athletes.

15.2 PLANNING BREAKFAST, LUNCH, DINNER, AND SNACKS

15.2.1 BASIC COMPONENTS OF A BALANCED PLATE AT MEALS

Just like an automobile, an athlete's body must have enough fuel to drive optimal athletic performance and recovery. In addition, an athlete needs the optional combination of ingredients so the engine runs as efficiently as possible and does not break down before the trip has been completed (or even begun). A winning plate at any meal includes carbohydrates, lean proteins, and healthy fats. *Carbohydrates* are "A" key ingredient for maximal energy, speed, stamina, concentration, recovery, and fluid balance. Plan a plate with colorful carbohydrates from fruits, vegetables, and whole grains. Carbohydrates should fill up one-half to two-thirds of your plate depending upon how hard you train. *Proteins* are needed by your body to supply amino acids to your various tissues to build and rebuild the hundreds of thousands of proteins found throughout our body as well as the trillions of cells. Protein-rich foods such as low-fat dairy, nuts, beans, soy, eggs, chicken, turkey, pork, and lean beef help to repair and build muscles and are important for immune function. Protein-rich foods should fill up one-quarter of your plate at each meal. Fats are not all bad much to popular belief. Fats are needed for proper cell function, vitamin and nutrient absorption, immune function, energy, and insulation. Healthy fats such as nuts, nut buttervs, seeds (chia or flax), avocado, and oils should be included at every meal. A little bit of a healthy fat goes a long way. Figure 15.1 is a diagram provided by the United States Olympic Committee (USOC) (http://www.teamusa.org) that is intended to provide a visual depiction of what quantities of each macronutrient (carbohydrates, proteins, and fats) are recommended.

15.2.2 BREAKFAST, LUNCH, AND DINNER OF "CHAMPIONS"

15.2.2.1 Breakfast

Breakfast is a must for optimal performance on the field and in the classroom. Eating breakfast is important, but eating high-quality breakfast foods sets up each athlete for optimal fueling,

How to Fuel Your Day

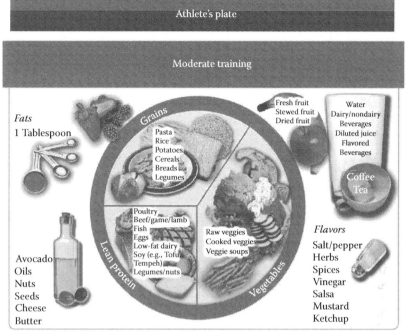

The athlete's plates are a collaboration between the United States Olympic Commitee Sport Dietitians and the University of Colorado (UCCS) Sport Nutrition Graduate Program.

FIGURE 15.1 The athlete's plate. A visual depiction of what quantities of each macronutrient (carbohydrates, proteins, and fats) are recommended. (Data from http://www.teamusa.org/About-the-USOC/Athlete-Development/Sport-Performance/Nutrition/Resources-and-Fact-Sheets)

performance, and recovery. Research shows that kids who choose filling, fiber-rich breakfast foods perform better in the classroom compared to those who eat high sugar breakfast foods such as sugar-coated cereal (Mahoney et al. 2005).

Each breakfast should include the following: protein + fiber-rich food + fruit. These three foods provide a mixture of carbohydrates ("necessary for brain and muscle energy") and protein ("important for muscle growth after a long night's sleep"). To help with planning and variety, consider that including just three different foods at each meal everyday means that 35 different foods are consumed by the end of the week!

15.2.2.1.1 A+ Breakfast Ideas

- *The Banana Dog*: Peanut butter on a whole-wheat hot dog bun with a banana sandwiched inside. Drizzle honey on top
- *The Greek Parfait*: Greek yogurt + whole-grain cereal + berries
- *Chunky Monkey Smoothie*: Milk + vanilla yogurt + frozen banana + peanut butter
- *The Protein Pita*: Whole-wheat pita + egg + low-fat cheese + sliced apple on the side
- *The Better Bowl*: Oatmeal made with milk or soy milk + dried fruit + sliced almonds

Early morning practices call for *not one, but two morning meals*. Prepractice meals or snacks should include carbohydrates and be easily digested especially if the time between waking up and starting practice is limited. Postpractice breakfast should include protein and carbohydrate to help repair and recover muscles and also provide the energy needed to support learning until lunch.

15.2.2.1.2 Lunch: (Protein + Whole Grain + Fruit/Vegetable)

- *Waffle Sandwich:* Peanut butter, banana, honey, and cinnamon on whole-grain waffles
- *Turkey and Pesto Wrap:* Turkey, Swiss cheese, pesto sauce in flatbread wrap
- *Pizza Muffins:* Whole-wheat English muffin, topped with marinara sauce, mozzarella cheese, and grilled chicken
- *Tuna Salad with a Health Kick:* Tuna fish salad made with 1/2 light mayo and 1/2 plain Greek yogurt, dried cranberries and walnuts in whole-wheat pita
- *Bento Box Lunch:* Yogurt parfait with fruit and whole-grain cereal, sugar snap peas to dip in hummus, frozen grapes

Consider that most high school baseball, softball, soccer, tennis, and track and field matches are in the afternoon; thus your lunch is likely going to serve as your pregame meal, so do not skimp on much high-quality food you consume for lunch. If you compete in the early evening, then a pregame meal needs to be consumed very soon after school is over. Waiting too long and eating too much food might upset your stomach come the start of the competition. As a result, plan ahead and have a meal ready at home or bring a large snack to eat when school lets out or on the bus ride or walk home. Energy is needed for both the muscles and brain to perform optimally.

15.2.2.1.3 Dinner: (Protein + Whole Grain + Vegetable/Fruit)

- *Tuna Melt*: Low-fat tuna fish salad with melted Swiss cheese on whole-wheat English muffin fruit, baby carrots
- *Veggie Burger*: Topped with low-fat cheddar, lettuce and tomato, whole-wheat roll, raw veggies, fruit
- *Soup's Up!*: Lentil soup, low-fat Swiss cheese, whole-wheat crackers
- *Bean Burrito*: Refried black beans, cheese, and salsa in whole-wheat tortillas
- *Shrimp Fried Rice*: Stir-fried shrimp, brown minute rice, frozen mixed veggies
- *Baked Potato Bar*: Large baked potato, broccoli in low-fat cheese salsa, sliced turkey, and salsa

15.2.2.1.3.1 Dinner Tip
Before you choose your meal, briefly think about what you have eaten so far that day. If you had fruit at breakfast, lunch, and your afternoon snack, then make sure to load up on vegetables at dinner. In order to meet the 3–5 servings of vegetables daily, most athletes need to include a vegetable at lunch and dinner.

15.2.3 FLUID NEEDS AND CHOICES

Water is always an ideal fluid fuel for an athlete at meal times, but low-fat milk, 100% fruit juice, and sports drinks can play a role as well, particularly for athletes who may struggle with their appetite or get enough fuel across the day. The best-fitting beverage depends on when it is consumed, training volume, and environmental conditions:

- *Water*: All day and any time!
- *Low-Fat Milk:* Great option with meals (for optimal health: serve up to 2 cups a day for kids aged 2 to 4; 2½ cups for kids 4 to 8; and 3 cups for kids 9 and older)
- *Sports Drinks:* During practice or competition lasting >60 min; sports drinks might offer a quick source of carbohydrate immediately before practice/competition. Sipping on a sports drink leading up to the start of competition is an excellent strategy! Sports drinks take on an even greater level of importance when environmental conditions are hot and humid and the athlete will be sweating a good bit in an effort to cool their body.
- *100% Juice:* An acceptable beverage with a meal—The American Academy of Pediatrics recommends no fruit juice servings for children under the age of 6 months; 4–6 oz of

100% fruit juice for children aged 6 months to 6 years, and 8–12 oz for kids aged 7 and older (Committee on Nutrition 2001). Juice with meals may help an underweight athlete gain weight.
- *Low-Fat Chocolate Milk:* Great post recovery drink for practice/training after a hard training or competition. As highlighted throughout Chapter 16, scientific studies have supported the use of chocolate milk as an excellent choice to rehydrate and refuel the body (Potter and Fuller 2015, Pritchett et al. 2009).

15.2.3.1 Helpful Tips to Meet Fluid Needs
- *Make sure fluids taste good*: Water is an ideal way to hydrate, but when children are offered water alone, they often only meet 50% of their fluid needs. Spruce up regular water with fruit-flavored ice cubes by freezing 100% juice in ice cube trays.
- *Offer fluids often*: It is important to make fluids convenient. Freezing water bottles and packing them with lunch will not only provide them with the fluids, but will also keep a lunch box cold.
- *Follow the 20-min rule*: Hydrate every 20 min when a child is engaged in outside activity. The American Academy of Pediatrics suggests children weighing approximately 88 lb should drink 5 oz of water or a sports drink every 20 min and adolescents weighing approximately 132 lb should drink about 9 oz every 20 min. An ounce is about two kid-size gulps (Committee on Nutrition 2001). Once again, the child will more likely meet their fluid needs when offering them a sports drink or flavored water. Similar guidelines are outlined in a position statement by the National Athletic Trainers Association (Casa et al. 2000).
- *Hydrate through food*: Water in food also contributes to daily water intake. Fruit and vegetables are 80%–90% water by weight and are a great way to keep an active child hydrated. Offer up slices of oranges, watermelon, cantaloupe, or honeydew melon when players come off the field, or frozen grapes as a true fruit popsicle!

15.2.4 SNACK ATTACK: WHAT TO PACK AND WHY

Snacks are an important mini meal for athletes. Nutritious snacks serve as an opportunity to fill in nutrient gaps, crowd out less healthy options, and serve as pre/posttraining between main meals.

15.2.4.1 Three W's of Snacking
1. WHAT
   a. Use snacks to fill in nutrient gaps with whole foods.
   b. Think in pairs.
2. WHEN
   c. Structure snacks as part of an eating schedule.
3. WHERE
   d. Create mindful snacking habits.
   e. Ideal: at the kitchen table on a plate.
   f. Plate snacks and avoid eating out of large packages.

Snack duo power:
You pick two:

1. Whole-grain rich carbohydrate (energy)
2. Healthy fat (staying power)
3. Lean protein (staying power)

15.2.4.2 Example Snack Duo Power
- Apple + string cheese
- Baby carrots + hummus
- Whole-wheat bread + peanut butter
- Hardboiled egg + pistachios
- Greek yogurt + blueberries

Healthy dips make snacking more nutritious and more fun! Research proves that children eat more fruits and vegetables when produce is paired with a dip (Savage et al. 2013).

15.2.4.3 Five Favorite Dips
1. *Fruit Dip*: Plain yogurt/Greek yogurt + peanut butter + honey
2. *Veggie Dip*: Premade/homemade hummus
3. *Mexi Dip*: Refried beans + shredded cheese + plain yogurt/Greek yogurt
4. *Cali Dip*: Mashed avocado with lemon and yogurt
5. *Tomato Dip*: Marinara sauce—goes great with breaded zucchini sticks or string cheese!

15.3 HEALTHY EATING ON THE ROAD

Setting a plan for eating on the road is very important, and should be done ahead of time. You can find most restaurant menus and nutritional information online or by downloading applications on a smartphone. Use the following tips below to help keep your young athletes well fueled every 3–4 h while traveling.

15.3.1 Planning Fueling Opportunities before Travel

15.3.1.1 Eating on the Road Checklist
- Plan meal stops before traveling
  - Look for
    - Grain-based options (sandwiches, rice dishes, pasta items)
    - Lean proteins (chicken, fish, turkey, beans, vegetarian options)
    - Produce-filled options (fruit and vegetable side dish options)
    - Low-fat options (i.e., marinara sauce over alfredo sauce and grilled chicken over breaded/fried)
- Pack nonperishable snacks as well as balanced meal options in a cooler if possible.
- Buffets can be a nice way of offering a variety of healthy foods—teach kids to fill their plates with the "athlete's plate" approach
- Try user-friendly applications such as healthydiningfinder.com or calorieking.com to guide your choices

15.3.2 Choosing the Healthiest Options When Eating Out

- *Plan ahead*: Check out the menu options online before dining out. Take your time to review the entire menu to ensure you make the most nutrient-dense choice.
- *Be proactive in ordering*—mix and match menu items: Replacing a side of French fries with a baked potato or vegetable side is usually always an option. Do not be afraid to ask your waiter for healthier substitutions on menu items.
- *Order plain/simple items and familiar foods*: Spicy, high-fat, and/or salty foods are not ideal, especially in the pregame meal. Stomach irritation and abdominal bloating may

occur, which can cause some discomfort and potentially interfere with performance. While variety and moderation are important concepts in balancing nutrient intake, never try new foods before competition.
- *Foods/drinks to look for on the menu*: Baked potatoes, broth-based soups, grilled chicken sandwich, low-fat milk, fruit and yogurt smoothie, granola bars, hardboiled eggs, thin cheese or veggie pizza, salad, fruit, and raw veggies with dip.

15.3.3 Questions Parents/Coaches Should Ask Regarding Individual Orders
- Can you leave off a heavy cream-based (i.e., alfredo sauce)?
- Does the restaurant accommodate all team members' diet needs? That is, gluten, vegetarian, allergies, and intolerances.
- Can they add sides of vegetables or fruit?
- Can they double something? (Two orders of rice instead of one)
- Can gravies, sauces, butter, dressings be served on the side?
- How is the food prepared? (Breaded, fried, etc.)

15.3.3.1 When Ordering Out, Keep in Mind
- High-fat items tend to crowd out needed carbohydrates
    - Select grilled/broiled foods and avoid fried foods
    - Order low-fat milk or 100% juice
    - Choose a salad or baked potato instead of fries
    - Use high-fat dressings and white sauces sparingly
    - Ask for veggies on your pizza, go easy on the cheese, or choose chicken over higher-fat meats such as pepperoni and sausage

15.3.4 Favorite Meal Ideas
Below are the best choices when dining out at various restaurant cuisines:
- American restaurant:
    - Turkey or veggie burger with fruit side
    - Fish with rice and vegetables
    - Small hamburger with salad and fruit
    - BBQ sandwich with baked potato and vegetables
- Mexican restaurant:
    - Fish tacos
    - Bean tostado or burrito
    - Chicken tacos
    - Chicken fajitas
- Burger joint:
    - Plain single patty burger
    - Plain grilled chicken sandwich
    - Veggie burger
    - Turkey burger
    - Baked potatoes, salads, fruit, milk as sides
- Chinese/Vietnamese:
    - Rice/noodle dishes with light sauces including lean choices such as chicken, pork, tofu vegetables
    - Spring rolls versus egg rolls
    - Avoid fried dishes and be aware of how spicy the dish is seasoned

- Sub shop:
  - Turkey, ham, roast beef, veggie subs
  - Avoid heavier choices (tuna salads, meatballs, bacon subs)
  - Go with vegetables and fruits over chips and cookies
  - Choose light mayonnaise options or even go for vinegar and oil as your dressing
- Italian:
  - Pastas with red sauce
  - Choose pastas or salads that include beans
  - Salads
  - Lean meats such as chicken or fish
  - Avoid creamy sauces and fried foods

15.3.4.1 Our Five Favorite Fast Food Picks

1. *Subway Veggie Delite Sandwich*
   Get it on wheat bread without cheese, and plenty of veggies. Picking out your toppings can be fun. Pair with a fruit and dairy.
2. *Subway Roast Beef Sandwich*
   Get it on wheat bread. Roast beef is a good source of iron. Turkey breast could also be a good choice. Pair with apple slices.
3. *Burger King Macaroni and Cheese*
   Get the apple slices (no caramel dipping sauce) and fat-free milk for only 285 cal. Burger King has a portioned sized out mac and cheese. Combine with apples slices and fat-free milk.
4. *KFC Grilled Chicken Drumstick*
   Pair with corn on the cob, unsweetened tea, and a cheese stick. This is a well-balanced meal with a veggie, grilled meat, and dairy.
5. *Sonic Junior Burger*
   Smaller size of burger makes for appropriate portion size. Pair with apple slices and water.

15.3.5 Air Travel

Planning meals and snacks for air travel can be more challenging than for car travel. Fluids cannot be carried through security at airports, but empty water bottles are acceptable. This way the athletes can refill their water as many times as they like without having to purchase expensive bottled water. Pack snacks that are rich in carbohydrate and protein that will clear security, such as homemade trail mix, fruit, cheese sticks, veggies, granola bars, instant oatmeal packets (ask for hot water), and premade peanut butter and jelly sandwiches.

If travel plans require meals in the airport, look for "do it yourself" sandwich or salad shops that will allow you to mix and match items. Try downloading the "gate guru" application, which will display available food choices based on your airport, terminal, and gate.

Variety of food or beverage choices at hotels may be limited, which is why you want to call and find out the meal options (i.e., what is available at the continental breakfast) ahead of time. If possible, request an in-room refrigerator and microwave, so you can stock plenty of balanced snacks in your room. Try filling your storage space with fruits and veggies, sandwich materials, hummus, nuts, edamame, and air-popped popcorn. Take it one step further by bringing your own mini plastic bags to prepare portion-controlled snacks that can be taken to go.

15.4 END OF THE DAY EATING: HOW TO EAT HEALTHY AT NIGHT

While the bulk of an athletes' eating occurs during the light of day, many athletes will need to eat at night to refuel after an evening practice/event. Eating at night provides the necessary energy and nutrients for both the body and brain. A well-balanced evening meal supports energy for after-training activities (i.e., homework), maintenance of lean muscle mass, and restful sleep.

While an exhausted athlete might feel too fatigued to prepare and sit down to a late night meal, skipping this fueling opportunity could result in inadequate recovery. Chronic underfueling results in a loss of muscle mass, slower recovery, and inadequate energy for the next day's training. The optimal mix of late night fuel includes nutrient-dense carbohydrates and lean proteins. Late night meals need not be complicated, and can be assembled in minutes if preplanned and accessible. Examples of ready-to-eat proteins include hard boiled eggs, cheese, deli meat, cottage cheese, yogurt, vegetable burgers, and leftover grilled meats. Pair proteins with whole grains such as whole-grain breads (wraps, pita, waffles, English muffins) pastas, rice, and whole-grain cereals to quickly convert them into an evening meal.

Below are five example meal ideas that provide the calories, carbohydrates, and proteins necessary to maintain a healthy body weight and muscle mass, improve performance for next day training, and naturally boost the sleep hormone serotonin for a restful night's sleep. Round out any evening meal with a piece of fruit or side of vegetables.

1. *Rainbow "Fried" Rice*: Cooked brown rice combined with one chopped hard boiled egg, cooked edamame, and carrots.
2. *Yogurt Parfait*: Plain Greek yogurt with mixed fruit, and whole-grain cereal. Cold cereals should be 8 g of sugar or less and at least 3–4 g of fiber.
3. *Turkey and Apple Wrap*: Whole-grain wrap filled with low-fat Swiss cheese, thinly sliced apple or pear, and turkey breast.
4. *Cinnamon Cottage Cheese Toast*: Combine low-fat cottage cheese with 2 tbsp. raisins and cinnamon. Place on top of whole-grain toast and warm in toaster oven.
5. *Chicken Pizza Pita*: Fill whole-wheat pita with low-fat mozzarella cheese, marinara sauce, and chicken breast. Melt in microwave.

15.4.1 Evening Eats to Avoid

To ensure good sleep and a comfortably content stomach, avoid caffeine, high-fat foods, and spicy foods in your evening meal. While most individuals know that caffeine is found in tea or coffee, they might not recognize sneaky sources of caffeine such as chocolate, coffee-flavored ice creams or yogurts, noncola sodas such as root beer or citrus sodas, pain relievers, and energy waters. The effects of caffeine can last at least 3–4 h depending on the individual, and if consumed, should be consumed earlier in the day.

Eating high-fat foods at night interferes with digestion and sleep quality. Fried foods, heavily sauced items, full-fat dairy, high-fat meats such as sausage and pepperonis, cookies and chips are all examples of high-fat foods that should be limited or avoided. Finally, spicy foods with hot sauces or peppery spices can cause indigestion and interfere with sleep. It is best to avoid these foods at night. Here are 10 ideas for light and nutrient-dense evening snacks:

1. Italian popcorn: Light or air-popped popcorn sprinkled with parmesan cheese and Italian seasoning
2. Apple wheels: Sliced apples light topped with peanut butter and raisins
3. Banana soft-serve: In a blender, combine one frozen banana with 2 tbsp. milk and 1/2 tsp. vanilla
4. String cheese with pear slices
5. Whole-grain toast topped with 1 tablespoon (T) sunflower seed butter (or any nut butter)
6. Frozen grapes
7. Hummus wrap—whole-grain wrap filled with any flavor of hummus
8. Carrots, red bell peppers, sugar snap peas with low-fat ranch dip

9. Sliced fruit with peanut butter yogurt dip (dip: combine 1 T nut butter + 2 T yogurt + 1 tsp. honey)
10. Whole-grain crackers topped with slight Swiss cheese and dried apricots

In summary, a well-planned late night meal can be the day's dining finale contributing to the energy and nutrient needs for a growing athlete.

15.4.2 Ten Grocery/Gas Station Snacks

1. String cheese + fruit
2. Granola bar + fruit
3. Yogurt + whole-grain cereal
4. Whole-grain cereal and low-fat milk
5. Crackers and cheese
6. Popcorn
7. Oatmeal cookie with nut butter
8. Turkey sandwich
9. Low-fat chocolate milk and fruit
10. Peanut butter sandwich

15.4.3 Eating at Night Myths

Myth 1: Eating at night will lead to weight gain. For active athletes, eating at night will not negatively impact weight. Eating a snack including carbohydrates and protein before bed can promote better recovery, and actually help an athlete sleep better.

Myth 2: Metabolism shuts down at night. An athlete's metabolism still runs while they sleep!

Myth 3: Eating at night leads to bad dreams. Avoid eating spicy, high-fat foods that might interfere with sleep. Enjoying a carbohydrate and protein-rich snack should actually aid in hormone functions conducive to sleep.

15.5 TACKLING THE GROCERY STORE

15.5.1 Before You Shop

Going to the grocery store can be a daunting task, especially for parents buying snack and meal items for the week. Use the following five tips to help you plan for a budget-friendly and pleasant grocery shopping trip.

1. *Grocery shopping starts in your kitchen.* Take inventory to prevent overbuying and wasting food. About 40% of food purchased is thrown away, and 90% of us throw out food prematurely. When reading the expiration date, keep in mind that "use by" or "best by" refer to the food's peak date for use. For example, eggs can be good for 3 to 5 weeks after purchase, and pantry items can be used up to a year after the "use by" date. Start your shopping at home by planning a "use what you have" night, and take the time to clean up and organize space in your cold and dry storage.
2. *Plan meals.* Set a tentative meal schedule for the week, so you know exactly what you need to include on your grocery list. If you buy and cook in bulk, be creative with your meals. For example, if you plan to make meatloaf for dinner on Monday, try to use the leftovers for a ground meat and rice stir fry on Tuesday.
3. *Make a list.* How do you keep track of what you need? Your best bet is to map it out. Arrange items on your grocery list by category to reflect the layout of your local store. Make sure to include your kitchen staples and scan the week's recipes for additional ingredients.

4. *Eat!* Always eat before you head to the grocery store. If it has been three or more hours since your last meal or snack, you should and will feel hungry, as your blood sugar levels lower. Studies show that people do not just buy more food when hungry, but select more foods that are less nutritionally dense.
5. *Do not forget your bags.* Bringing reusable shopping bags with you to the grocery store is similar to bringing plastic containers to a party to take home leftovers: you are planning to take home only what you intend to fit. Additionally, most grocery stores will offer discounts to customers that bring their own bags, and it is great for the environment!

15.5.2 Navigating the Store Aisle by Aisle

Once you have planned the week's meals and completed your grocery list, tackling the grocery store is the next step. If possible, bring your athletes to the store with you. Get them involved in all stages of meal planning, including the grocery shopping and food preparation. Follow our aisle-by-aisle guide below, as well as ideas to get your kids involved!

15.5.2.1 Aisle by Aisle

- *Produce:* Make produce a priority. Walk through *every* produce aisle. Anything sold by the pound can be customized, so make it work for you.
  - Soft produce (avocados, bananas):
    – Choose a mix of ripe/unripe
  - Grab sturdy staples
    – Apples, carrots, potatoes
  - Fresh is not always the best
    – Frozen or dried is just as nutritious!
  - Try something new!
    – What looks fresh? On sale?
- *Bread/bread products:*
  - The *first* ingredient should be 100% whole grain
  - Look for the 100% Whole Grain Stamp
  - "Made with whole grains" does not mean it contains a substantial amount of whole grains
  - Do not judge a loaf by its color
    – May contain caramel coloring that gives it a brown color
  - Aim for 2–3 g of fiber per slice
- *Dairy:*
  - Choosing a yogurt:
    – Check the label for sugar. Many yogurts are high in added sugars (i.e., Brand A: 26 g sugar/6 oz versus Brand B: NF Greek Vanilla: 12 g/5.3 oz serving)
    – Regular versus Greek: Greek is higher in protein, but lower in calcium
    – Kefir milk is drinkable yogurt with healthy strains of good bacteria
- Cheese
  - Quantity: low fat (cheese slices)
  - Quality: flavorful cheeses pack big flavor in a small serving (a sprinkle of goat cheese on salad)
- Milk
  - Cow's milk: opt for low fat or skim
  - Soy milk: Look for calcium and vitamin D fortified, and watch for added sugars
  - Almond milk and rice milk: Mostly water, low in protein (1 g per cup), and watch for added sugars
  - Coconut milk: 50% of calories come from saturated fat

- *Protein:*
  - Lean meats: Chicken, turkey, lean beef
  - Seafood: Canned tuna, salmon
  - Deli: Opt for low-sodium lean meats
  - Vegetarian sources:
    – Canned beans
    – Lentils
    – Nuts
    – Eggs
  - Tofu is a common and excellent alternative protein option
- *Cart Worthy Convenience Foods:*
  - Rotisserie chicken
  - Frozen meals
    – 500 cal or less
    – 600 mg of sodium or less
    – 2 g of saturated fat or less
    – Bulk up with extra veggies or a salad
    – Vegetable and grain steam bags: limit added sauces

15.5.3 Getting Kids Involved

1. *Empower*: Get kids involved in the meal preparation process. Teaching kids how to cook empowers them with life-long skills. The more involved children are in the meal preparation process, the more likely they will try new foods and enjoy healthier options.
2. *Equip*: Stock the fridge with grab-and-go healthy food options. Cut up fruits and vegetables and store in plastic containers. Place grab-and-go produce front and center in the refrigerator. Offer dips with produce, as kids love to dip foods. Studies show kids eat more veggies when offered a dip. Offering your kids fun, healthy, and creative dips can be a great way to boost nutrition. Load up on dips such as hummus, light salad dressings, and Greek yogurt.
3. *Engage*: The kitchen is an amazing classroom. Kids can practice their math skills by measuring ingredients in a recipe. They can improve their language and vocabulary by reading and following recipes. Furthermore, talk to your kids about the science of food, like why one would use baking soda over baking powder in a muffin recipe. Even toddlers can help snap beans or shuck corn, which engages small and large muscle control.
4. *Excite*: Turn your grocery list into a "treasure hunt" game. Be creative! Try adding a new fruit or vegetable to the list every week. Encourage kids to pick out ingredients for a "DIY" trail mix or snack mix, or select healthier sundae toppings, such as berries, graham crackers, and chia seeds.

15.5.4 Label Reading

When trying to make a decision between two food items at the grocery store, reading the label and comparing nutrient information is a great way to ensure you choose the healthier of the two items. Portion size and nutrient content (limit fat, sodium and sugar content; encourage fiber, protein, and micronutrient content) of a food item can easily be determined by reading the food label. Filling your grocery cart with nutrient-dense foods and beverages is just as important as loading your cart with budget-friendly foods and beverages.

15.5.4.1 Beware of Health Halo Labeling

As more and more Americans have turned to lower-fat, lower-sugar foods and beverages to maintain a healthy diet, more and more companies have expanded their package front marketing claims to make their products more appealing to consumers. It is very important to beware of health halo labeling: overestimating the value of a food because of a specific quality or feature. For example, reduced-fat peanut butter has less fat and calories compared to regular peanut butter, but if you consume a greater portion of the reduced-fat peanut butter in place of the regular version, it can lead to more calories and more fat. Below are five examples of common health halo labels and a "smart swap" option for each.

1. *Vegetable chips.* Nutritional value is lost in the processing and you still get a hefty dose of fat and salt in most brands.
   Smart swap: Bean and lentil chips, which offer more protein and fiber, and contain less salt.
2. *Nutrient-enhanced waters.* The four main ingredients: water + sugar + vitamins + a lot of hype.
   Smart swap: Tap water and a varied diet and/or a daily multivitamin.
3. *"Gluten free."* While individuals with celiac disease or gluten intolerance must remove all products that contain gluten (wheat, rye, barley, and sometimes oats), following a gluten-free diet has recently become more of a fad diet. Just because something is gluten-free does not mean it is healthy.
   Smart swap: Instead of replacing wheat bread with gluten-free bread, try making sandwiches as lettuce wraps or serve lunchmeat and shredded cheese over a baked potato.
4. *"Multigrain."* This term simply means that the product is made from more than one type of grain. It does not mean the product is whole grain.
   Smart swap: Look for "whole grain" as first ingredient and aim for 5 g of fiber per serving.
5. *"Natural."* Natural does not mean organic. Items that are labeled 100% organic, organic, or "made with organic ingredients" have to meet government-approved standards. Natural, on the other hand, does not have to follow rules or regulations, and therefore a product labeled "natural" could very well contain processed ingredients.
   Smart swap: Choose 100% organic or organic products.

15.6 NAVIGATING THE CAFETERIA

For most young athletes, lunch is a prepractice or precompetition meal. And because most 6- to 18-year-olds eat lunch in the school cafeteria, it is important to educate children and adolescents regarding lunch selections, specifically what to eat and how much. See Table 15.1 for an example of a cafeteria meal replacement.

TABLE 15.1
Cafeteria Meal Makeover

Before	After
Large French fries, diet coke, and brownie	Deli Turkey sandwich, baked potato with 1 tbsp. sour cream, 8 oz skim milk, and an orange
Calories: 660	Calories: 520
Protein: 8 g (16%)	Protein: 44 g (90%)
Fat: 32 g (49%)	Fat: 10 g (16%)
Carbohydrates: 85 g	Carbohydrates: 63.5 g
Vitamin A: 3%	Vitamin A: 50%
Vitamin C: 30%	Vitamin C: 140%
Calcium: 4%	Calcium: 46%
Iron: 10%	Iron: 24%

15.6.1 Building a "Champions" Plate

- Step 1—*Prioritize produce*: Review the school menu and identify which fruits and vegetables your child is willing to choose. Teach them to fill 1/3 to 1/2 of their plate with fruits and vegetables.
- Step 2—*Get grainy*: Encourage your child to look for whole grains at their cafeteria if offered (brown rice, wheat pasta, quinoa, whole-wheat breads, and whole-wheat tortillas). Aim to fill 1/4 to 1/3 of their plate with whole grains.
- Step 3—*Go lean on protein*: Top grains with lean animal protein (grilled chicken, pulled pork, lean beef patty, deli turkey) and/or vegetable protein (peanut butter, baked tofu, beans).
- Step 4—*Put on your creative cap*: Make the cafeteria work for you by combining foods from different areas of the dining hall.
- Step 5—*Less is sometimes more*: The more processed a food is, the more salt, fat, and calories are often added.
- Step 6—*Think in 3's*: Aiming for three food groups each time you eat will provide a more balanced diet.

15.6.2 Brown Bag Lunches

If possible, encourage your child to bring his or her lunch to school. Packing a balanced, portion-controlled lunch guarantees your child will get the calories and nutrients he or she needs. Many parents or children usually pack their lunch on a full stomach after a meal such as dinner or breakfast, and usually put a little thought into it, like adding a yogurt or some fruit. On the flipside, when your child is in the cafeteria trying to make a decision when they are starving, they might be more likely to choose a less healthy meal. Below are great ideas for building a healthy, balanced, and creative lunch for your child athlete.

1. *Shake it up.* Food ruts are easy to fall into. Coming up with new ideas can be as simple as preparing old favorites in new ways. For example, instead of a regular peanut butter and jelly sandwich on white bread, make pinwheel PB&J's by rolling up the PB&J in a flour tortilla and slicing it into pinwheels. Table 15.2 lists more brown bag makeover ideas for lunches.

TABLE 15.2
Healthy Brown Bag Makeovers

Old Boring Lunch	Fun, Parent Makeover
Peanut butter and jelly	Peanut butter and jelly pin-wheels
	Spread peanut butter and 100% fruit jelly on a whole-wheat tortilla, roll up, and cut into bite-size pieces
Lunch-able: pizza style	Pizza muffins—kid assembly
	Whole-wheat English muffin, side of marinara, mozzarella cheese, and grilled chicken
Side of pretzels or goldfish	DUNK IT
	Cut up assorted veggies with ranch or hummus
	Kids love to dip foods
Bag of chips	DUNK IT
	Cut up fruits and provide either peanut butter or a yogurt dip
Chocolate chip cookies	Chocolate pudding with sliced bananas
Capri-sun	1% Chocolate or strawberry milk
Ham and cheese sandwich	Pita bread with ham and hummus

2. *Get them to pitch in.* Packing a balanced lunch takes a bit of planning ahead, and if you include your child in the process, you improve the odds that his/her lunch gets eaten! In addition, many kids have a short amount of time to eat. Pack a lunch that can be eaten quickly (i.e., apple slices versus unpeeled orange). You can begin the packing process by offering a range of healthy foods for them to choose from. For example, instead of choosing fruit for them, offer up dried apples, applesauce, or sliced apples; which would they prefer?
3. *Theme of the week.* Surprise your kids by incorporating a new lunch theme every few weeks, such as serving all red foods. Pair strawberry Greek yogurt with fresh strawberries, cherry tomatoes, and low-fat ranch dressing with cherry Jell-O for dessert. They could come up with the theme or you could have them try and guess the theme.
4. *Give it a new name.* Put on your creative cap and tell your young ones that you packed them some monster fingers and little trees to dunk into their favorite dip. They will look forward to your creativity, and might come up with some good names on their own. Believe it or not, actions like these can encourage healthy eating.
5. *Skewer it and combine with a dip.* There is something about a skewer that gives ordinary foods a magical makeover. Cut the end off so it is not sharp and fill it with two to three different food groups, with at least one of them being a fruit or vegetable. Pair your skewers with dips. Kids love to be interactive with food and studies show that kids eat more veggies when offered a dip. Dips can also be a great way to boost nutrition. For example, make an Italian skewer with precooked spinach ravioli, cheese, and tomatoes, with a light Italian dressing or a pineapple, yellow bell pepper, and teriyaki tofu skewer with a tomato-based BBQ sauce.
6. *Think outside the bread box.* Bread can get boring day after day. Instead, lean on sandwiching your protein with fruits and vegetables. Here are three of our favorites:
Spread hummus and cheese between two cucumber slices.
Combine banana and honey and put on mini whole-grain waffles or pancakes.
Spread nut butter on two apple slices with raisins.
Your kids will not even realize all of the fruits and vegetables they are eating!
7. *Enhance it.* Enhancing your lunch means simply dressing up what you have already prepared. For instance, keep a variety of cookie cutters on hand, which work great to transform whole-wheat soft bread into something fun. Turn apples or bananas into a funny face by adhering googly candy eyeballs. Or, use edible markers to write a sweet note onto fruit or vegetable slices. Spruce up your brown bag with a Bento box, which kids tend to love because they are an easy way to send a hodgepodge of small, snack size portions.

15.6.3 Other Meal Suggestions for a Healthy Brown Bag

- Peanut butter sandwich wedges with jelly or honey. Add raisins, sliced bananas, strawberries, applesauce, grated carrots, or zucchini to the peanut butter.
- Make a yogurt parfait with plain or vanilla yogurt and cut up fresh fruit. Have them sprinkle with raisins or granola as a topping. Pack in an insulated food jar thermos.
- Bake or buy a cooked chicken in the beginning of the week, shred and slice it to use for lunches the rest of the week.
- Hard boiled eggs or egg salad sandwiches. Add grated vegetables to the egg salad.
- Pasta. Add chopped spinach, tomatoes, cucumbers, and a favorite dressing for a cold pasta salad. Tortellini filled with spinach and a touch of olive oil or flaxseed oil.
- Rice. Make a cold rice salad by chopping up vegetables, pineapples, apples, chicken or fish.

15.7 HELPFUL RESOURCES FOR PARENTS/COACHES

- United States Olympic Committee—Team USA (http://www.teamusa.org/About-the-USOC/Athlete-Development/Sport-Performance/Nutrition)
- Australian International Sports Commission (http://www.ausport.gov.au/ais/nutrition)

- Bonci, L. 2009. *Sport Nutrition for Coaches*. Human Kinetics, Champaign, Illinois.
- United States Department of Agriculture: Food and Nutrition Information Center (http://fnic.nal.usda.gov/lifecycle-nutrition/teen-nutrition)
- Nemours Center for Children's Health Media: Kids Health (http://kidshealth.org/teen/food_fitness/sports/eatnrun.html)

REFERENCES

Casa, D. J., L. E. Armstrong, S. K. Hillman, S. J. Montain, R. V. Reiff, B. S. Rich, W. O. Roberts, and J. A. Stone. 2000. National Athletic Trainers Association position statement: Fluid replacement for athletes. *J Athl Train* 35 (2):212–224.

Committee on Nutrition. 2001. American Academy of Pediatrics: The use and misuse of fruit juice in pediatrics. *Pediatrics* 107 (5):1210–1213.

Mahoney, C. R., H. A. Taylor, R. B. Kanarek, and P. Samuel. 2005. Effect of breakfast composition on cognitive processes in elementary school children. *Physiol Behav* 85 (5):635–645. doi: 10.1016/j.physbeh.2005.06.023.

Potter, J. and B. Fuller. 2015. The effectiveness of chocolate milk as a post-climbing recovery aid. *J Sports Med Phys Fitness* 55 (12):1438–1444.

Pritchett, K., P. Bishop, R. Pritchett, M. Green, and C. Katica. 2009. Acute effects of chocolate milk and a commercial recovery beverage on postexercise recovery indices and endurance cycling performance. *Appl Physiol Nutr Metab* 34 (6):1017–1022, doi: 10.1139/H09-104.

Savage, J. S., J. Peterson, M. Marini, P. L. Bordi, Jr., and L. L. Birch. 2013. The addition of a plain or herb-flavored reduced-fat dip is associated with improved preschoolers' intake of vegetables. *J Acad Nutr Diet* 113 (8):1090–1095, doi: 10.1016/j.jand.2013.03.013.

16 How to Fuel Your Workouts and Games

Jennifer McDaniel and Elizabeth Fox

CONTENTS

Abstract 281
16.1 Introduction 282
16.2 Fueling before Exercise 282
    16.2.1 Pre-Exercise Fueling Strategies 282
    16.2.2 Top 10 Pre-Exercise Meals 283
16.3 Fueling during Exercise 283
    16.3.1 Fluids Tips to Avoid Dehydration and Overheating 283
    16.3.2 Which Fluids Are Best? 284
    16.3.3 Easy Ways to Increase Fluid Intake 284
    16.3.4 Fluid and Carbohydrate Needs for Different Types of Training 285
        16.3.4.1 Nonendurance Sports: Events of Less than 30 Minutes of Duration 285
    16.3.5 Fuel Options during Exercise 285
16.4 Fueling after Exercise 285
    16.4.1 Fueling after Exercise: Recovery Options 286
    16.4.2 Liquid Food Options 286
    16.4.3 Solid Food Options 286
16.5 Planning Considerations for All-Day or Multiday Events 287
    16.5.1 Fast Carbs for Pre-Loading or Refueling Prior to the Next Game 287
    16.5.2 Multiple Sport Example Day 287
    16.5.3 All/Multigame Day Checklist 287
16.6 Helpful Resources for Parents/Coaches 288
    16.6.1 Sports Nutrition Fact Sheets 288
    16.6.2 Sports Nutrition Professional Resources 288
    16.6.3 Scientific Reviews 288
References 288

ABSTRACT

This chapter provides specific food, fluid, and timing recommendations for young athletes and their parents, coaches, and other interested parties before, during, and after exercise. Pre-exercise meals and snacks, including carbohydrate and fluid requirements, are discussed in detail. Practices to prevent dehydration and overhydration are outlined, as well as types and amount of fluids to consume. Based on mode and duration of exercise, some sports or activities will require fueling during training. This chapter details carbohydrate and fluid recommendations for different types of exercise, including multiday and all-day sporting events. Within 30 minutes to an hour after exercise, refueling practices should include carbohydrate, protein, and fluids. Recovery nutrition for young athletes using solid or liquid fuel sources is provided, and an example "champions" day of fueling is included.

16.1 INTRODUCTION

This chapter is designed to provide young athletes, coaches, parents, and other health professionals with food and fluid recommendations before, during, and after training. Meals and snacks must be planned in advance and timed appropriately with exercise. Knowing *what* and *when* to feed your active child is critical for improving performance, reducing injury risk, and maintaining a happy, healthy body.

16.2 FUELING BEFORE EXERCISE

Breakfast should be a part of every athlete's training and race-day nutrition plan. You cannot race like a beast if you eat like a bird. When and what one eats should be tailored to the individual. Eating 3–4 hours before your feet hit the playing field will allow you to get adequate fuel and fluids. However, if time does not allow, you can eat closer to exercise, but meals should be lighter, primarily carb-centered, and maybe even in liquid form.

Studies have shown that athletes often eat far below the optimal level of carbohydrate calories (Costill et al. 1988, Guest and Barr 2005, Hinton 2005, Stevenson et al. 2005). As a result, many players *begin* competitions with glycogen levels (fuel tank) that are nowhere near topped off. What race car driver do you know starts a race with their fuel tank only half full? Players who start a match with low glycogen (stored fuel) usually have little carbohydrate left in their muscles by the time the second half starts. If competition requires high-intensity exercise performance, the athlete might not have enough fuel available to support a win.

16.2.1 Pre-Exercise Fueling Strategies

- Days leading up to a competition should include a plate that is 2/3 covered with whole grains, fruits, and vegetables, and the remaining 1/3 comprising lean proteins with 1 serving of dairy.
- Avoid eating right before practice. Allow sufficient time for digestion, at least 2–3 hours. Every athlete's digestive system and tolerances are unique. Therefore, an athlete should personally experiment with meal size and timing. It may be appropriate and necessary to include a small, easily digestible snack 60–90 minutes prior to practice. For sensitive stomachs, a liquid carbohydrate food source is optimal. Table 16.1 lists recommended carbohydrate amounts based on what time the meal is being consumed along with sample food ideas.
- Foods, snacks, and/or meals should be primarily starchy carbohydrates such as pasta, rice, potatoes, breads, etc. Foods or drinks high in sugar should be consumed in limited amounts.
- Protein intake should be modest, approximately 10%–15% of total calories. Protein is typically more difficult to digest and some sources may also provide appreciable amounts of fat and possibly slow digestion.

TABLE 16.1
Pre-Event Meal Ideas

Pre-Event Timing	Carbohydrate Dose (g/kg Body Mass)	Recommended Amount for 150-Pound (68 kg) Athlete (g)	Foods That Fulfill Requirement
4 hours before	4	270	Bagel w/peanut butter, banana, yogurt and granola, sports drink
3 hours before	3	200	Bagel w/peanut butter, banana, sports drink
2 hours before	2	130	Bagel w/peanut butter, sports drink
1 hour before	1	70	Sports drink and banana

How to Fuel Your Workouts and Games

- Limit heavy foods high in fats, oils, or cream-based sauces to ease digestion.
- Limit high-fiber foods that cause stomach distress or cramping.
- Avoid trying new foods prior to competition—stick to tried and true pre-workout meals for competition meals.
- If traveling, make sure to bring familiar food staples, or visit a nearby grocery store to stock up on necessary items.
- For athletes who tend to lose appetite with pre-race jitters, lean on liquid carbs such as—sports drinks, low-fat cold chocolate milk, smoothies, yogurts, and gels.
- Do not forgo the fluids! Athletes wake in a dehydrated state. The slightest amount of dehydration can negatively impact performance and be detrimental to both the working body and mind. Place a full glass of water by the bedside and drink before bouncing out of bed. Always have a water bottle nearby.

16.2.2 Top 10 Pre-Exercise Meals

- *Raise the bar*: Pair a whole food bar with a piece of fruit and pre-portioned yogurt
- *Breakfast bowl*: Yogurt base + whole-grain cereal + sliced banana + drizzle honey
- *Monkey wrap*: Whole-grain tortilla with nut butter + sliced banana + cinnamon and honey
- *It is in the bag*: Place dried whole-grain cereal, dried fruit, and nuts in a plastic baggie and eat on the way to practice
- *Waffle sandwich*: Two whole-grain waffles with an egg, sliced avocado, and cheese
- *Mexi wrap*: Whole-grain tortilla with shredded cheese, refried beans, and an egg
- *Almond joy oats*: Oatmeal combined with 1/2 scoop vanilla protein powder, 1 T. almond butter, 1 tsp. cocoa powder, and sliced almonds
- *Egg cups*: Eggs microwaved in a cup with + spinach + cheese on a whole-grain English muffin
- *Easy start*: Cooked rice with little butter + hard boiled egg + banana
- *Four-part smoothie*: Liquid base (soy milk, regular milk, almond milk) + protein source (protein powder, Greek yogurt, regular yogurt) + produce (frozen fruits and vegetables) + healthy fat (nut butter, nuts, avocado, chia/hemp/flaxseeds)

16.3 FUELING DURING EXERCISE

Carbohydrate consumption and fluid intake should be the two areas of focus for optimizing nutritional status during exercise. What and when to eat and/or drink during exercise is dependent on the individual plus temperature and humidity, intensity of practice, clothing/equipment worn, and other factors. General recommendations for carbohydrate feedings and fluid needs are provided below, but keep in mind that individual needs will vary based on age, body surface area, body composition, training status, and environmental conditions.

16.3.1 Fluids Tips to Avoid Dehydration and Overheating

- Drink plenty of fluids. Consume fluids during every timeout, break in action, etc. Sports drinks are acceptable as they also provide sodium and other electrolytes.
- Small amounts of easily digested foods can be considered, particularly during halftime of certain sports. Gels, blocks, or bars cut up into small pieces are foods employed with success. Be wary of the size of the solid food and how easily it can be digested.
- Drink fluids by a schedule
  - If possible, every 15–20 minutes. Set a timer for nutrition—in the heat of competition, it is easier to be forgetful about fuel, enlist parents to serve as reminders to fuel and hydrate or set a timer on the child's watch. This is even a good practice for coaches to employ so they get used to providing necessary fluids on a schedule and to train their athletes that regular, quick water breaks will be offered during practice.

- Replace water weight
  - Weigh yourself both before and after a workout.
  - Replace each pound of weight lost with 3 cups of water or sports drink.
  - Consider the weight of your clothes.
  - Coaches, nurses, and athletic trainers should consider holding athletes out of the next practice if they do not return their pre-practice weight by the time the next practice starts.
- Check the color of urine—urine should look like pale lemonade, not clear or dark in color.
- Be especially diligent with hydration when the humidity is high.
- Swimmers should be equally concerned about fluid loss even though it may not feel they are sweating.
- Drink the water. Water cools one most efficiently when consumed versus poured over the head.

16.3.2 Which Fluids Are Best?

- Less than 30 minutes? Water is always best
  - Temperature of water does not matter.
- Sports drinks: Activities >1 hour in duration
  - 6%–8% carbohydrate = 6–8 g of carbohydrate per 100 mL fluid.
- Avoid high sugar beverages such as fruit juice or soda can cause stomach/GI distress.
- Additional fluid tips:
  - Kids are more susceptible to dehydration because they are smaller than adults and do not adjust to hot temperatures as well meaning they sweat less and do not respond to thirst as well.
- Prevention: Remember these hydration "3's"—pre-hydrate, hydrate, and rehydrate.

16.3.3 Easy Ways to Increase Fluid Intake

1. Tempt with taste
   - Fluids should have flavor: Water is the best way to hydrate, but in one study, voluntary consumption of fluids increased by 48% when grape flavoring was added (Wilk and Bar-Or 1996).
     - Spruce up plain water with: 100% juice ice cubes, a splash of juice, and a frozen fruit.
2. Make H_2O an easy-access beverage
   - It is important to provide a convenient source of water to ensure easy access to fluids.
   - Freeze a couple of water bottles to pack in the lunch. This will keep lunch items cold as well as be a source of fluids to drink.
3. Follow the 20 minute rule
   - Hydrate every 20 minutes when a child is engaged in activity outside.
   - The American Academy of Pediatrics suggests children weighing approximately 88 pounds (40 kg) should drink 5 ounces of water or a sports drink every 20 minutes and adolescents weighing approximately 132 pounds (60 kg) should drink about 9 ounces every 20 minutes. An ounce is about the two kid-size gulps. Once again, the child will more likely meet their fluid needs when offering them a flavored drink that meets their taste preference (Rowland 2011).
4. Hydrate through food
   - Fruit and vegetables are 80%–90% water by weight, and contribute to a child's hydration needs.

16.3.4 Fluid and Carbohydrate Needs for Different Types of Training

16.3.4.1 Nonendurance Sports: Events of Less than 30 Minutes of Duration

Primary concern: minimal interference to competition

- Begin exercise in a well-hydrated condition.
- Replace fluid losses as completely as possible between competition/exercise sessions.
- No real benefit to drink fluids during exercise of less than 30 minutes.
- Athletes competing in tournament situations or multiple events should aim to rehydrate between sessions to avoid a progressive dehydration over the competition.

Events of 30–60 Minutes of Duration

Primary concern: fluid intake, some support for carbohydrate provision

- Begin exercise in a well-hydrated condition.
- Use a fluid replacement plan that has been practiced in training; drink as much as is practical and comfortable in attempting to match sweat loss.
- Use water, flavored water, or a sports drink that is cool, palatable, and provides some carbohydrate if exercise is intense or ≥60 minutes.
- Ingest beverage every 15–20 minutes to maintain gastric volume and increase fluid availability.
- Make the most of opportunities to drink within the confines of the sport.
- Replace fluid losses as completely as possible between competition sessions.

Sports: Events of 1–3 Hours

The primary concern at the time point should be fluid replacement plus carbohydrate provision.

- Begin exercise in a well-hydrated state.
- Use a fluid replacement plan that has been practiced in training, drink as much as is practical and comfortable in attempting to match sweat losses.
- Choose a sports drink that is cool, palatable, and provides carbohydrate.
- Begin ingesting fluid early in the exercise and continue to ingest beverage regularly to maintain gastric volume and increase fluid availability.
- Plan to consume 30–60 g of carbohydrate per hour of exercise.

16.3.5 Fuel Options during Exercise

Fruit: Bananas/orange slices/watermelon cubes/dried fruit
Cookie: Animal cookies, figure newtons, gingersnaps
Sports products: Sports gels, sport blocks
Salty carbs for hot weather: Hard and soft pretzels, goldfish, store-bought peanut butter, and crackers
Mixed meal foods options: 1/2 peanut butter and jelly sandwiches, granola bars, 1/2 plain turkey sandwich
Semiliquid options: Yogurt sticks, sports drinks, gels

16.4 FUELING AFTER EXERCISE

It is very important that athletes include carbohydrate, protein, and fluids in their fueling strategies after exercise. Carbohydrates act as the "muscle replenisher." Athletes must refill their fuel tank (muscle glycogen) with plenty of nutrient-dense carbohydrates, to ensure that they are not running on an empty tank for their next training session. Protein acts as the "muscle repairer." Consuming protein after exercise helps with tissue repair and recovery. Lastly, 150% of fluid losses need to be replaced after exercise. Fluids with electrolytes, in particular sodium, can help with rehydration practices.

16.4.1 Fueling after Exercise: Recovery Options

Post-exercise recovery is an important consideration, particularly for those athletes who may compete multiple times each day or for athletes who train or practice multiple times per day. Both liquid and solid food options have the potential to offer an excellent balance of carbohydrates and protein along with some healthy fats. Liquid options are good because many athletes have little to no desire to eat solid food when it is hot after a tough workout. Outlined below are some sample ideas and suggestions for athletes to consider. Each of the food options below contains a combination of carbohydrate and protein as well as additional nutrients and healthy fats. It is important to consider that many fruits, vegetables, high-fiber foods, beans, etc. can lead to digestive and intestinal gas, causing stomach cramps, discomfort, and poor performance. As a general rule, do not try anything new in the day of an important practice or competition.

16.4.2 Liquid Food Options

1. *Low-fat chocolate milk*: Studies have been conducted on chocolate milk as a recovery drink and it was observed that not only did athletes perform well, but they also performed better compared to other formulated sports recovery products (Pritchett et al. 2009). Low-fat chocolate milk has an impressive nutritional resume for recovery (Potter and Fuller 2015). It contains a nearly ideal carb-to-protein ratio of 3:1, both slow- (casein) and fast- (whey) digesting proteins for quick and sustaining protein fuel, and important vitamins and minerals that American's diets tend to fall short in: calcium, vitamin D, and potassium.
2. *Smoothie*: A four-part smoothie is an excellent consideration:
Part I comprises the liquid, commonly either skim, soy, or almond milk.
Part II comprises the protein source, commonly whey protein powder, Greek yogurt, or other yogurt.
Part III is a serving of fruits and/or vegetables.
Part IV is a healthy fat source such as a nut butter, chopped nuts, flax, or chia seeds.

This formula provides you with the carbs and protein you need for recovery, anti-inflammatory healthy fats, and variety of nutrients and antioxidants from fruits and vegetables.

16.4.3 Solid Food Options

1. *Egg, avocado, whole-wheat wrap*: The yolk of an egg is a nutrient gold mine and contains nutrients such as choline that tend to decrease with endurance training. Intense, endurance training decreases levels of choline in the body. Choline is an essential nutrient that plays a role in mental function, energy levels, and muscle contraction. Therefore, eggs are also a good option to include in a pre-workout meal. The fat in the avocados will help you feel full after your workout, and the fat + fiber formula also helps maintain even energy levels post-workout.
2. *Whole-wheat toast topped with cottage cheese and fruit*: Great mix of carbs and high-quality protein. Cottage cheese tends to be higher in sodium and can help replace lost sodium from a hot summer workout.
3. *Protein bar + fruit*: This food combination serves as a quick grab and go snack. Look for a food bar that contains mostly whole ingredients, at least 3 g of fiber, 8–10 g of protein,

and is low in saturated fats. Avoid "coatings" on bars and bars with long ingredient lists. You can find great recipes for homemade bars online, which include whole grains such as quinoa, brown rice, oats, etc. Make a huge batch and freeze!

16.5 PLANNING CONSIDERATIONS FOR ALL-DAY OR MULTIDAY EVENTS

Weekends with multiple sporting events in one day can make it very difficult to adequately and effectively feed young athletes. As discussed in Chapter 15, planning meals and snacks ahead of time for competition days is a must! Below are some simple ways to prepare for feeding an athlete during all-day or multiday events.

- Pack a cooler, purchase ice, storage bags, and containers.
- Plan ahead. Have plenty of fluids and sports drink. Do not assume suitable performance foods will be available on site, as it is usually hamburgers, hot dogs, and French fries.
- Scout out a place in the shade. Bring a sunshade/canopy or tent.
- Pack small bags of trail mix, dried fruit, nuts, granola bars, yogurt pouches, and ready-to-drink beverages.
- Cut and peel fruit ahead of time.

16.5.1 Fast Carbs for Pre-Loading or Refueling Prior to the Next Game

- Pasta, pancakes, waffles, toast, breads, potatoes, soft pretzels.
- Most dry cereals not highly concentrated with whole grains. (Not 100% bran flakes, but rather corn- or rice-based/processed cereal.)
- Bananas, oranges, and grapes are high sugar fruits and are good.
- Sports drinks, strawberry, and chocolate milk as well as the new V8 Fusion Fruit drinks.
- Snack crackers and cookies are a good filler and a snack that can be taken anywhere/thrown into a soccer bag with a sports drink.

16.5.2 Multiple Sport Example Day

- *Breakfast*: Cream of wheat (made with milk), white toast topped with thin spread of nut butter, banana, and honey and orange juice
- *Pre-Game*: 8 ounces sports drink
- *Post-Game 1*: Fruit yogurt with cereal and banana
- *Lunch*: Turkey sub with fruit, pretzels, and a sport drink
- *Post-Game 2*: Graham crackers with honey and peanut butter and chocolate milk
- *Dinner*: Grilled chicken with baked potato, zucchini, and Italian bread
- *Post-Dinner*: Angel food cake with strawberries and whipped cream

16.5.3 All/Multigame Day Checklist

- Packing equipment: Mentioned earlier
- Fluids and fluid-carrying containers: Water, sports drinks, smoothie/recovery drinks/chocolate milk
- Pre/during competition foods: Fresh and dried fruit, pretzels, cookies, dry cereals, wraps with little nut butter and honey, rice, baked potatoes, granola bars
- Post-competition foods: Sandwiches, yogurt with granola, chicken pizza, wraps, smoothies, slushy sports drinks for hot days
- Nervous stomach foods: Sports drinks, chocolate milk, yogurt, gels

16.6 HELPFUL RESOURCES FOR PARENTS/COACHES

16.6.1 SPORTS NUTRITION FACT SHEETS

Sports, Cardiovascular, and Wellness Nutrition—Dietetic Practice Group of the Academy of Nutrition and Dietetics (http://www.scandpg.org/sports-nutrition/sports-nutrition-fact-sheets/)

16.6.2 SPORTS NUTRITION PROFESSIONAL RESOURCES

Sports, Cardiovascular, and Wellness Nutrition—Dietetic Practice Group of the Academy of Nutrition and Dietetics (http://www.scandpg.org/sports-nutrition/sports-nutrition-professional-resources/)

16.6.3 SCIENTIFIC REVIEWS

- Burke, L. M., J. A. Hawley, S. H. Wong, and A. E. Jeukendrup. 2011. Carbohydrates for training and competition. *J Sports Sci* 29 (Suppl 1):S17–27. doi: 10.1080/02,640,414.2011. 585,473.
- Casa, D. J., L. E. Armstrong, S. K. Hillman, S. J. Montain, R. V. Reiff, B. S. Rich, W. O. Roberts, and J. A. Stone. 2000. National Athletic Trainers' Association position statement: Fluid replacement for athletes. *J Athl Train* 35 (2):212–24.
- Kerksick, C. M. and M. G. Kulovitz. 2013. Requirements of protein, carbohydrates and fats for athletes. In *Nutrition and Enhanced Sports Performance: Recommendations for Muscle Building*, edited by D. Bagchi, S. Nair and C.K. Sen. Elsevier Publishers, Waltham, MA.
- Phillips, S. M. 2004. Protein requirements and supplementation in strength sports. *Nutrition* 20 (7–8):689–95. doi: 10.1016/j.nut.2004.04.009.
- Rodriguez, N. R., N. M. Di Marco, and S. Langley. 2009. American College of Sports Medicine position stand. Nutrition and athletic performance. *Med Sci Sports Exerc* 41 (3):709–31. doi: 10.1249/MSS.0b013e31890eb86, 00,005,768-200,903,000-00,027 [pii].
- Sawka, M. N., L. M. Burke, E. R. Eichner, R. J. Maughan, S. J. Montain, and N. S. Stachenfeld. 2007. American College of Sports Medicine position stand. Exercise and fluid replacement. *Med Sci Sports Exerc* 39 (2):377–90. doi: 10.1249/mss.0b013e31802ca597.

REFERENCES

Burke, L. M., J. A. Hawley, S. H. Wong, and A. E. Jeukendrup. 2011. Carbohydrates for training and competition. *J Sports Sci* 29 (Suppl 1):S17–27. doi: 10.1080/02,640,414.2011.585,473.

Casa, D. J., L. E. Armstrong, S. K. Hillman, S. J. Montain, R. V. Reiff, B. S. Rich, W. O. Roberts, and J. A. Stone. 2000. National Athletic Trainers' Association position statement: Fluid replacement for athletes. *J Athl Train* 35 (2):212–24.

Costill, D. L., M. G. Flynn, J. P. Kirwan, J. A. Houmard, J. B. Mitchell, R. Thomas, and S. H. Park. 1988. Effects of repeated days of intensified training on muscle glycogen and swimming performance. *Med Sci Sports Exerc* 20 (3):249–54.

Guest, N. S. and S. I. Barr. 2005. Cognitive dietary restraint is associated with stress fractures in women runners. *Int J Sport Nutr Exerc Metab* 15 (2):147–59.

Hinton, P. 2005. Running on empty. *Training and Conditioning* 15 (6).

Kerksick, C. M. and M. G. Kulovitz. 2013. Requirements of protein, carbohydrates and fats for athletes. In *Nutrition and Enhanced Sports Performance: Recommendations for Muscle Building*, edited by D. Bagchi, S. Nair and C.K. Sen. Elsevier Publishers, Waltham, MA.

Phillips, S. M. 2004. Protein requirements and supplementation in strength sports. *Nutrition* 20 (7–8):689–95. doi: 10.1016/j.nut.2004.04.009.

Potter, J. and B. Fuller. 2015. The effectiveness of chocolate milk as a post-climbing recovery aid. *J Sports Med Phys Fitness* 55 (12):1438–44.

Pritchett, K., P. Bishop, R. Pritchett, M. Green, and C. Katica. 2009. Acute effects of chocolate milk and a commercial recovery beverage on post exercise recovery indices and endurance cycling performance. *Appl Physiol Nutr Metab* 34 (6):1017–22. doi: 10.1139/H09-104.

Rodriguez, N. R., N. M. DiMarco, S. Langley, Association American Dietetic, Canada Dietitians of, Nutrition American College of Sports Medicine, and Performance Athletic. 2009. Position of the American Dietetic Association, Dietitians of Canada, and the American College of Sports Medicine: Nutrition and athletic performance. *J Am Diet Assoc* 109 (3):509–27.

Rowland, T. 2011. Fluid replacement requirements for child athletes. *Sports Med* 41 (4):279–88. doi: 10.2165/11,584,320-000,000,000-00,000.

Sawka, M. N., L. M. Burke, E. R. Eichner, R. J. Maughan, S. J. Montain, and N. S. Stachenfeld. 2007. American College of Sports Medicine position stand. Exercise and fluid replacement. *Med Sci Sports Exerc* 39 (2):377–90. doi: 10.1249/mss.0b013e31802ca597.

Stevenson, E., C. Williams, G. McComb, and C. Oram. 2005. Improved recovery from prolonged exercise following the consumption of low glycemic index carbohydrate meals. *Int J Sport Nutr Exerc Metab* 15 (4):333–49.

Wilk, B. and O. Bar-Or. 1996. Effect of drink flavor and NaCl on voluntary drinking and hydration in boys exercising in the heat. *J Appl Physiol (1985)* 80 (4):1112–7.

Index

A

AA, *see* Arachidonic acid (AA)
AAP, *see* American Academy of Pediatrics (AAP)
AAU, *see* Amateur Athletic Union (AAU)
Academy of Nutrition and Dietetics (AND), 18, 207, 210
Acceptable macronutrient distribution ranges (AMDR), 36, 65, 194, 207
Accessory growth factors, 99
Acclimation, 119–120
Acclimatization, 124
Acetyl-CoA, 81
ACSM, *see* American College of Sports Medicine (ACSM)
Action compound, 60–61
Active adolescent athlete, 5–6
Activities of daily living (ADL), 83
Acute alcohol consumption, 143
Acute lymphoblastic leukemia (ALL), 224
Adenosine triphosphate (ATP), 49, 81, 103
Adequate intake (AI), 10
ADL, *see* Activities of daily living (ADL)
Adolescents, 5–6, 114
Adolescents Training and Learning to Avoid Steroids (ATLAS), 158, 167, 232
Aerobic conditioning and power, 243–244
Aerobic power, *see* VO_2 max
AI, *see* Adequate intake (AI)
Air travel, 272
Aisle by aisle, navigating store, 275–276
Albumin, 62
Alcohol (EtOH), 136; *see also* Caffeine; Marijuana; Nicotine
    effects on health and performance, 142–144
    history, 142
    legal status, 144
    overview, 142
    summary, 144–145
ALL, *see* Acute lymphoblastic leukemia (ALL)
Alpha-linolenic acid, 10, 80, 81
Alternative smokeless tobacco (snus), 140
Amateur Athletic Union (AAU), 88
AMDR, *see* Acceptable macronutrient distribution ranges (AMDR)
American Academy of Pediatrics (AAP), 225
American College of Sports Medicine (ACSM), 37, 121, 144, 205, 207, 210, 212
Anabolic–androgenic steroids, 154, 155
    anabolic steroid use among U.S. adolescents, 155
    body composition, 164
    legal considerations and testing, 166–167
    management, 158
    performance benefits for strength, power, endurance athletes, 162–164
    physiological adaptations, 159–162
    prevalence of use, 154–155
    prevention and education, 158
    reasons for use, 155–157
    related drug use, 157
    side effects, 164–166
AND, *see* Academy of Nutrition and Dietetics (AND)
Androgen effects, 160
Androstenedione, 157
Anthropometrics, 20
    BMI, 23
    contribution of select constituents of FFM, 23
    FFM, 22
    population-specific Db, 22
    prediction equations, 21
    SKF, 20
    2C models, 24
Apocrine glands, 119
Arachidonic acid (AA), 80
Artificial Trans Fats, 92
Asthma, 88, 124–125
ATHENA, *see* Athletes Targeting Healthy Exercise and Nutrition Alternatives (ATHENA)
Athletes' burnout, 256
Athletes, nutrients for, 211; *see also* Weight-conscious athlete
"Athlete's plate" approach, 270
Athletes Targeting Healthy Exercise and Nutrition Alternatives (ATHENA), 158, 167, 232
Athletes Training and Learning to Avoid Steroids, *see* Adolescents Training and Learning to Avoid Steroids (ATLAS)
ATLAS, *see* Adolescents Training and Learning to Avoid Steroids (ATLAS)
ATP, *see* Adenosine triphosphate (ATP)
Avocado, 286

B

Bariatric surgery, 197–198
BCAAs, *see* Branched-chain amino acids (BCAAs)
"Beer and Whiskey League", 142
"Beer Ball League", 142
Beta-oxidation (β-oxidation), 81
BIA, *see* Bioelectrical impedance analysis (BIA)
Bigorexia, 157
Bioelectrical impedance analysis (BIA), 24
Biological maturation, 119
Biological value (BV), 69
Blood markers, 121
Blood pressure (BP), 227
BMD, *see* Bone mineral density (BMD)
BMI, *see* Body mass index (BMI)
Body composition, 20, 119, 164; *see also* Energy intake
    anthropometrics, 20–24
    body composition and weight with diet and exercise, 211
    body water, 24–26
    multiple-component models, 26–30
    recommendations regarding body fatness of child and adolescent athletes, 30–31
    and weight management, 204

Body mass index (BMI), 4, 22, 23, 64, 181, 197
Body mass measurement, 121
Body proteins, 61
Body water, 24–26
Bone mineral density (BMD), 106
BP, *see* Blood pressure (BP)
Branched-chain amino acids (BCAAs), 68, 229
Breakfast, 266–267
Brown bag
    lunches, 278–279
    meal suggestions for healthy, 279
Burger king macaroni and cheese, 272
BV, *see* Biological value (BV)

C

Cafeteria navigation, 277
    brown bag lunches, 278–279
    building "champions" plate, 278
    meal suggestions for healthy brown bag, 279
Caffeine, 136, 225; *see also* Alcohol (EtOH); Marijuana; Nicotine
    effects on performance, 137, 139
    ergogenic and nonergogenic outcomes, 226
    history, 136
    legal status, 138
    negative effects, 228
    overview, 136–137
    summary, 138, 139
    supplementation and youth, 226–228
    use and energy drink consumption, 228–229
Calcium, 12, 105–106
Cannabis (*Cannabis sativa*), 145
Carbohydrate intake, 36
    child–adult metabolic differences, 39–40
    of current levels in young athletes, 37–38
    days and hours before endurance exercise, 40–42
    during endurance exercise, 42–47
    estimated daily total energy, 37
    examples of reported CHO intakes in young athletes, 38
    health, glycemic index, and insulin sensitivity, 50–52
    performance, 42–45
    postexercise, 47–49
    recommended values for young athletes, 36–37
    short-duration high-intensity exercise and skill performance, 49
    sports drinks and hydration, 49–50
    substrate oxidation, 45–47
Carbohydrates (CHO), 8–9, 36, 266, 285
    availability, 67
    consumption, 283
    loading, 40, 41, 178
    as muscle replenisher, 285–286
    supplementation, 51, 52
Carbon skeleton, 63
Cardiovascular exercise, 240
    advanced training guidelines for performance, 243–246
    benefits, 240
    example of cardiovascular/endurance training intensities, 245
    example of progression, 246
    guidelines to promoting fitness, 241–242

Carnitine palmitoyltransferase (CPT1), 40
Casein, 229–230
"Cause and effect" relationship, 156
Celiac disease, 179
Central nervous system (CNS), 36, 80, 134
Certified sports dietitian (CSSD), 211
cGMPs, *see* current good manufacturing practices (cGMPs)
"Champions" plate, building, 278
Child, 5–6, 114
Child–adult metabolic differences, 39–40
Child and adolescent athlete
    clinical considerations, 174
    eating disorders, 184–189
    T1D, 174–180
    T2D, 180–184
Childhood obesity, 240
CHO, *see* Carbohydrates (CHO)
Choline, 286
Chronic alcohol abuse, 145
Chronic health conditions, hydration considerations in
    lung conditions, 124–125
    metabolic conditions, 125–126
Chronic muscle spasms, 107
Chronological age, 119
Cigarettes, 139
Citric acid cycle, *see* Krebs cycle
CLAs, *see* Conjugated linoleic acids (CLAs)
Clothing, 120–121
CNS, *see* Central nervous system (CNS)
Combat sport modalities, 117
Competitive adolescent athlete, 5–6
Conjugated linoleic acids (CLAs), 84, 88–89
Continual protein turnover, 64
Continuous subcutaneous insulin infusion (CSII), 177
CPT1, *see* Carnitine palmitoyltransferase (CPT1)
Creatine, 221
    ergogenic effects, 223
    negative effects of supplementation, 224–225
    skeletal muscle, 221
    supplementation in youth, 225
    supplementation research in youth, 223–224
CSII, *see* Continuous subcutaneous insulin infusion (CSII)
CSSD, *see* Certified sports dietitian (CSSD)
current good manufacturing practices (cGMPs), 231
Cystic fibrosis, 125
Cytokines, 88

D

Daily value (DV), 91
DBP, *see* Diastolic blood pressure (DBP)
Deamination, 63
DEBQ, *see* Dutch Eating Behavior Questionnaire (DEBQ)
Dehydration, 117, 206, 212; *see also* Hydration
Dehydroepiandrosterone (DHEA), 157
Deoxyribonucleic acid (DNA), 103
DHEA, *see* Dehydroepiandrosterone (DHEA)
Diabetes, 126
Diabetes prevention program (DPP), 205
Diagnostic and Statistical Manual of Mental Disorders-Fifth edition (DSM-V), 186
Diastolic blood pressure (DBP), 257
Diet(ary), 68

fats, 19
protein, 19
status and challenges of young people, 6
survey methods, 10
Dietary Guidelines for Americans, 210
Dietary reference intake (DRI), 8, 36–37, 81
    for fats, 81–82
Dietary supplement, 219, 220
    among young athletes, 221
    caffeine, 225–229
    considerations for choosing, 230
    creatine, 221–225
    ergogenic aid classifications, 220
    good manufacturing practices, 231–232
    proteins, 229–230
    selected dietary supplement resources, 232–233
    third-party testing, 231–232
    use in youth and adolescent athletes, 12–13
    by youth and adolescent athletes, 221, 222–223
Dietary Supplement Health and Education Act (DSHEA), 220, 230
Diets for weight loss in youth, 196–197
Dilution method, 25
Dinner, 268
Disordered eating, 209
DMD, *see* Duchenne muscular dystrophy (DMD)
DNA, *see* Deoxyribonucleic acid (DNA)
Doubly labeled water, 25
DPP, *see* Diabetes prevention program (DPP)
DRI, *see* Dietary reference intake (DRI)
Drugs, 154, 163; *see also* Anabolic–androgenic steroids
    interactions, 146–147
DSHEA, *see* Dietary Supplement Health and Education Act (DSHEA)
DSM-V, *see* Diagnostic and Statistical Manual of Mental Disorders-Fifth edition (DSM-V)
Dual-energy x-ray absorptiometry (DXA), 27
Duchenne muscular dystrophy (DMD), 224
Dutch Eating Behavior Questionnaire (DEBQ), 38
DV, *see* Daily value (DV)
DXA, *see* Dual-energy x-ray absorptiometry (DXA)

E

Eating disorders, 184
    assessment, 185–186
    case study, 189
    exercise and, 184–185
    female athlete triad, 186
    medical diagnosis, 186–187
    medical interventions, 187
    monitoring and evaluation, 188
    nutrition diagnosis, 187
    nutrition intervention, 187–188
    responsibilities, 188–189
Eccrine sweat glands, 119
ECW, *see* Extracellular water (ECW)
Educational intervention, 123–124
EER, *see* Estimated energy requirement (EER)
EFA, *see* Essential fatty acids (EFA)
Egg, 286
EIA, *see* Exercise-induced asthma (EIA)
"Elixir of life", *see* Alcohol (EtOH)
Endocrine Society's thresholds, 102

Endopeptidases, 61
Energy balance, 194
"Energy dense" foods, 6
Energy drinks, 123
Energy intake, 17; *see also* Body composition
    energy needs estimation, 18
    macronutrient recommendations, 18–19
Energy needs, estimation of, 18
Environmental factors, 118, 120–121
EPO, *see* Erythropoietin (EPO)
Ergogenic effects, 137
Ergogenic outcomes, 164
Erythropoietin (EPO), 154
Essential amino acids, 60, 68
Essential fatty acids (EFA), 79
Estimated energy requirement (EER), 194, 210
Ethanol, *see* Alcohol (EtOH)
EtOH, *see* Alcohol (EtOH)
Euhydration, 115, 117
Excessive caloric restriction, 206–207
Excessive exercise, 184
Excreting sweat, 125
Exercise
    benefits, 205
    factors, 118, 120
    intensity, 120
    and nutritional timing, 213–214
    proper exercise prescription, 205–206
Exercise-induced asthma (EIA), 88
Exercise prescription and strength
    cardiovascular exercise, 240–246
    healthy training for performance, 255–258
    muscular strength and endurance, 246–253
    physical activity in school-aged children, 240
    stretching and flexibility, 253–255
    in youth and adolescents, 241
Exertional heat illness, 115, 116
Explosive type skills, 255
Extracellular water (ECW), 24

F

FAD, *see* Flavin dinucleotide (FAD)
Fast food, 272
Fat-free mass (FFM), 20, 224
Fat(s), 10–11, 266
    fat-soluble vitamins, 99
    free, 78
Fat mass (FM), 204
Fat needs, 78, 80; *see also* Protein needs of young athletes
    alpha-linolenic acid, 80, 81
    created equally, 79–80
    differences between adults and children, 83
    DRI, 81–82
    fat as fuel, 81
    fat supplements and human performance, 84–89
    favorable functions of, 78–79
    female athletes, 94–95
    fueling young athlete, 82–84
    guidelines for young athletes, 95
    linoleic acid, 80
    lipids, 78, 79
    omega-3 and omega-6 fatty acid teams, 80, 81

Fat needs (*Continued*)
  quarterback of children's metabolic playing field, 83–84
  reading food labels for fat, 90–92
  snacks and meal recommendations, 93–94
  vegetarian athletes, 94
  young athletes should avoid and ways to avoid, 89–90
Fat supplements and human performance, 84
  CLA, 88–89
  fats and testosterone, 89
  fish oils, 86–88
  LCT, 86
  MCT, 84–86
  popular claims, 85
FDA, *see* Food and Drug Administration (FDA)
Federal Drug Administration (FDA), 197
Federal Trade Commission (FTC), 230, 231
Female athlete(s)
  fats for, 94–95
  triad, 186
FFA, *see* Free fatty acid (FFA)
FFM, *see* Fat-free mass (FFM)
Fibrinogen, 62
Field methods, 24
Fish oils, 86
  asthma and EIA, 88
  muscle damage, inflammation, and immune function, 88
  RBC deformability and VO_2 max, 87
Fitness
  duration and frequency, 251
  examples of resistance exercises, 250
  guidelines to promoting, 241–242, 248
  health-related fitness program for beginners, 252
  intensity and volume, 249
  principles of resistance training for youth, 249
  progression of activities, 251–252
  resistance training considerations for youth, 249
  type of activity, 248–249
Five-component models (5C models), 27
Flavin dinucleotide (FAD), 62
Fluid, 285
  intake, 283
  status and needs, 11
Fluid replacement recommendations and strategies, 122
  during exercise, 122–123
  before exercise, 122
  after exercise, 123
FM, *see* Fat mass (FM)
Follicle-stimulating hormone (FSH), 207
Food and Drug Administration (FDA), 85, 230, 231
Four-component models (4C models), 27
Free fatty acid (FFA), 40, 81
FSH, *see* Follicle-stimulating hormone (FSH)
FTC, *see* Federal Trade Commission (FTC)
Fueling, 281, 282
  before exercise, 282–283
  during exercise, 283–285
  after exercise, 285–287
  helpful resources for parents/coaches, 288
  planning considerations for all-day, 287

G

GAMT, *see* Guanidinoacetate methyltransferase (GAMT)
Gastric emptying, 122
Gatorade™, 154
Generally recognized as safe (GRAS), 85
Globulins, 62
Gluconeogenesis, 67
Glucose–electrolyte solution, 154
Glycemic index, 50–52
Gonadotropin-releasing hormone (GnRH), 207
Good manufacturing practices, 231–232
GRAS, *see* Generally recognized as safe (GRAS)
Grocery/gas station snacks, 274
Grocery store, tackling, 274
  getting kids involving, 276
  label reading, 276–277
  navigating store aisle by aisle, 275–276
  before shop, 274–275
Growth hormone, 161–162
Guanidinoacetate methyltransferase (GAMT), 224

H

HDL, *see* High-density lipoprotein (HDL)
Health, 50–52
  halo labeling, 276–277
Healthy eating
  air travel, 272
  choosing healthiest options, 270–271
  favorite meal ideas, 271–272
  at night, 272–274
  planning fueling opportunities before travel, 270
  questions parents/coaches, 271
  on road, 270
Healthy training regimen
  benefits, 257
  consequences of unhealthy training regimen, 256–257
  considerations for, 258
  for performance, 255
Heart rate (HR), 227, 241
Heat acclimatization, 119–120
Heat acclimatization/acclimation process, 124
Heat production during exercise, 119
Heme iron, 103
Hemoglobin, 103
HGI, *see* High glycemic index (HGI)
High-CHO diet, 40, 41
High-density lipoprotein (HDL), 165
High-intensity interval training (HITT), 205
High glycemic index (HGI), 48
High protein intake, 207
  benefits, 207
  protein needs based on varying body weights, 208
  safety, 207–209
HITT, *see* High-intensity interval training (HITT)
HR, *see* Heart rate (HR)
HRmax, *see* Maximal heart rate (HRmax)
Hydration, 49–50, 115; *see also* Dehydration
  considerations in chronic health conditions, 124–126
  educational intervention, 123–124
  energy drinks, 123
  fluid replacement recommendations and strategies, 122–123
  sports drinks, 123
  status estimation, 121
  sweating responses, 121
Hyperhydration, 115

Index

Hypoglycemia, recognizing and treating, 178
Hypohydration, 115
    and aerobic performance, 115–116
    and cognitive function, 117
    and high-intensity intermittent efforts and strength performance, 116–117

I

ICDH, *see* Isocitrate dehydrogenase (ICDH)
IDDM, *see* Insulin-dependent diabetes mellitus (IDDM)
IGF-1, *see* Insulin-like growth factor-1 (IGF-1)
Illegal substances, 154
Immune function, 88
IMTAG, *see* Intramuscular triacylglycerol (IMTAG)
Individual factors, 118, 119–120
Inflammation, 88
Ingested performance-enhancing substances, 154
Institute of Medicine (IOM), 7, 102
Institutes of Medicine for Obese Youth (IOM-OY), 194
Insulin
    resistance, 181
    sensitivity, 50–52
Insulin-dependent diabetes, *see* Type 1 diabetes (T1D)
Insulin-dependent diabetes mellitus (IDDM), 51
Insulin-like growth factor-1 (IGF-1), 161
Intensity, 241–242, 244–245
International Olympic Committee (IOC), 146, 228
Intramuscular triacylglycerol (IMTAG), 40
Involuntary dehydration, 115
IOC, *see* International Olympic Committee (IOC)
IOM-OY, *see* Institutes of Medicine for Obese Youth (IOM-OY)
IOM, *see* Institute of Medicine (IOM)
Iron, 12, 103–105
Isocitrate dehydrogenase (ICDH), 39

J

Janus/signal transducer and activator of transcription pathway (JAK/STAT pathway), 161–162
Juvenile-onset diabetes, *see* Type 1 diabetes (T1D)

K

Ketoacidosis, 175
KFC grilled chicken drumstick, 272
Krebs cycle, 63

L

Label reading, 276–277
Lactate dehydrogenase (LDH), 39
Lactate increase above baseline (LIAB), 39
LBM, *see* Lean body mass (LBM)
LCTs, *see* Long-chain triglycerides (LCTs)
LDH, *see* Lactate dehydrogenase (LDH)
LDL, *see* Low-density lipoprotein (LDL)
Lean body mass (LBM), 204
Legally available substances, 154
Leucine, 68
LH, *see* Luteinizing hormone (LH)
LIAB, *see* Lactate increase above baseline (LIAB)
Linoleic acid, 10, 80

Lipids, 78, 79
Lipolysis, 81
Liquid food options, 286
"Loading" phase, 223
Long-chain triglycerides (LCTs), 84, 86
Long, slow distance training (LSD training), 244
Loughborough Intermittent Shuttle Test, 49
Low-density lipoprotein (LDL), 165
Low-fat
    chocolate milk, 286
    versions, 78
LSD training, *see* Long, slow distance training (LSD training)
Lunch, 268
Luteinizing hormone (LH), 207

M

Macronutrient considerations, 8
    carbohydrates, 8–9
    fat, 10–11
    protein, 9–10
Macronutrient needs, 194–195
Macronutrient recommendations, 18–19
Magnesium, 106–107
Magnetic resonance imaging (MRI), 163
Maladaptive perfectionism, 256
mammalian target of rapomyosin (mTOR), 161
Marijuana, 136; *see also* Alcohol (EtOH); Caffeine; Nicotine
    effects on performance, 145–146, 147
    history, 145
    legal status, 146
    overview, 145
    summary, 146, 147
Maturation, 247
"Maudsley" method, 187
Maximal heart rate (HRmax), 241
MCTs, *see* Medium-chain triglycerides (MCTs)
Medical diagnosis
    eating disorders, 186–187
    T1D, 175
    T2D, 181, 182
Medical interventions
    eating disorders, 187
    T1D, 176–177
Medications, 197
Medium-chain triglycerides (MCTs), 84–86
Meta-analysis, 140
Metformin, 182
3-(1-Methyl-2-pyrrolidinyl) pyridine, *see* Nicotine
Micronutrient concerns and considerations, 11–12
milliliters per kilogram per minute (mL/kg/min), 243
Minerals, 11, 102; *see also* Vitamins
    calcium, 105–106
    iron, 103–105
    key functions and food sources, 104
    magnesium, 106–107
    RDA for, 103
    zinc, 107–108
mL/kg/min, *see* milliliters per kilogram per minute (mL/kg/min)
Monounsaturated fatty acids (MUFAs), 79
MRI, *see* Magnetic resonance imaging (MRI)

mTOR, *see* mammalian target of rapomyosin (mTOR)
MTU, *see* Muscle-tendon units (MTU)
MUFAs, *see* Monounsaturated fatty acids (MUFAs)
Multiple-component models, 26
    of body composition assessment, 26
    FFM, 28
    low level of body fat, 29
    repetitive/no-impact sport athletes, 30
    2C model, 26
    3C models, 27
    4C models, 27
Multiple-frequency analyzers, 24
Muscle
    contraction effect, 114
    damage, 88
    growth process, 160
Muscle-tendon units (MTU), 253
Muscular strength and endurance, 246
    advanced training guidelines, 252–253
    benefits, 247–248
    guidelines to promoting fitness, 248–252
    muscular injury, 247
Myoglobin, 103

N

NaCl, *see* Sodium chloride (NaCl)
NAD+, *see* Nicotinamide dinucleotide (NAD+)
NATA, *see* National Athletic Trainer's Association (NATA)
National Athletic Trainer's Association (NATA), 122
National Basketball Association (NBA), 166
National Collegiate Athletic Association (NCAA), 146, 154, 228
National Federation of State High School Associations (NFHS), 225
National Football League (NFL), 166
National Institute on Drug Abuse, 155
National Strength and Conditioning Association, 158
Natural Trans Fats, 91–92
NBA, *see* National Basketball Association (NBA)
NCAA, *see* National Collegiate Athletic Association (NCAA)
Negative perfectionism, *see* Maladaptive perfectionism
Net protein balance, 63
Neutrophilia, 88
NFHS, *see* National Federation of State High School Associations (NFHS)
NFL, *see* National Football League (NFL)
Nicotinamide dinucleotide (NAD+), 62
Nicotine, 136; *see also* Alcohol (EtOH); Caffeine; Marijuana
    effects on performance, 139–141
    history, 138–139
    legal status, 141
    overview, 139
    summary, 141
Nitrogen, 62
Nonendurance sports, 285
Nonessential amino acids, 68
Nutrient(s)
    for athletes, 211
    partitioning, 64
Nutrition
    education, 182
    during exercise, 214
    for postexercise recovery, 214
    for weight modification, 212–213
Nutritional diagnosis
    eating disorders, 187
    T1D, 175, 177
    T2D, 181–182
Nutritional interventions
    eating disorders, 187–188
    energy balance, 194
    macronutrient needs, 194–195
    predictive equations in obese youth, 195
    T1D, 177–179
    T2D, 182–183
Nutritional recommendations for athletes
    dietary guidelines, 210
    nutrients for athletes, 211
    predicted and measured energy needs, 210

O

Obesity, 125–126
Oligopeptides, 61
Omega-3 fatty acid teams, 80
Omega-6 fatty acid teams, 80
Omega-6 PUFA, 88
One-repetition maximum (1RM), 162, 249
Optimal energy, 6
    deficiency of energy results, 6–7
    estimated daily caloric needs, 7, 8
    TEE, 7
Orlistat, 197
Overuse injury, 256–257
Overweight, 193; *see also* Weight-loss
    diets for weight loss in youth, 196–197
    health and performance consequences of extreme weight control behaviors, 196

P

PADS, *see* Professionals Against Doping in Sports (PADS)
PAL, *see* Physical activity level (PAL)
Parathyroid hormone (PTH), 105
PCr, *see* Phosphocreatine (PCr)
PDCAAS, *see* Protein digestibility-corrected amino acid score (PDCAAS)
Pediatric assessment, 181
Pepsin, 61
Peptidases, 61
Peptones, 61
PER, *see* Protein efficiency ratio (PER)
Performance-enhancing substance, 154
Performance climate, 256
PFK, *see* Phosphofructokinase (PFK)
Pharmacological therapy, 182
Phosphocreatine (PCr), 221
Phosphofructokinase (PFK), 39
Physical activity level (PAL), 7
Physical training, 120
Physiological adaptations
    general effects of testosterone and androgens, 160
    growth hormone, 161–162
    testosterone and testosterone analogs, 159–160

PNF, *see* Proprioceptive neuromuscular facilitation (PNF)
Polypeptides, 61
Polyunsaturated fatty acids (PUFAs), 79
Portion control, 183
Positive net protein balance, 66
Post-exercise recovery, 286
    nutrition for, 214
Postexercise, 47–49
Powerade™, 154
Preexercise, 214
    fueling strategies, 282–283
    meals, 281, 283
Professionals Against Doping in Sports (PADS), 232–233
Proper body fluid balance, 114
Proprioceptive neuromuscular facilitation (PNF), 254
Protein(s), 9–10, 207, 229–230, 266, 286
    balance, 64
    digestion, 61
    foods, 68
    intake safety, 71
    metabolism, 62–64, 67
    protein-rich foods, 266
    sources, 69–71
Protein digestibility-corrected amino acid score (PDCAAS), 69, 70
Protein efficiency ratio (PER), 69, 70
Protein needs of young athletes, 59; *see also* Fat needs
    action compound, 60–61
    essential, nonessential, and conditionally essential amino acids, 60
    highs and lows of protein quality, 69–71
    need-to-eat basis, 64–67
    not all proteins created equal, 67–69
    physiological roles of protein, 61–62
    protein digestion, 61
    protein intake safety, 71
    protein metabolism, 62–64
    protein sources, 69–71
Protein quality, highs and lows of, 69–71
Proteoses, 61
PTH, *see* Parathyroid hormone (PTH)
PUFAs, *see* Polyunsaturated fatty acids (PUFAs)
Purine alkaloid, 136

R

Ratings of perceived exertion (RPE), 45, 242
RBC, *see* Red blood cell (RBC)
RD, *see* Registered dietitian (RD)
RDA, *see* Recommended daily allowance (RDA)
Recommended daily allowance (RDA), 26, 37, 64, 66, 102, 207
Recommended dietary allowance, *see* Recommended daily allowance (RDA)
Recovery drinks, 52
Red blood cell (RBC), 87
    deformability, 87
REE, *see* Resting energy expenditure (REE)
Refractometer, 121
Registered dietitian (RD), 195
RER, *see* Respiratory exchange ratio (RER)
Resistance-training program, 66

Respiratory exchange ratio (RER), 39, 227
Resting energy expenditure (REE), 7, 194
Resting metabolic rate (RMR), 210
1RM, *see* One-repetition maximum (1RM)
RMR, *see* Resting metabolic rate (RMR)
Road checklist, eating on, 270
"Roid rage", 165
RPE, *see* Ratings of perceived exertion (RPE)

S

Saturated fats, 79
SBP, *see* Systolic blood pressure (SBP)
Scientific reviews, 288
SDH, *see* Succinate dehydrogenase (SDH)
Secondary male-sex characteristics, 159
Segmental analyzers, 24
Serum 25 (OH)D, 102
Sex, 119
Sex hormone-binding globulin (SHBG), 159
SHBG, *see* Sex hormone-binding globulin (SHBG)
Short-duration high-intensity exercise, 49
Skeletal muscle, 67, 221
SKF, *see* Skinfold (SKF)
Skill performance, 49
Skinfold (SKF), 20
Slow protein, *see* Casein
Smoked tobacco, 139
Smoothie, 286
Snack attack, 269–270
Snacks and meal recommendations, 93–94
snus, *see* Alternative smokeless tobacco (snus)
Sodium chloride (NaCl), 49
Solid food options, 286–287
Somatotropin, *see* Growth hormone
Sonic junior burger, 272
Soy protein, 230
Sporting activity, 4
Sport nutrition and youth, 4
    child and adolescents, 5–6
    dietary status and challenges of young people, 6
    dietary supplement use in youth and adolescent athletes, 12–13
    fluid status and needs, 11
    macronutrient considerations, 8–11
    micronutrient concerns and considerations, 11–12
    optimal energy, 6–8
    percentage of youth, 4, 5
    youth sport participation, 6
Sport performance, 118
Sports drinks, 49–50, 123
Sports nutrition; *see also* Young athletes
    fact sheets, 288
    professional resources, 288
SSCs, *see* Stretch-shortening cycles (SSCs)
Stable isotope tracer techniques, 45
Strength and Conditioning professionals, 158
Stretch-shortening cycles (SSCs), 255
Stretching and flexibility, 253
    benefits, 253–254
    considerations, 255
    guidelines, 256
    recommendations, 254–255
    types of exercises, 254

Substrate oxidation, 45
    exercise metabolism, 47
        higher exogenous CHO oxidation, 46
        stable isotope tracer techniques, 45
Subway roast beef sandwich, 272
Subway veggie delite sandwich, 272
Succinate dehydrogenase (SDH), 39
Sugar-sweetened beverages, 51
"Sustained-release" protein, 229
Sweating patterns affecting factors, 118
    environmental factors, 118, 120–121
    exercise factors, 118, 120
    individual factors, 118, 119–120
    physical training, 120
Sweating responses, 120, 121
Sweat volume, 119
Sympathoadrenal system, 140
Systolic blood pressure (SBP), 257

T

T1D, see Type 1 diabetes (T1D)
T2D, see Type 2 diabetes (T2D)
T3, see Triiodothyronine (T3)
T4, see Thyroxine (T4)
TBI, see Traumatic brain injury (TBI)
TEE, see Total energy expenditure (TEE)
T/E ratio, see Testosterone/estrogen ratio (T/E ratio)
Testosterone, 89, 159
    and analogs, 159–160
    effects, 160
Testosterone/estrogen ratio (T/E ratio), 162
Tetrapolar BIA estimation equations, 25
Third-party testing, 231–232
Three-component models (3C models), 27
Three W's of snacking, 269
Thyroid-stimulating hormone (TSH), 206
Thyroxine (T4), 206
Total energy expenditure (TEE), 7
Trace element, 103
Training volume, 249
Transamination, 63
Trans fats, 79–80, 91
Traumatic brain injury (TBI), 224
Triglycerides, 78, 81
Triiodothyronine (T3), 206
TSH, see Thyroid-stimulating hormone (TSH)
20-min rule, 269
Two-component models (2C models), 24, 26
Type 1 diabetes (T1D), 174
    assessment, 175
    case study, 179–180
    change in growth, 176
    exercise physiology and, 174–175
    laboratory tests, 177
    medical diagnosis, 175
    medical interventions, 176–177
    monitoring and evaluation, 179
    nutrition diagnosis, 175, 177
    nutrition interventions, 177–179
    recognizing and treating hypoglycemia, 178
    responsibilities, 179
Type 2 diabetes (T2D), 174, 180
    assessment, 180–181
    case study, 183
    exercise and, 180
    medical diagnosis, 181
    medical intervention, 182
    monitoring and evaluation, 183
    nutritional diagnosis, 181–182
    nutrition intervention, 182–183
    responsibilities, 183

U

UL, see Upper limit (UL)
Unhealthy training regimen consequences, 256–257
United States Olympic Committee (USOC), 266
Unsaturated fats, 79
Upper limit (UL), 65
U.S. Anti-Doping Agency (USADA), 231
USOC, see United States Olympic Committee (USOC)

V

Vegetarian athletes, fats for, 94
Vertical analyzers, 24
Visceral proteins, 61
Vitamins, 11, 99; see also Minerals
    classifications, 99
    key functions and food sources for, 101
    RDA, functions, and food sources, 100
    Vitamin D, 100–102
VO_2 max, 87, 243

W

WADA, see World Anti-Doping Agency (WADA)
WAnT, see Wingate anaerobic tests (WAnT)
Water, 268
    and hydration, 122
    loss through sweating, 120
    water-soluble vitamins, 99
Weight-conscious athlete
    exercise and nutritional timing, 213–214
    fluid needs, 212
    nutrition during exercise, 214
    nutrition for postexercise recovery, 214
    nutrition for weight modification, 212–213
    recommendations for, 211
Weight gain, 209
    principles, 213
Weight-loss
    bariatric surgery, 197–198
    diets for weight loss in youth, 196–197
    guidelines for healthy weight control/loss practices, 198
    healthy eating tips, 197
    medications, 197
    principles, 213
    psychological considerations, 198–199
    remedies, 197
    resources for parents and health educators, 199
    weight recommendations to age and BMI percentile, 199
Weight management, 182–183
    assessing successful weight change, 209
    benefits of exercise, 205
    body composition and, 204, 211

Index

dehydration and, 206
disordered eating and, 209
excessive caloric restriction, 206–207
high protein intake, 207–209
proper exercise prescription, 205–206
unsafe weight management practices, 204–205
Weight modification, nutrition for, 212–213
Whey, 229
Whey protein concentrate (WPC), 229
WHO, *see* World Health Organization (WHO)
Whole-wheat wrap, 286
"Win at all cost" mentality, 156–157
Wingate anaerobic tests (WAnT), 49
World Anti-Doping Agency (WADA), 136, 162, 228
World Health Organization (WHO), 180
WPC, *see* Whey protein concentrate (WPC)

X

Xenical, *see* Orlistat

Y

Young athletes, 154
    adaptation, 122
    athlete's plate, 267
    breakfast, lunch, dinner, and snacks planning, 266–270
    carbohydrate intake recommended values for, 36–37
    current levels of carbohydrate intake in, 37–38
    dehydration versus euhydration, 117
    difficulties in maintaining euhydration, 116
    eat healthy at night, 272–274
    examples of reported CHO intakes in, 38
    fluid replacement recommendations and strategies, 122–123
    food and fluid recommendations for, 266
    healthy eating on road, 270–272
    helpful resources for parents/coaches, 279–280
    navigating cafeteria, 277–279
    tackling grocery store, 274–277
Young people, dietary status and challenges of, 6
Youth-specific equations, 7
Youth sport participation, 6

Z

"Zero" Trans Fat, 90
Zinc, 107–108